Prāṇāyāma, the yogic art of breathing, leads to a control of the emotions which in turn brings stability, concentration and mental poise. Prāṇāyāma is a bridge which helps the student of yoga to cross from the realm of purely physical development to that of the spirit and forms a crucial stage in his journey towards self-realisation.

Light on Prāṇāyāma is a worthy companion and sequel to the author's *Light on Yoga* which is now widely recognised as a classic text on the practice of Hatha Yoga. The present book is also practical and thorough, offering a trustworthy guide to all who wish to develop the art of yogic breathing.

The respiratory system is discussed from the points of view of both modern anatomy and the ancient yoga texts. The 14 basic types of Prāṇāyāma are analysed in such a way as to offer the reader a programme of 82 carefully graded stages from the simplest breathing patterns to the most advanced. These stages have been tabulated for easy reference and the tables are a unique feature of the book.

Light on Prāṇāyāma provides the student with a comprehensive background of yoga philosophy and discusses such allied topics as the Nāḍīs, Bandhās, Chakras and Bija Mantra. For the serious student there is a full progressive course lasting 200 weeks with special emphasis on the difficulties and dangers that are to be avoided in the practice of Prāṇāyāma.

LIGHT ON PRĀNĀYĀMA

By the same author

CONCISE LIGHT ON YOGA
LIGHT ON YOGA
THE ART OF YOGA
LIGHT ON YOGA SUTRA OF PATANJALI

Light on Prāṇāyāma

Prāṇāyāma Dīpikā

B. K. S. Iyengar

Introduction by Yehudi Menuhin

HarperCollins *Publishers* India
a joint venture with
THE INDIA TODAY GROUP
New Delhi

HarperCollins *Publishers* India
a joint venture with
The India Today Group
by arrangement with
HarperCollins *Publishers* Limited

Published 1993 by
HarperCollins *Publishers* India

Twenty second impression, 2008

Published in 1992 by the Acquarian Press
an imprint of HarperCollins *Publishers*, London

First published by George Allen & Unwin in 1981

ISBN 13: 978 -81-7223-541-7
ISBN 10: 81-7223-541-0

HarperCollins Publishers
A-53, Sector 57, NOIDA, Uttar Pradesh - 201301, India
77-85 Fulham Palace Road, London W6 8JB, United Kingdom
Hazelton Lanes, 55 Avenue Road, Suite 2900, Toronto, Ontario M5R 3L2
and 1995 Markham Road, Scarborough, Ontario M1B 5M8, Canada
25 Ryde Road, Pymble, Sydney, NSW 2073, Australia
31 View Road, Glenfield, Auckland 10, New Zealand
10 East 53rd Street, New York NY 10022, USA

Printed and bound at
Thomson Press (India) Ltd.

This book is dedicated
to the memory of my beloved wife
Ramāmaṇi

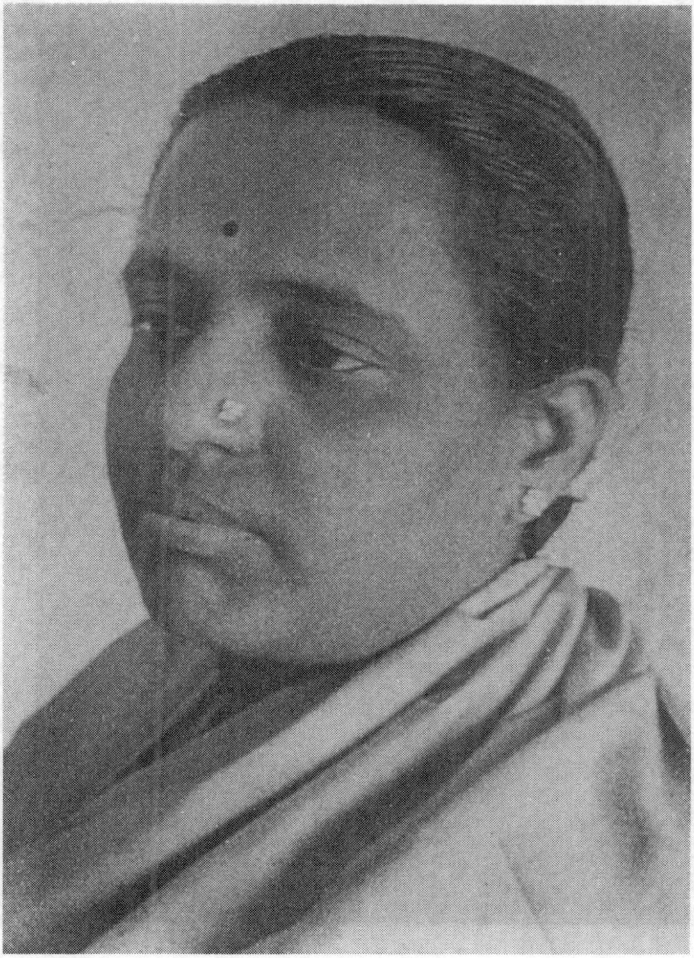

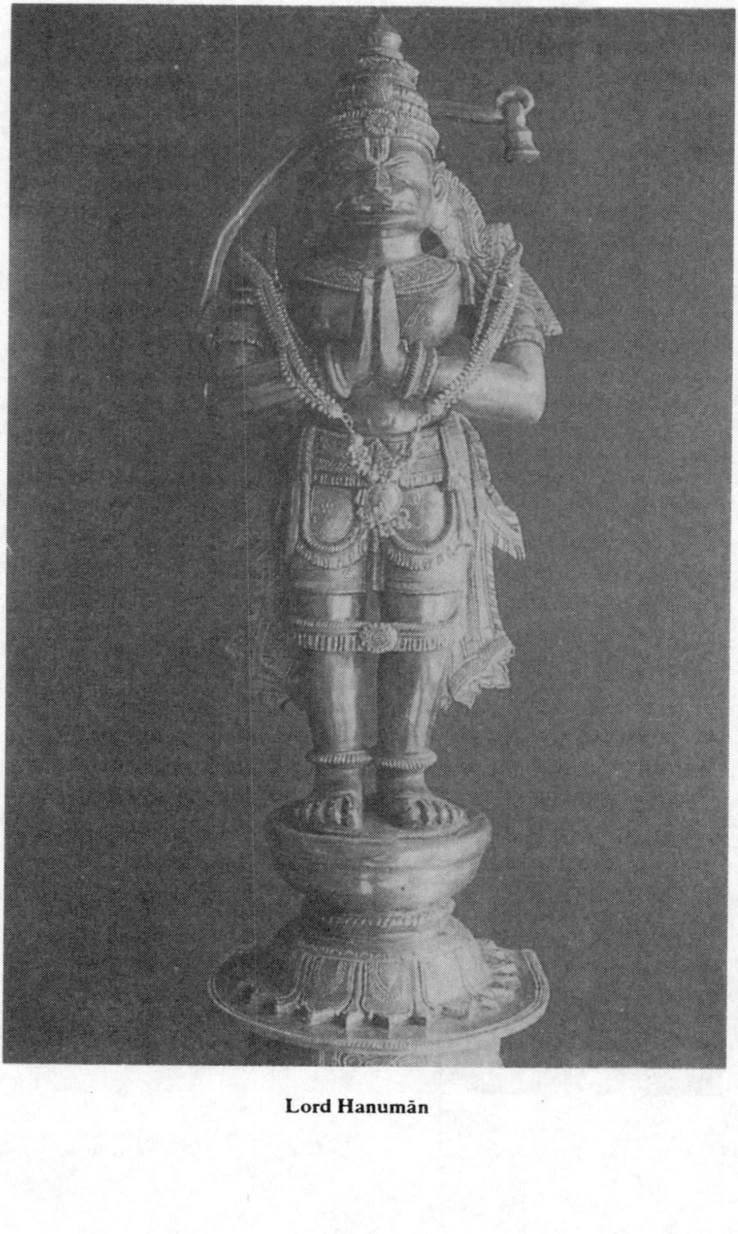

Lord Hanumān

INVOCATIONS

To Lord Hanumān

I salute Lord Hanumān, Lord of Breath, Son of the
Wind God –
who bears five faces and dwells within us
In the form of five winds or energies
pervading our body, mind and soul,

Who re-united Prakṛti (Sîtā) with Puruṣa (Rāma) –
May He bless the practitioner
By uniting his vital energy – prāṇa –
With the Divine Spirit within.

* * *

To Sage Patanjali

I bow before the noblest of sages, Patanjali –
Who brought serenity of mind by his work on Yoga,
Clarity of speech by his work on grammar, and
Purity of body by his work on medicine.

* * *

Where there is Yoga,
There is prosperity, success, freedom,
and bliss.

TRIBUTE FROM MY GURUJĪ

B. K. Sundrarājēna rachitā nūtnayuktibihi
Yogasāstram samālaṃbhya prāṇāyāma pradīpīkā 1

Vividhai prāṇasaṃchāra vṛtti rodha vibhodhanaihi
Ṣaṭchakranikare nāḍījāle lohita śodhakaihi 2

Panchaprāṇa prasāraiścha nirodhānāṅcha bhodhakaihi
Yuktādhyānānukūlācha Prāṇāyāmābhilāṣiṇāṃ 3

Ālokitācha sasvartham mayā śrī kṛṣṇayoginā
Ādriyerannimaṃ grantharatnam bhuvi vipaśchitaha 4

1 June 1979 *T. Kṛṣṇamāchārya*

1. *Light on Prāṇāyāma* written by B. K. Sundara Raja Iyengar, is a fresh, up-to-date presentation of the ancient science of Yoga.

2. It deals with subtle functioning of the breath, various techniques of inhalation, retention and exhalation and of the filtration of the crimson coloured fluid – the Life Force – with unchecked flow through the network of channels (nāḍīs) and the subtle centres (chakras)

3. It explains the vitalising of the cosmic energy as it makes itself manifest in five forms, while emphasis is laid on do's and don'ts. The work is of immense value to ardent practitioners of prāṇāyāma.

4. Scholars will surely be interested by this thought-provoking treatise, a precious gem in the firmament of yoga.

T. Kṛṣṇamāchārya

Introduction by Yehudi Menuhin

B. K. S. Iyengar has done for the more elusive prāṇāyāma, that is the movement of air which is said to determine life on earth, the same service that he has rendered to the physical features of haṭha yoga. He has moved into a more ethereal, subtle aspect of our very existence. He has placed in the hands of the layman a book which contains, in some respects, more information, more knowledge and more wisdom in a more integrated way than is available to our most brilliant students of conventional medicine, for it is a medicine of health and not of sickness, it is an understanding of spirit, body and mind that is as healing as it is invigorating. Not only can the individual be restored to wholeness but the whole progress of a lifetime is seen in powerful perspective. He teaches us in line with the ancient Indian philosophy that life is not only dust to dust, but air to air, that, as with the process of fire, matter is transformed into heat, light and radiation from which we may gather strength. But strength is more than the transformation of matter into other forms of matter, it is the transformation of the whole cycle of air and light into matter and back again. In fact, it completes Einstein's equation of matter and energy and translates it into the human, the living incarnation. It is no longer an atomic bomb, it is no longer the explosion of the atom, the harnessing of matter, it is the irradiation of the human being with light and power, the very sources of energy.

I believe that this treatise, drawn from ancient, classical Indian texts, will provide illuminating guidelines to the reconciliation of various practices of medicine from acupuncture to touch and sound therapy to the mutual and reciprocal benefit of them all. It will also teach us to respect those elements which we have treated with such contempt – air, water and light – without which life cannot survive. With this book, Mr Iyengar, my guru in yoga, has added a new and greater dimension to the life of the people of the West, urging us to join our brothers of every colour and every creed in the celebration of life with due reverence and purpose.

Yehudi Menuhin

Foreword

'Yoga is nothing but the total experience of
human life; it is a science of the integral man!'
Jaques S. Masui.

Yogāchārya Sri B. K. S. Iyengar, the author of *Light on Yoga* hardly needs an introduction to the seekers of light on Prāṇāyāma. The science and art of Yoga, as presented by Patanjali centuries before Christ, begins by moral and other precepts for physical, vital and mental health, potency and purification. It proceeds to postures – āsanas, which influence the aspirant beneficially through the neurophysiological system and the endocrine glands. Sri Iyengar has dwelt with them in his book *Light on Yoga* in such a thorough and detailed manner, with about six hundred photographs, that there is scarcely any other work on that subject so encyclopaedic, precise and lucid. The book gives the complete theory of Yoga and treats the subject of āsanas fully, with a peep into prāṇāyāma. Published by George Allen and Unwin, Ltd, the book is so popular that it has run into many editions and has been translated into several languages. It is being used as a practical guide by people all over the world.

Sri Iyengar, impelled by nature and driven by circumstances, learnt Yoga the hard way at the feet of his guru Sri Krishnamāchārya. Sri Iyengar has been himself a teacher of Yoga, and a good task-master at that, all the time. What he speaks and writes about Yoga is like an abundant overspill from all his rich and meaningful personal experiences. The demonstration lecture on āsanas that he gave in Bombay last December on the occasion of his sixty-first birthday, with his daughter Geetā and son Prashānta, was a marvellous revelation of his control over every nerve and muscle of his supple body. Hundreds of his disciples from abroad witnessed the performance and wondered how he retained such plasticity and vigour at that age. To him it was child's play, a mere routine. One of his close disciples remarked that he has trained his body 'to twist, to twine, to turn, to bend, to wriggle, to pull, to flex' and much besides!

It is but logical that one should expect from Sri Iyengar an equally exhaustive and instructive book on Prāṇāyāma, which is the next step in Yoga, namely, the science and art of breath-control. Though there are several yogas practised, such as haṭha-yoga, rāja-yoga, jñāna-yoga, kuṇḍalini-yoga, mantra-yoga, laya-yoga and so on, basically and in essence Yoga is a scientific and systematic discipline for a successful organisation of all the energies and faculties of the integral human being with a view to attaining the highest ecstatic communion with the cosmic reality or God. Breath-control is helpful in every one of the yogas mentioned above. All the texts on Yoga as well as the experience of ages testify to the fact that breath-control is an important factor in the control of the mind as well. However, breath-control, that is prāṇāyāma, is not merely deep-breathing or breathing exercises, normally a part of physical culture. It is something far more, involving exercises which affect not only the physical, physiological and neural energies but also the psychological and cerebral activities, such as memory-training and creativity. Sri Aurobindo, the sage and seer of Pondicherry, has recorded that after practising prāṇāyāma he could compose and retain in his memory about two hundred lines of poetry, while earlier he could not handle even a dozen.

In recent decades, western medicine, after experimentation, has come to recognise and use the health-giving and invigorating effects of what is called voluntary respiration. Yoga teaches and practises prāṇāyāma, ascribing to it indisputable educative, regulative and spiritual value. Wladimir Bischler, in Chapter 14 of *The Forms and Techniques of Altruistic and Spiritual Growth*, says that medical science has now reconciled itself to some of the methods borrowed from the orient and studied the multiple effects of correct voluntary respiration. He has detailed the multiple effects of it not merely on the lungs but on the whole metabolism of the human body. He has said that spirotherapy, the name he gives to the method, opens new and broad horizons to medicine, to hygiene and to therapeutics. He has ended by saying that investigations of modern science have only confirmed the empirical intuitions of the oriental sages and philosophers.

Prāṇāyāma, as an essential ingredient of yogic discipline, might well bestow a number of benefits other than mental and spiritual. But the main aim of Yoga is self-realisation, communion of the self with the Self; the exercise of prāṇāyāma involves the control of the mind and of the whole of human consciousness, which is the basis of all cognition and awareness. A human being consists of his body, his life, including all biological activities, and his mind, which is the seat of what we call the ego – the 'I', and all cerebral activities centred round the 'I'. The goal of Yoga is to empty the whole of one's basic power of consciousness of all memory, ideation, sensual urges and desires and try to be aware of pure consciousness, as a spark of the cosmic energy itself, which is of the nature of the self-conscious principle of Supreme Intelligence. For a person who wants to tread the path of Yoga, his first effort will have to be to cease to identify himself with the body-life-mind complex completely and to look upon those three elements as tools for transcending the ego, in order to identify his inner being with the pure, unmixed power of consciousness whose very nature is all-peace, harmony and creative joy.

Prāṇāyāma therefore has a special meaning and significance in Yoga. Prāṇa means the breath, the air and life itself. But in Yoga, prāṇa (in all its five aspects in man of prāṇa, apāna, vyāna, udāna and samāna) is the very essence of the energising principle of the animate and inanimate world. It pervades the whole universe. And prāṇāyāma means the full control of that energising principle in one's own being by a certain discipline. This discipline aims not only at good health, an equilibrium in the physical and vital energies, but also the purification of the whole nervous system in order to make it more capable of responding to the will of the Yogi in controlling the sense-urges, and in making the mental powers more subtle and sensitive to the call of the evolutionary urge, the higher divine nature in man.

It is not often that prāṇāyāma is treated as an independent subject. Most of the ancient texts on Yoga, beginning with Patanjali, treat it as an essential part of yogic discipline. Recently however, there have been publications on this subject independently, though they are few when compared with the wilderness of books on āsanas. A full scientific treatment, based on a lifetime experience of teaching in all aspects of Yoga has, however, been long-awaited. Every lover of Yoga will therefore welcome Sri Iyengar's book.

When I took up Sri Iyengar's manuscript in order to write the Foreword, I could see how difficult and challenging a task it must have been for him to write on this subject for westerners in the English language. Unlike many other writers on such a subject, he has been a householder and has followed the tradition of invoking his Iṣṭa Devatā (chosen deity) as well as quoting the Gīta and relevant texts. Here I would assert that Yoga is not a part of any religion with a theology and ritualism. It has no hierarchy. It is a cultural and spiritual discipline open to all mankind without any distinction of caste, creed, colour, race, sex or age. Perhaps the only essential qualification is a belief in the potentialities of one's own consciousness and an aspiration to reach its summit by following the laws of consciousness itself. Another very unorthodox and striking characteristic of Sri Iyengar is that instead of looking upon a family as a burden, and a wife as an obstacle to yogic life, he has named his Yoga Institute in Pune after his departed life-mate Shrimati Ramāmaṇi and dedicated this book to her. By these acts Sri Iyengar abundantly proves that Yoga is *for* life and not *away* from it, as Sri Aurobindo has so often repeated.

Another difficulty concerns terminology and the use of words which are all in Sanskrit in the original. Sri Iyengar has done his best to be as precise and accurate as possible in his choice of English equivalents and has tried to convey the sense of the original. He is a master of detail and is never satisfied till he feels that the reader has understood what he has wanted to tell him. Take the word Prāṇāyāma itself: it is so rich in its connotation that to convey its meaning by saying 'breath-control', 'voluntary respiration' or 'the science of breathing' would not be adequate at all. For instance, none of these phrases can include the idea of kumbhaka, nor of breathing through alternate nostrils in different measures. Much less can they indicate the different types of breathing such as ujjāyī, śeetalı and so on, or these in combination with mūdras and bandhas. Sri Iyengar has taken special care to see that even the use of the thumb and fingers for holding the nostrils in position is accurately and adequately described. This care in the use of words, together with necessary precautions and combined with the illustrations, are calculated to guide the aspirant in following the art of prāṇāyāma as closely as the written word can achieve.

Sri Iyengar knows full well that the science and art of Yoga is not complete without dhāraṇa, dhyāna and samādhi. This triune is the crown of Yoga and is called saṁyama. It leads the yogi step by step to transcend the region of the senses and the reign of the ego for the gradual transformation of the integral being into a new life of unitive living with the Supreme Spirit in unmixed joy and harmony. He has therefore given in this book an inkling of what is called meditation or dhyāna. He has ended by providing a few hints about śavāsana, the posture which leads to utter relaxation with faint awareness. He rounds off this great effort of writing on prāṇāyāma by offering the reader the secret of real relaxation, so that he may be ready for the next and final ascent to the summit of meditative samādhi. Let us look forward for the completion in due course of the trio: *Light on Yoga*, *Light on Prāṇāyāma* and *Light on Dhyāna*, so that while Sri Iyengar's life would be one of fulfillment, that of others would have a triple illumination for their journey to the Everest of spirituality.

R. R. Diwakar

Bangalore
14 June 1979

Preface

My first book, *Light on Yoga*, captured the minds and hearts of ardent students and even changed the lives of many who at first were curious about this noble art, science and philosophy. I hope that *Light on Prāṇāyāma* will also enhance their knowledge.

With respect and reverence to Patanjali and the Yogis of ancient India who discovered Prāṇāyāma, I share with fellow men and women the nectar of its simplicity, clarity, subtleness, fineness and perfection. In the recent past, during my practices, a new light of inner awareness dawned on me which I had not experienced when I wrote *Light on Yoga*. My friends and pupils pressed me to put my experiences as well as my oral teachings down on paper; hence this attempt to explain the subtle observations and reflections that I made to help students in their search for refinement and precision.

Many western scholars have accepted the ancient conception that man is a trinity of body, mind and spirit. Various techniques of physical exercises, athletics and sports were devised to keep men and women healthy. They were designed to supply the needs of the body (annamaya kośa) with its bones, joints, muscles, tissues, cells and organs. Indian scholars call this discipline the 'conquest of matter'. This I have explained fully in my book *Light on Yoga*. Only recently have western savants become aware of the techniques developed in ancient India for examining the systems of breathing, blood-circulation, digestion, assimilation, nourishment, the endocrine glands and the nerves, the subtle forms of which are collectively known as the Conquest of Life Force (prāṇamaya kośa).

Yoga Vidyā is a codified system which has laid down eight phases for self-realisation. They are: Yama, Niyama, Āsana, Prāṇāyāma, Pratyāhāra, Dhāraṇā, Dhyaṅa and Samādhi. In this book emphasis is laid on Prāṇāyāma to keep the involuntary or autonomous controlling systems of the human body in a balanced state of health and perfection.

There were no scholars, saints or yogis in my home to inspire me to take up Yoga. As a child I was afflicted with many diseases, and as destiny would have it, this led me to Yoga in 1934 in the hope of regaining my health. Since then it has been my way of life. It has taught me to be punctual and disciplined despite hardships which frequently disrupted my daily practices, learning and experiences.

In the beginning, Prāṇāyāma was a struggle. Over-indulgence in the daily practice of āsanas shook my inner body many times within minutes of starting Prāṇāyāma. Each morning I got up to practise, and it was a strain to hold my breath and keep to the rhythm. I struggled on, hardly doing three or four cycles, by which time I was gasping for air. I would rest for a few minutes and then try again until it was impossible to continue. I asked myself why I could not do so. I could find no answer. I had no-one to guide me. Failures and errors taunted my body, mind and self for a number of years, but I steadfastly continued to improve my standards. Today, I still devote daily one hour at a stretch to Prāṇāyāma and find that even this is inadequate.

Words can hypnotise and attract a reader towards a religious practice (sādhana) and make him think that he understands a spiritual experience. Reading, however, only makes him more learned, while practice (sādhana) in what he has read brings him nearer to truth and clarity. Fact is truth and clarity is purity. The present age is one of scientific advancement and new words flood the dictionaries. Being a pure sādhaka and not a man of words, I find it difficult to choose the correct technical terms to express all I want to write. I can only do my inadequate best to present to my readers all that I have experienced in my practice of this finest of arts.

Prāṇāyāma is a vast subject with illimitable potentialities. It is psychosomatic, since it explores the intimate relationship between the body and the mind. It may appear quite simple and easy, but the moment one sits down to practise, one quickly realises that it is a difficult art. Its subtleties are little known and much more remains to be explored. In the past, writers of Yoga texts dealt more with the effects of Prāṇāyāma than with its practical application. This may be because Prāṇāyāma used to be widely practised and the majority were familiar with it. Their explanations of its effects give some idea of their experiences, which surpass their words.

Many of the movements in Prāṇāyāma are infinitely subtle. For example, the deliberate and fine movements of the skin in opposing directions appears objectively impossible, but is a process developed in Yoga. With training the skin can be moved in this way, and this plays a major role in Prāṇāyāma practices. Thus Prāṇāyāma is in many respects a subjective art. When this skill is used to maximum effect, where skin movements synchronise with those of inhalation, exhalation and retention, the flow of energy (prāṇa) is harmonious.

Modern scientists have verified the efficacy of the intuitive knowledge of yogis by using electronic instruments. The effects of Prāṇāyāma are definite and not illusory. I am confident that in the not too distant future the pole of objective knowledge (science or experimentation) and the other of subjective knowledge (art or participation) will play their part in unifying the study of Prāṇāyāma and its benefits.

Owing to the development of technology, modern life has become endlessly competitive, resulting in increased strain on both men and women. It is difficult to maintain a balanced life. Anxieties and diseases affecting the nervous and circulatory systems have multiplied. In despair, people become addicted to psychedelic drugs, smoking and drinking or indiscriminate sex to find relief. These activities allow one to forget oneself temporarily, but the causes remain unsolved and the diseases return.

Only Prāṇāyāma gives real relief from these problems. It cannot be learnt by arguments and discussions, but must be mastered with patient and cautious effort. It starts by giving relief to sufferers from ordinary ailments like common colds, headaches and mental disharmony. Its nadir is the elixir of life.

This book is in two parts. The first covers three sections dealing with the theory, the art and the techniques of Prāṇāyāma. The second part, entitled 'Freedom and Beatitude' is concerned with the conquest of the soul (ātma jaya). It deals with meditation (dhyāna) and relaxation (śavāsana).

In the first part, I have tried to integrate Prāṇāyāma with all the different aspects of Yoga. Prāṇāyāma is the connecting link between the body and the soul of man, and the hub in the wheel of Yoga.

I have tried to bring out hidden techniques, so that the reader may derive maximum benefit without being beset by doubt and confusion. I have incorporated tables analysing different stages of important varieties of Prāṇāyāma. The tables give detailed information of the methodology for ready reference. They also give the reader some idea of the infinite number of permutations and combinations possible in this noble art and science. Even the uninitiated sādhaka can practise independently without fear of ill-effects. The information contained in the tables will make the sādhakas cautious and bold.

In the appendix I have introduced five courses, arranging them stage by stage for the practitioner to follow according to his capacity. Each of the courses may be extended by additional weeks if the standard given cannot be completed within the stipulated time. Though Prāṇāyāma is essentially to be learnt at the feet of a guru (master), I have endeavoured with all humility to guide the reader – both teacher and student – to a safe method of perfecting this art.

I shall be happy if my work helps people to achieve peace in body, poise in mind and tranquillity in the self. Prāṇāyāma is a vast subject. Since my knowledge in this field has its limitations, I shall welcome suggestions for incorporation in future editions.

The *Yogachūdāmaṇi Upaniṣad* says that Prāṇāyāma is an exalted knowledge (mahā vidyā). It is a royal road to prosperity, freedom and bliss.

Read, re-read and digest Part I of this book before starting to practise.

I am indebted to my guruji Śri T. Krishnamacharya for his tributes to the book. I am sincerely grateful to Mr Yehudi Menuhin for his Introduction and Mr R. R. Diwakar for his Foreword and support. I am indebted to my children Geeta and Prashant and to my pupils B. I. Taraporevala, M. T. Tijoriwala, S. N. Motivala, and Dr B. Carruthers,

MD, CM, FRCP, who gave their valuable time in the preparation of the work. Their patience in editing and re-editing this book over and over again gave it its final shape. I am grateful to Kumari Srimathi Rao for typing the script innumerable times. I thank Mr P. R. Shinde for taking innumerable photographs for the book and Miss Robijn Ong for providing the anatomical drawings.

I express my sincere gratitude to Mr Gerald Yorke for his constructive suggestions and encouragement. But for his persistent guidance, this book would not have come to light. I am permanently indebted to him for the care he took in editing the entire script.

B. K. S. Iyengar

Contents

Part One

Section I

The Theory of Prāṇāyāma

Chapter 1

What is Yoga?

1. Nobody knows the timeless, primeval absolute One, nor when the world came into existence. God and nature existed before man appeared, but as man developed he cultivated himself and began to realise his own potential. Through this came civilisation. Words were evolved with this, concepts of God (Puruṣa) and nature (prakṛti), religion (dharma) and Yoga developed.

2. Since it is so difficult to define these concepts, each man has to interpret them according to his understanding. When man was caught in the web of worldly joys, he found himself separated from God and nature. He became a prey to the polarities of pleasure and pain, good and evil, love and hatred, the permanent and the transient.

3. Caught in these opposites, man felt the need of a personal divinity (Puruṣa), who was supreme, unaffected by afflictions, untouched by actions and reactions, and free from the experience of joy and sorrow.

4. This led man to seek the highest ideal embodied in the perfect Puruṣa or God. Thus the Eternal Being, whom he called Īśvara, the Lord, the guru of all gurus, became the focus of his attention, and of his concentration and meditation. In this fundamental quest of reaching Him, man devised a code of conduct whereby he could live in peace and harmony with nature, his fellow beings and himself.

5. He learnt to distinguish between good and evil, virtue and vice, and what was moral and immoral. Then arose a comprehensive concept of right action (dharma) or the science of duty. Dr S. Radhakrishnan wrote that '*it is Dharma which upholds, sustains, supports*' and guides mankind to live a higher life irrespective of race, caste, class or faith.

6. Man realised that he should keep his body healthy, strong and clean in order to follow Dharma and to experience the divinity within himself. Indian seers in their search for light distilled the essence of the Vedas in the Upaniṣads and Darśanas (mirrors of spiritual perception). The Darśanas or schools are: sāṃkhya, yoga, nyāya, vaiśesika, pūrva mīmāṁsa and uttara mīmāṁsa.

7. *Sāṃkhya* says that all creation takes place as a product of the twenty-five essential elements (tattvas) but does not recognise the Creator (Īśvara). Yoga recognises the Creator. *Nyāya* stresses logic and is primarily concerned with the laws of thought, relying on reason and analogy. It accepts God as the result of inference. *Vaiśeṣika* stresses notions such as space, time, cause and matter, and is supplementary to nyāya. It, too, endorses the Nyāya view of God. *Mīmāṁsa* is dependent on the Vedas and has two schools – pūrva mīmāṁsa, which deals with the general concept of the Deity but stresses the importance of action (karma) and rituals; and uttara mīmāṁsa, which accepts God on the basis of the Vēdas, but lays special stress on spiritual knowledge (jñāna).

8. *Yoga* is the union of the individual self (jīvātmā) with the Universal Self (Paramātmā). The sāmkhya philosophy is theoretical while Yoga is practical. Sāṁkhya and Yoga combined give a dynamic exposition of the system of thought and life. Knowledge without action, and action without knowledge do not help man. They must be intermingled. So sāṁkhya and Yoga go together.

9. According to Yoga, Yājñavalkya Smṛti, the Creator (Brahmā) as Hiraṇyagarbha (the Golden Foetus) was the original propounder of the Yoga system for the health of the body, control of the mind and attainment of peace. The system was first collated and written down by Patanjali in his *Yoga Sūtras* or aphorisms. These are directive rather than discursive, revealing the means and the end. When all the eight disciplines of Yoga are combined and practised, the yogi experiences oneness with the Creator and loses his identity of body, mind and self. This is the Yoga of integration (saṁyama).

10. The *Yoga Sūtras* consist of 195 aphorisms divided into four chapters. The first deals with the theory of Yoga. It is aimed at those who have already attained a poised mind and lays down what they should do to maintain their poise. The second chapter on the art of Yoga initiates the beginner into his practices. The third is concerned with internal discipline and the powers (siddhis) he gains. The fourth and the last chapter deals with emancipation or freedom from the shackles of this world.

11. The word 'Yoga' is derived from the Sanskrit root 'yuj' which means to bind, join, attach and yoke, to direct and concentrate the attention in order to use it for meditation. Yoga, therefore, is the art which brings an incoherent and scattered mind to a reflective and coherent state. It is the communion of the human soul with Divinity.

12. In nature's heritage to man are the three characteristics or qualities (guṇas), namely, illumination (sattva), action (rajas) and inertia (tamas).

Set on the wheel of time (kālachakra: kāla = time, chakra = wheel), like a pot on the potter's wheel (kulālachakra), man is moulded and remoulded in accordance with the predominating order of these three fundamental intermingling characteristics.

13. Man is endowed with mind (manas), intellect (buddhi) and ego (ahaṁkāra), collectively known as consciousness (chitta), which is a source of thinking, understanding and acting. As the wheel of life turns, consciousness experiences the five miseries of ignorance (avidyā), selfishness (asmitā), attachment (rāga), aversion (dveṣa) and love of life (abhiniveśa). These in turn leave the chitta in five different states which may be dull (mūḍha), wavering (kṣipta), partially stable (vikṣipta), one-pointed attention (ekāgra) and controlled (niruddha). Chitta is like fire, fuelled by desires (vāsanas), without which the fire dies out. Chitta in that pure state becomes a source of enlightenment.

14. Patanjali evolved eight stages on the path of realisation, which are dealt with in the next chapter. Chitta in a state of dullness is purified through yama, niyama and āsana through which the mind is spurred to activity. Āsana and Prāṇāyāma bring the wavering mind to a state of some stability. The disciplines of prāṇāyāma and Pratyāhāra make the chitta attentive and focus its energy. It is then restrained in this state by dhyāna and samādhi. As it progresses the higher stages of Yoga become predominant, but the preceding stages which lay the foundation should be neither ignored nor neglected.

15. Before exploring the unknown 'Ātmā', the sādhaka has to learn about his known body, mind, intellect and ego. When he knows the 'known' in its totality, these merge into the 'unknown' like rivers merging into the sea. At that moment he experiences the highest state of joy (ānanda).

16. First, Yoga deals with health, strength and conquest of the body. Next, it lifts the veil of difference between the body and the mind. Lastly, it leads the sādhaka to peace and unalloyed purity.

17. Yoga systematically teaches man to search for the divinity within himself with thoroughness and efficiency. He unravels himself from the external body to the self within. He proceeds from the body to the nerves, and from the nerves to the senses. From the senses he enters into the mind, which controls the emotions. From the mind he penetrates into the intellect, which guides reason. From the intellect, his path leads to the will and thence to consciousness (chitta). The last stage is from consciousness to his Self, his very being (Ātmā).

18. Thus, Yoga leads the sādhaka from ignorance to knowledge, from darkness to light and from death to immortality.

Chapter 2

Stages of Yoga

1. The stages of Yoga are eight: yama, niyama, āsana, prāṇāyāma, pratyāhāra, dhāraṇā, dhyāna and samādhi. They are all integrated, but for the sake of convenience they are dealt with as independent components.

2. A tree has roots, trunk, branches, leaves, bark, sap, flowers and fruits. Each one of these components has a separate identity, but each component cannot by itself become a tree. It is the same with Yoga. As all the parts put together become a tree, so all the eight stages put together form Yoga. The universal principles of Yama are the roots and the individual disciplines of Niyama form the trunk. Āsanas are like various branches spreading in different directions. Prāṇāyāma, which aerates the body with energy, is like the leaves which aerate the entire tree. Pratyāhāra prevents the energy of the senses flowing outwards, just as the bark protects a tree from decay. Dhāraṇā is the sap of the tree that holds the body and intellect firm. Dhyāna is the flower ripening into the fruit of samādhi. Even as the fruit is the highest development of a tree, the realisation of one's true self (ātma-darśana) is the culmination of the practice of Yoga.

3. Through the eight stages of Yoga, the sādhaka develops understanding of his own self. He proceeds step by step from the known – his body – to the unknown. He proceeds from the outer envelope of the body – the skin – to the mind. From the mind (manas), he goes to the intellect (buddhi), the will (saṁkalpa), discriminating consciousness (viveka-khyāti or prajñā), conscience (sad-asad-viveka) and lastly the Self (Ātmā).

Yama

4. Yama is a collective name for universal moral commandments. These commandments are eternal, irrespective of class, time and place. These great vows (mahāvratas) are non-violence (ahiṁsā), truth (satya), non-stealing (asteya), continence (brahmacharya) and non-covetousness (a-parigraha). Non-violence is withdrawal from the infliction of any type of injury, whether physical or mental, in thought or deed. When hatred and animosity are abandoned, an all-embracing love remains. The yogi is ruthlessly truthful and honest with himself, and whatever he thinks or speaks turns out to be true. He controls his desires and reduces his wants, so that he becomes richer without stealing and things come to him without his

asking. Continence (brahmacharya) is enjoined in all matters of sex, whether in imagination or in fact. This discipline brings in its wake virility and the ability to see divinity in all forms without sexual arousal. One should not desire things that are not necessary to maintain life, for desire is followed by avarice which leads to sorrow if one cannot get what one wants. When desires multiply, right conduct is destroyed.

Niyama

5. Niyamas are the rules for self-purification, namely, purity (śaucha), contentment (santoṣa), austerity (tapas), study of the scriptures (svādhyāya) and surrender to the Lord of all our actions (Īśvara praṇidhāna). The yogi knows that his body and senses are susceptible to desires, which prejudice the mind, so he observes these principles. Purity is of two kinds, internal and external, and both must be cultivated. The latter means purity of behaviour and habits, cleanliness of person and surroundings. The former is the rooting out of six evils, namely, passion (kāma), anger (krodha), greed (lobha), infatuation (moha), pride (mada), malice and envy (mātsarya). This eradication is achieved by occupying the mind with good constructive thoughts, leading to divinity. Contentment reduces desires, makes one cheerful and gives balance of mind. Austerity enables one to discipline the body and to endure hardship and adversity, thus directing the mind towards the Self within. Study here is the education of oneself by searching for truth and self-realisation. Finally it is the surrender of all our actions to the Lord and abiding entirely in His will. Thus the niyamas are the virtues which calm the disturbed mind, leading towards peace both within and around the sādhaka.

Āsanas

6. Before dealing with the āsanas, it is essential to know about puruṣa and prakṛti. Puruṣa (literally 'person') is the universal psychic principle, which though unable to perform any action by itself, animates and vitalises nature (prakṛti or the producer), the universal physical principle, which through its three qualities and evolutionary powers (guṇas) produces intellect (buddhi) and mind (manas).

Puruṣa and prakṛti acting together stir the material world to activity. Both are limitless, without beginning or end. Prakṛti consists of five gross elements (pancha mahābhūtas) namely, earth (pṛthvi), water (ap), fire (tejas), air (vāyu) and ether (ākāśa). Their five subtle counterparts (tanmātras) are smell (gandha), taste (rasa), form (rūpa), touch (sparśa) and sound (śabda). These gross elements and their counterparts merge with the three qualities and evolutionary powers (guṇas) of prakṛti, namely, illumination (sattva), activity (rajas) and dormancy (tamas) to form the cosmic intellect (mahat). Ego (ahaṁkāra), intellect (buddhi) and mind (manas) form consciousness (chitta), the individual counterpart of mahat.

Mahat is the unevolved primary germ of nature or productive principle whence all phenomena of the material world are developed. There are five organs of perception (jñānendriyas) – ears, nose, tongue, eyes and skin – and five sense of action (karmendriyas) – legs, arms, speech, excretory and reproductive organs. Prakṛti, the five gross elements, their five subtle counterparts, the ego, intellect and mind, the five organs of perception, the five organs of action and puruṣa make up the twenty-five basic elements (tattvas) of sāṁkhya philosophy. A pitcher cannot be made without a potter, nor can a house without a mason. Creation cannot take place without puruṣa, the Primeval Force, coming into contact with the tattvas. All existence revolves around purusa and prakrti.

7. Life is a combination of the body, organs of perception and action, mind, intellect, ego and soul. The mind acts as a bridge between the body and the soul. The mind is imperceptible and intangible. The self fulfils its aspirations and pleasures through the mind acting as a mirror and the body as an instrument of enjoyment and attainment.

8. According to the Indian system of medicine (Āyurveda) the body is made up of seven constituent elements (dhātus) and three humours (doṣas). The seven elements are so called because they sustain the body. They are chyle (rasa), blood (rakta), flesh (māṁsa), fat (medas), bones (asthi), marrow (majjā) and semen (śukra). These keep the body immune from infection and diseases.

9. Chyle is formed by the action of gastric juices on food. Blood produces flesh and refreshes the entire body. Flesh protects the bones and produces fat. Fat lubricates and brings firmness to the body. Bones uphold the body and produce marrow. Marrow gives strength and produces semen. Semen not only procreates but, according to the ancient texts, in its subtle state flows throughout the subtle body in the form of certain vital energy.

10. The three humours (dosas) of wind (vāta), bile (pitta) and phlegm (śleṣma), when evenly balanced give perfect health. Imbalances in them cause diseases. The subtle or vital energy called wind prompts breathing, movement, action, excretion and procreation. It co-ordinates the functions of different parts of the body and human faculties. Bile creates thirst and hunger. It digests food and converts it into blood, keeping the body temperature constant. Phlegm lubricates the joints and muscles and helps to heal wounds. Mala is the waste matter, solid, liquid or gaseous. Unless it is excreted, diseases set in, disturbing the balance of the three humours.

The Kośas

11. According to Vedanta philosophy, there are three frames or types of body (śarīra) enveloping the soul. They consist of five inter-penetrating and inter-dependent sheaths (kośas).

The three śarīras are: (a) sthūla, the gross frame or the anatomical sheath, (b) sūkṣma, the subtle frame, consisting of the physiological, the psychological and intellectual sheaths, and (c) kāraṇa, the so-called causal frame – the spiritual sheath.

The sthūla śarīra is the sheath of nourishment (annamaya kośa).

The physiological (prāṇamaya), the psychological (manomaya) and the intellectual (vijñānamaya) sheaths make up the subtle body (sūkṣma śarīra).

Prāṇamaya kośa includes the respiratory, circulatory, digestive, nervous, endocrine, excretory and genital systems. Manomaya kośa affects the functions of awareness, feeling and motivation not derived from subjective experience. Vijñānamaya kośa affects the intellectual process of reasoning and judgement derived through subjective experience.

The kāraṇa śarīra is the sheath of joy (ānandamaya kośa). The experience of being aware of it is felt by the sādhaka when he wakes after a deep refreshing sleep and when he is totally absorbed in the object of his meditation.

The skin encloses all the sheaths and bodies. It should be firm and sensitive to the slightest movement. All the sheaths are inter-mingled on their different levels from the skin to the Self.

Aims in Life (Puruṣārthas)

12. Man has four aims in his life; dharma, artha, kāma and mokṣa. Dharma is duty. Without this and ethical discipline, spiritual attainment is impossible.

Artha is the acquisition of wealth for independence and higher pursuits in life. It cannot give lasting joy; nevertheless, a poorly nourished body is a fertile ground for worries and diseases.

Kāma means the pleasures of life, which depend largely on a healthy body. As the *Kaṭhopaniṣad* says, the 'self' cannot be experienced by a weakling.

Mokṣa is liberation. The enlightened man realises that power, pleasure, wealth and knowledge pass away and do not bring freedom. He tries to rise above his sāttvic, rājasic and tāmasic qualities and so escape from the grasp of the guṇās.

13. The body is the abode of Brahman. It plays a vital part in attaining the four-fold aims of life. The sages knew that though the body wears out, it serves as an instrument to attain realisation and, as such, it has to be kept in good condition.

14. Āsanas purify the body and mind and have preventive and curative effects. They are innumerable, catering to the various needs of the muscular, digestive, circulatory, glandular, nervous and other systems of the body.

They cause changes at all levels from the physical to the spiritual. Health is the delicate balance of body, mind and spirit. By practising āsanas the sādhaka's physical disabilities and mental distractions vanish and the gates of the spirit are opened.

Āsanas bring health, beauty, strength, firmness, lightness, clarity of speech and expression, calmness of the nerves and a happy disposition. Their practice can be compared to the growth of a mango tree. If the tree has grown sound and healthy, its essence is to be found in its fruit. Likewise, the essence distilled from practising āsanas is the spiritual awakening of the sādhaka. He is free from all dualities.

15. There is a popular misconception that both āsanas and prāṇāyāma should be practised together from the time Yoga-sādhanā is begun. It is the author's experience that if a novice attends to the perfection of the postures, he cannot concentrate on breathing. He loses balance and the depth of the āsanas. Attain steadiness (sthiratā) and stillness (achalatā) in āsanas before introducing rhythmic breathing techniques. The range of bodily movements varies from posture to posture. The less the range of movement, the smaller will be the space in the lungs and the breathing pattern will be shorter. The greater the range of bodily movement in āsanas, the greater will be the lung capacity, and the deeper the breathing pattern. When Prāṇāyāma and āsanas are done together, see that the perfect posture is not disturbed. Until the postures are perfected, do not attempt prāṇāyāma. One soon realises that when āsanas are well performed, prāṇāyāmic breathing automatically sets in.

Prāṇāyāma

16. Prāṇāyāma is a conscious prolongation of inhalation, retention and exhalation. Inhalation is the act of receiving the primeval energy in the form of breath, and retention is when the breath is held in order to savour that energy. In exhalation all thoughts and emotions are emptied with breath: then, while the lungs are empty, one surrenders the individual energy, 'I', to the primeval energy, the Ātmā.

The practice of Prāṇāyāma develops a steady mind, strong will-power and sound judgement.

Pratyāhāra

17. This is a discipline to bring the mind and senses under control. The mind plays a dual role. On one hand it seeks to gratify the senses, and on the other, to unite with the Self. Pratyāhāra quietens the senses and draws them inwards, leading the aspirant to the Divine.

Dhāraṇā, Dhyāna and Samādhi

18. Dhāraṇā is concentration on a single point, or total attention on what one is doing, the mind remaining unmoved and unruffled. It stimulates the

inner awareness to integrate the ever-flowing intelligence, and releases all tensions. When it continues for a long time it becomes meditation (dhyāna), an indescribable state that has to be experienced to be understood.

19. When the state of dhyāna is maintained for a long time without interruption it merges into samādhi, where the sādhaka loses his individual identity in the object of meditation.

20. In samādhi, the sādhaka loses consciousness of his body, breath, mind, intelligence and ego. He lives in infinite peace. In this state, his wisdom and purity, combined with simplicity and humility, shine forth. Not only is he enlightened, but he illumines all those who come to him in search of truth.

21. Yama, Niyama, Āsana and Prāṇāyāma are essential parts of the Yoga of action (karma). They keep the body and mind healthy for performing all acts that please God. Prāṇāyāma, Pratyāhāra and Dhāraṇa are parts of the Yoga of knowledge (jñāna). Dhyāna and samādi help the sādhaka to merge his body, mind and intelligence in the ocean of the Self. This is the Yoga of devotion and love (bhakti).

22. These three streams of jñāna, karma and bhakti flow into the river of Yoga and lose their identity. Thus the path of Yoga alone takes every type of sādhaka, from the dull (mūḍha) to the restrained (niruddha), towards freedom and beatitude.

Chapter 3

Prāṇa and Prāṇāyāma

1. It is as difficult to explain Prāṇa as it is to explain God. Prāṇa is the energy permeating the universe at all levels. It is physical, mental, intellectual, sexual, spiritual and cosmic energy. All vibrating energies are prāṇa. All physical energies such as heat, light, gravity, magnetism and electricity are also prāṇa. It is the hidden or potential energy in all beings, released to the fullest extent in times of danger. It is the prime mover of all activity. It is energy which creates, protects and destroys. Vigour, power, vitality, life and spirit are all forms of prāṇa.

2. According to the Upaniṣads, prāṇa is the principle of life and consciousness. It is equated with the real Self (Ātmā). Prāṇa is the breath of life of all beings in the universe. They are born through and live by it, and when they die their individual breath dissolves into the cosmic breath. Prāṇa is the hub of the Wheel of Life. Everything is established in it. It permeates the life-giving sun, the clouds, the winds (vāyus), the earth (pṛthvi), and all forms of matter. It is being (sat) and non-being (asat). It is the source of all knowledge. It is the Cosmic Personality (the puruṣa) of Sāṁkhya philosophy. Therefore the Yogi takes refuge in prāṇa.

3. Prāṇa is usually translated as breath, yet this is only one of its many manifestations in the human body. If breathing stops, so does life. Ancient Indian sages knew that all functions of the body were performed by five types of vital energy (prāṇa-vāyus). These are known as prāṇa (here the generic term is used to designate the particular), apāna, samāna, udāna and vyāna. They are specific aspects of one vital cosmic force (vital wind), the primeval principle of existence in all beings. God is one, but the wise designate Him by various names, and so it is with prāṇa.

4. Prāṇa moves in the thoracic region and controls breathing. It absorbs vital atmospheric energy. Apāna moves in the lower abdomen and controls the elimination of urine, semen and faeces. Samāna stokes the gastric fires, aiding digestion and maintaining the harmonious functioning of the abdominal organs. It integrates the whole of the human gross body. Udāna, working through the throat (the pharynx and the larynx), controls the vocal cords and the intake of air and food. Vyāna pervades the entire body, distributing the energy derived from food and breath through the arteries, veins and nerves.

5. In prāṇāyāma, the prāṇa-vāyu is activated by the inward breath and the apāna-vāyu by an outward breath. Udāna raises the energy from the lower spine to the brain. Vyāna is essential for the function of prāṇa and apāna as it is the medium for transferring energy from the one to the other.

6. There are also five subsidiary divisions known as upaprāṇas or upavāyus, namely, nāga, kūrma, kṛkara, devadatta and dhanaṁjaya. Nāga relieves pressure on the abdomen by belching. Kūrma controls the movements of the eye-lids to prevent foreign matter entering the eyes; it also controls the size of the iris, thereby regulating the intensity of light for sight. Kṛkara prevents substances passing up the nasal passages and down the throat by making one sneeze or cough. Devadatta causes yawnings and induces sleep. Dhanaṁjaya produces phlegm, nourishes and remains in the body even after death and sometimes inflates a corpse.

7. According to Āyurveda, vāta, which is one of the three humours (doṣa), is another name of prāṇa. Charaka Saṁhitā explains the functions of vāta in the same manner as Yoga texts explain prāṇa. The only perceptible expression of the functioning of prāṇa is felt in the movements of the lungs activated by inner energy, causing respiration.

Chitta and Prāṇa

8. Chitta and prāṇa are in constant association. Where there is chitta there prāṇa is focused, and where prāṇa is there chitta is focused. The chitta is like a vehicle propelled by two powerful forces, prāṇa and vāsanā (desires). It moves in the direction of the more powerful force. As a ball rebounds when struck to the ground, so is the sādhaka tossed according to the movement of prāṇa and chitta. If breath (prāṇa) prevails, then the desires are controlled, the senses are held in check and the mind is stilled. If the force of desire prevails, the breathing becomes uneven and the mind gets agitated.

9. In the third chapter of *Haṭha Yoga Pradīpikā*, Swātmārāma states that as long as the breath and prāṇa are still, the chitta is steady and there can be no discharge of semen (śukra). In time the sādhaka's increased vigour is sublimated for higher and nobler pursuits. He then attains the state of ūrdhva-retas (ūrdhva = upwards; retas = semen), one who has sublimated his sexual energy and his chitta to merge in pure consciousness.

Prāṇāyāma

10. 'Prāṇa' means breath, respiration, life, vitality, energy or strength. When used in the plural, it denotes certain vital breaths or currents of energy (prāṇa-vāyus). 'āyāma' means stretch, extension, expansion, length, breadth, regulation, prolongation, restraint or control. 'Prāṇāyāma' thus means the prolongation of breath and its restraint. The Śiva Saṁhitā calls it

vāyu sādhana (vāyu = breath; sādhana = practice, quest). Patanjali in his *Yoga Sūtras* (Ch. 2, Sūtras 49–51) describes prāṇāyāma as the controlled intake and outflow of breath in a firmly established posture.

11. Prāṇāyāma is an art and has techniques to make the respiratory organs to move and expand intentionally, rhythmically and intensively. It consists of long, sustained subtle flow of inhalation (pūraka), exhalation (rechaka) and retention of breath (kumbhaka). Pūraka stimulates the system; rechaka throws out vitiated air and toxins; kumbhaka distributes the energy throughout the body. The movements include horizontal expansion (dairghya), vertical ascension (āroha) and circumferential extension (viśālata) of the lungs and the rib cage. The processes and techniques of prāṇāyāma are explained in later chapters.

This disciplined breathing helps the mind to concentrate and enables the sādhaka to attain robust health and longevity.

12. Prāṇāyāma is not just automatic habitual breathing to keep body and soul together. Through the abundant intake of oxygen by its disciplined techniques, subtle chemical changes take place in the sādhaka's body. The practice of āsanas removes the obstructions which impede the flow of prāṇa, and the practice of prāṇāyāma regulates that flow of prāṇa throughout the body. It also regulates all the sādhaka's thoughts, desires and actions, gives poise and the tremendous will-power needed to become a master of oneself.

Chapter 4

Prāṇāyāma and the Respiratory System

'As long as there is breath in the body, there is life. When breath departs, so too does life. Therefore, regulate the breath.'
(*Haṭha Yoga Pradīpikā* – Ch.2 : Ś.3.)

1. During normal inhalation, an average person takes in about 500 cubic centimetres of air; during deep inhalation the intake of air is about six times as great, amounting to almost 3000 cubic centimetres. The capacities of individuals vary according to their constitution. The practice of prāṇāyāma increases the sādhaka's lung capacity and allows the lungs to achieve optimum ventilation.

2. The second chapter of the *Haṭha Yoga Pradīpikā* deals with prāṇāyāma. The first three verses state: 'Being firmly established in the practice of āsanas, with his senses under control, the yogi should practice prāṇāyāma as taught by his Guru, observing moderate and nutritious diet. When the breath is irregular, the mind wavers; when the breath is steady, so is the mind. To attain steadiness, the yogi should restrain his breath. As long as there is breath within the body, there is life. When breath departs, life also departs. Therefore, regulate the breath.'

3. The practice of prāṇāyāma helps to cleanse the nāḍīs, which are tubular organs of the subtle body through which energy flows. There are several thousand nāḍīs in the body and most of them start from the areas of the heart and the navel. Prāṇāyāma keeps the nāḍīs in a healthy condition and prevents their decay. This in turn brings about changes in the mental attitude of the sādhaka. The reason for this is that in prāṇāyāma breathing starts from the base of the diaphragm on either side of the body near the pelvic girdle. As such, the thoracic diaphragm and the accessory respiratory muscles of the neck are relaxed. This in turn helps to relax the facial muscles. When the facial muscles relax, they loosen their grip over the organs of perception, namely, the eyes, ears, nose, tongue and skin, thereby lessening the tension in the brain. When tension there is lessened, the Sādhaka attains concentration, equanimity and serenity.

Why So Many Prāṇāyāmas?

4. Numerous āsanas have been evolved to exercise various parts of the anatomy – muscles, nerves, organs and glands – so that the entire organism works in a healthy and harmonious manner. Human environments, constitutions, temperaments and states of health and mind vary, and different āsanas help in different situations to alleviate human ills and develop harmony. Many types of Prāṇāyāmas have been devised and evolved to meet the physical, mental, intellectual and spiritual requirements of the sādhakas under fluctuating conditions.

Four Stages of Prāṇāyāma

5. The *Śiva Saṁhitā* discusses the four stages (avasthā) of prāṇāyāma in its third chapter. These are: (a) commencement (ārambha), (b) intent endeavour (ghaṭa), (c) intimate knowledge (pariċhaya) and (d) consummation (niṣpatti).

6. In the ārambha stage, the sādhaka's interest in prāṇāyāma is awakened. In the beginning he is hasty and by reason of his exertion and the speed with which he wants results, his body trembles and he perspires. When by perseverence he continues his practice, the tremors and perspiration cease and the sādhaka reaches the second stage of ghaṭāvasthā. Ghaṭa means a water pot. The body is compared to a pot. Like an unbaked earthen pot, the physical body wears away. Bake it hard in the fire of prāṇāyāma to gain stability. In this stage the five kośas and the three śarīras are integrated. After this integration, the sādhaka reaches the parichayāvasthā, where he obtains intimate knowledge of prāṇāyāma practices and of himself. By this knowledge he controls his qualities (guṇas) and realises the causes of his actions (karma). From the third stage, the sādhaka goes forth towards niṣpatti avasthā, the final stage of consummation. His efforts have ripened, the seeds of his karma are burnt out. He has crossed the barriers of the guṇas and becomes a guṇātīta. He becomes a jīvanmukta – a person who is emancipated (mukta) during his lifetime (jīvana) by the knowledge of the Supreme Spirit. He has experienced the state of ecstasy (ānanda).

Respiratory System

7. To enable the reader to have a clear picture of how prāṇāyāma benefits the body, it is essential to have some idea of the respiratory system. This is discussed below.

8. It is known that the basic energy needs of the human body are met predominantly by oxygen plus glucose. The former aids in the process of elimination by oxidising the waste matter, while glucose supplied with oxygen nourishes the body cells in the flow of respiration.

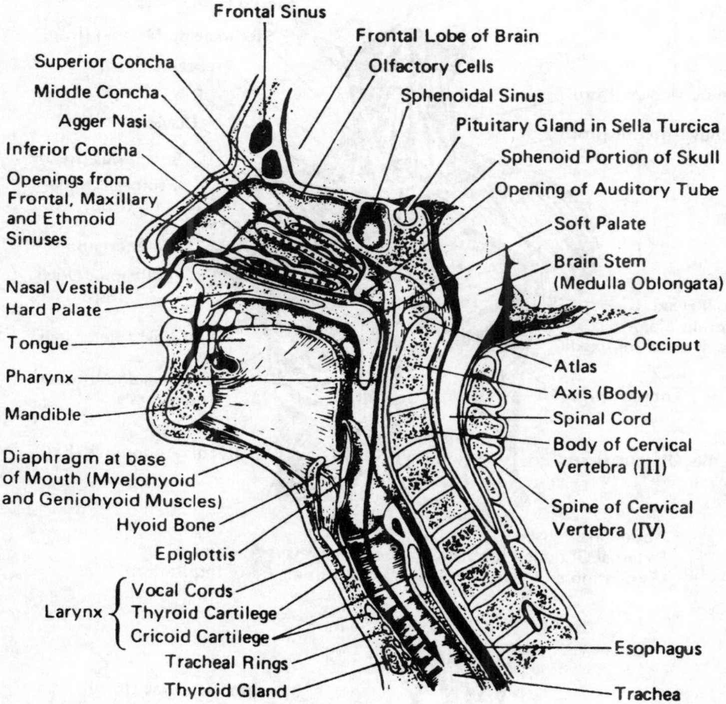

Fig. 1 ⟶ **Air passage during Inspiration through the Nose, Pharynx, Larynx and Trachea**

9. The purpose of prāṇāyāma is to make the respiratory system function at its best. This automatically improves the circulatory system, without which the processes of digestion and elimination would suffer. Toxins would accumulate, diseases spread through the body and ill-health becomes habitual.

10. The respiratory system is the gateway to purifying the body, mind and intellect. The key to this is prāṇāyāma.

11. Respiration is essential for sustaining all forms of animal life from the single-celled amoeba to man. It is possible to live without food or water for

Figs. 2 & 3 Front and back muscles of the torso used in respiration

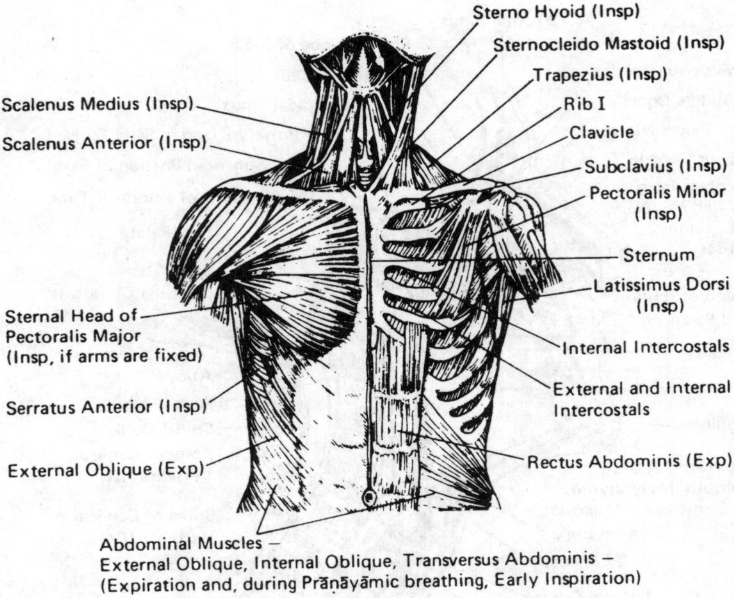
Sterno Hyoid (Insp)
Sternocleido Mastoid (Insp)
Trapezius (Insp)
Rib I
Clavicle
Subclavius (Insp)
Pectoralis Minor (Insp)
Sternum
Latissimus Dorsi (Insp)
Internal Intercostals
External and Internal Intercostals
Rectus Abdominis (Exp)
Scalenus Medius (Insp)
Scalenus Anterior (Insp)
Sternal Head of Pectoralis Major (Insp, if arms are fixed)
Serratus Anterior (Insp)
External Oblique (Exp)
Abdominal Muscles – External Oblique, Internal Oblique, Transversus Abdominis – (Expiration and, during Prāṇāyāmic breathing, Early Inspiration)

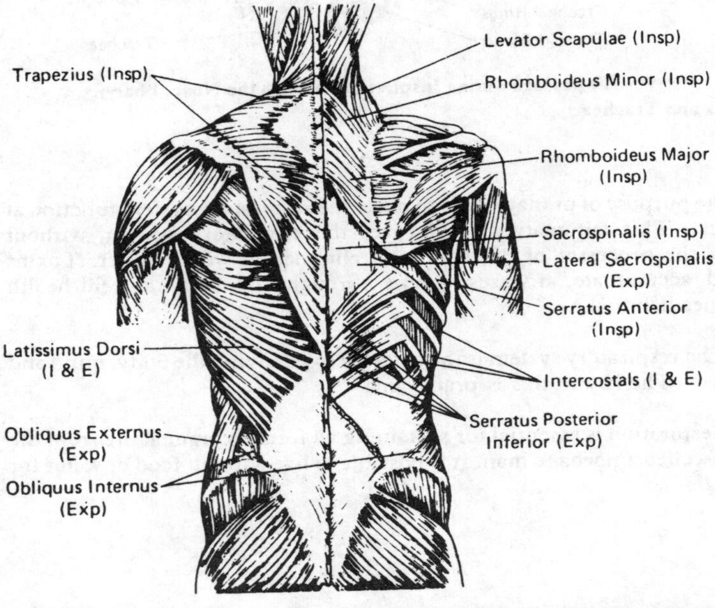
Levator Scapulae (Insp)
Trapezius (Insp)
Rhomboideus Minor (Insp)
Rhomboideus Major (Insp)
Sacrospinalis (Insp)
Lateral Sacrospinalis (Exp)
Serratus Anterior (Insp)
Latissimus Dorsi (I & E)
Intercostals (I & E)
Serratus Posterior Inferior (Exp)
Obliquus Externus (Exp)
Obliquus Internus (Exp)

a few days, but when respiration ceases so does life. In the *Chāndogyopaniṣad* it is said: 'Even as the spokes are fastened to the hub, so on this life breath, all is fastened. Life moves with the life breath, which gives life to a living creature. Life breath is one's father, . . . one's mother, . . . one's brother, . . . one's sister, and one's teacher, . . . the Brahman. . . . Verily, he who sees this knows and understands this becomes the excellent speaker.' (S. Radhakrishnan: *The Principal Upaniṣads*, VII, 15, 1–4.)

12. The *Kauṣītakī Upaniṣad* says 'One can live deprived of speech, for we see the dumb; one deprived of sight, for we see the blind; of hearing, for we see the deaf; and of mind, for we see the childish; one can live without arms and legs, for thus we see. But now it is the breathing spirit alone, the intelligence-self that seizes hold of this body and makes it rise up. This is the all obtaining in the breathing spirit. What is the breathing spirit, that is the intelligence-self. What is intelligence-self, that is the breathing spirit, for together they live in this body and together they go out of it.' (S. Radhakrishnan: *The Principal Upaniṣads*, III, 3.)

Fig.4

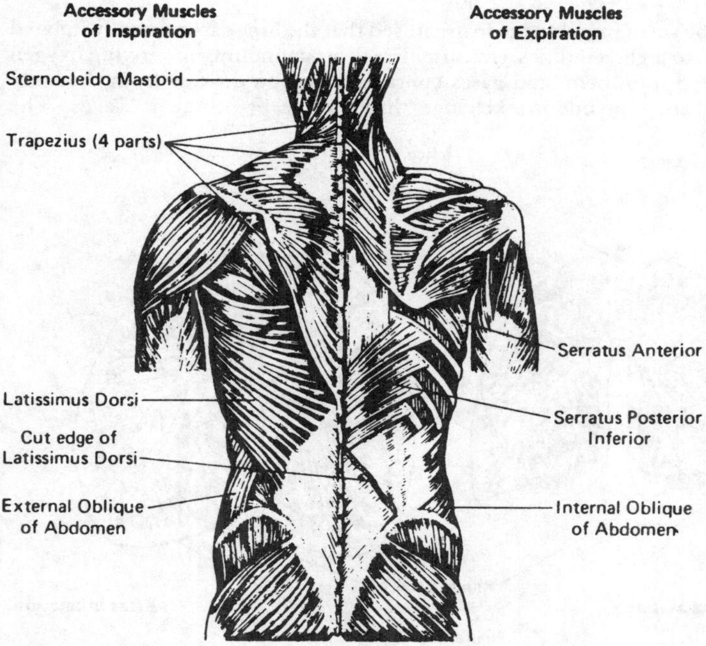

13. Breathing starts with independent life outside the mother and ends when life ceases. When the child is still in the womb its oxygen is supplied through its mother's blood, and its lungs are not required to function. When it is born, the first breath of life is started by command from the brain.

14. During most of one's life, the depth and rate of breathing are self-regulated through the nervous system to meet the purposes of breathing, to supply in a regulated and controlled way the fresh oxygen which is constantly needed by the cells and to discharge the carbon dioxide accumulated in them.

15. Most of us assume that because breathing is usually automatic, it is beyond our active control. This is not true. In prāṇāyāma by arduous training of the lungs and nervous system, breathing can be made more efficient by changing its rate, depth and quality. The lung capacity of great athletes, mountain climbers, and yogis is far greater than that of ordinary men, allowing them to perform extraordinary feats. Better breathing means a better and healthier life.

16. The act of breathing is so organised that the lungs are normally inflated sixteen to eighteen times a minute. Fresh air containing life-giving oxygen is sucked into them, and gases containing carbon dioxide from the body tissues are sent out in exchange through the breathing passages. The

Fig. 5 **Lungs**

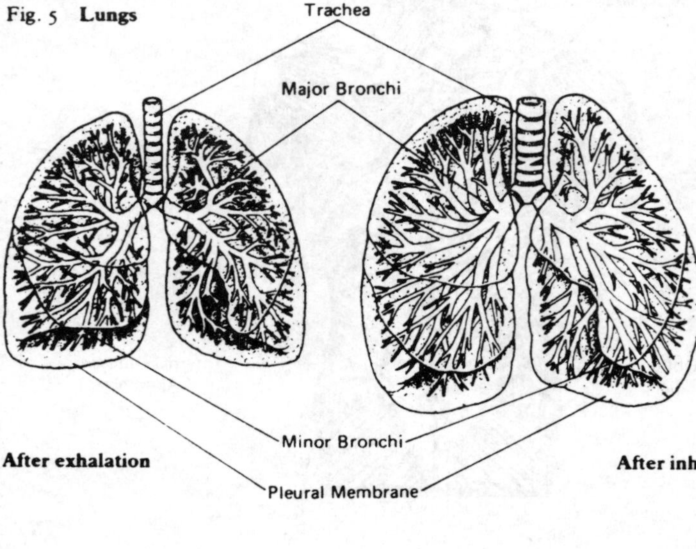

After exhalation **After inhalation**

rhythmic inflation of the soft, honey-combed bellows of the lungs is maintained by the movements of the rib-cage and diaphragm. The latter in turn are driven or powered by impulses sent down by the respiratory centre in the brain to the relevant muscles through the nerves. Thus the brain is the instigator through which the respiration and the three mental functions of thought, will and consciousness are regulated.

17. The breathing cycle consists of three parts: inhalation, exhalation and retention.

Inhalation is an active expansion of the chest by which the lungs are filled with fresh air. Exhalation is a normal and passive recoil of the elastic chest wall by means of which the stale air is exhaled and the lungs are emptied. Retention is a pause at the end of each inhalation and exhalation. These three form one cycle of breathing. The breathing affects the heart rate. During the prolonged holding of breath, a slowing of the heart rate is observed, which ensures increased rest to the heart muscle.

18. Respiration may be classified into four types:

(a) High or clavicular breathing, where the relevant muscles in the neck mainly activate the top parts of the lungs.
(b) Intercostal or midbreathing, where only the central parts of the lungs are activated.
(c) Low or diaphragmatic breathing, where the lower portions of the lungs are activated chiefly, while the top and central portions remain less active.
(d) In total or prāṇāyāmic breathing, the entire lungs are used to their fullest capacity.

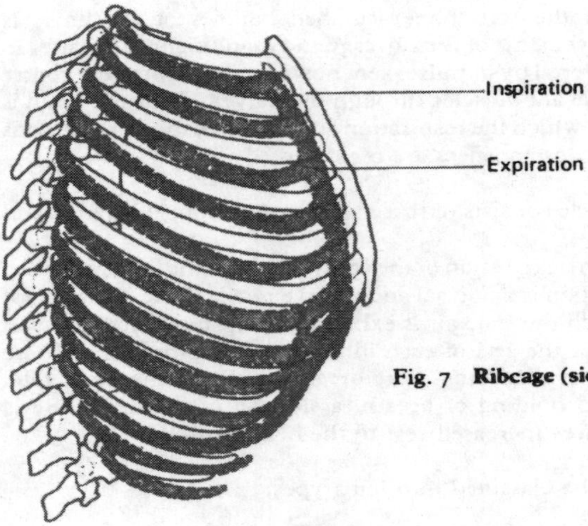

Fig. 7 Ribcage (side view)

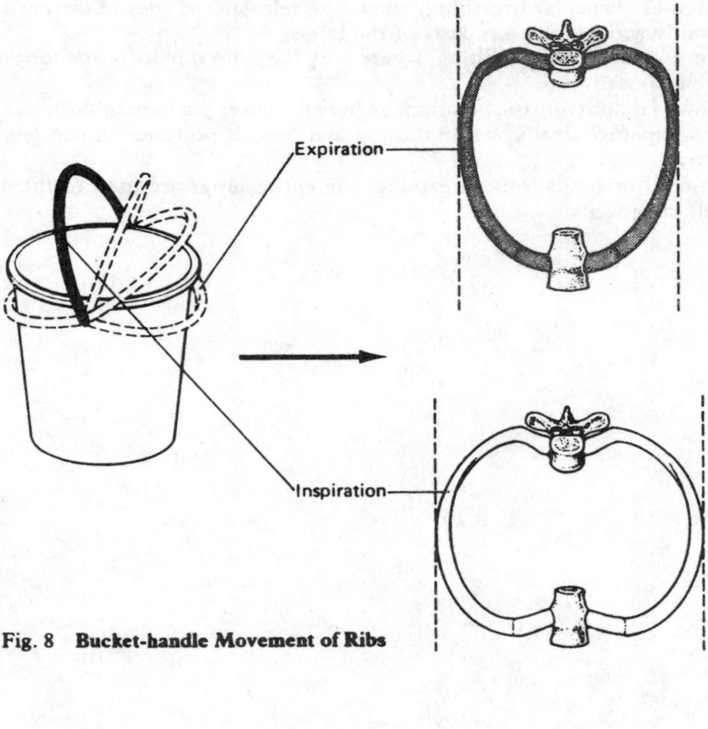

Fig. 8 Bucket-handle Movement of Ribs

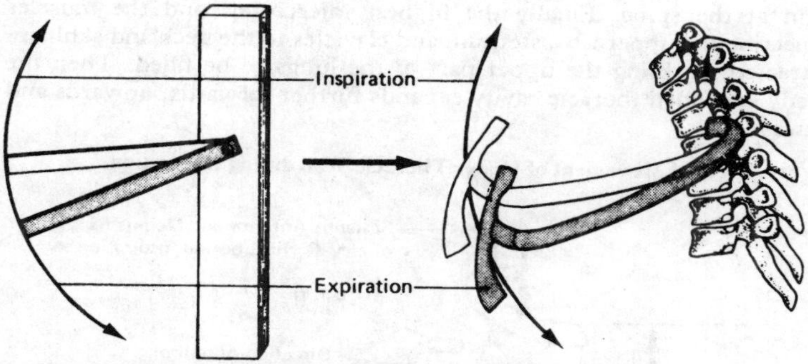

Fig. 9 **Antero-posterior Movement of Ribs in Respiration**

In prāṇāyāmic inspiration, diaphragmatic contraction is delayed until after the conscious contraction of the muscles of the anterior and lateral abdominal wall. These muscles are diagonally connected to the ribcage above and the pelvis below. This action lowers and stabilises the dome-shaped diaphragm which originates at the lower rib margin; it pushes up the abdominal organs and increases the capacity of the thorax. This prepares the diaphragm for a subsequent contraction of maximum extent and efficiency by reducing the centripetal pull. This minimises interference with the next action of the sequence, the elevation and expansion of the lower ribcage in ascending upwards. This is accomplished by the vertical pull of the diaphragm followed by the sequential activation of the intercostal muscles to allow the fullest caliper-like movements of the floating ribs, bucket-handle like movements of the individual ribs, elevation and full circumferential expansion of the ribcage as a whole from its

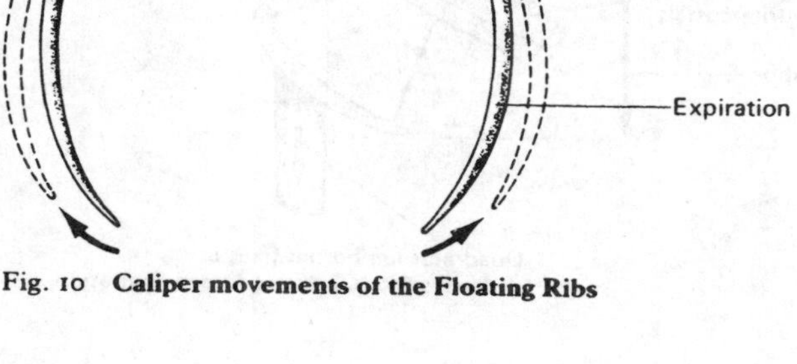

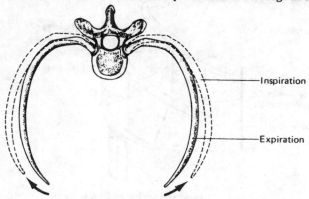

Fig. 10 **Caliper movements of the Floating Ribs**

origin at the spine. Finally the highest intercostals and the muscles connecting the upper ribs, sternum and clavicles to the neck and skull are contracted, enabling the upper part of the lungs to be filled. Then the already expanded thoracic cavity expands further forwards, upwards and sideways.

Fig. 11 **Upward Movement of Upper Thoracic Wall during Inspiration**

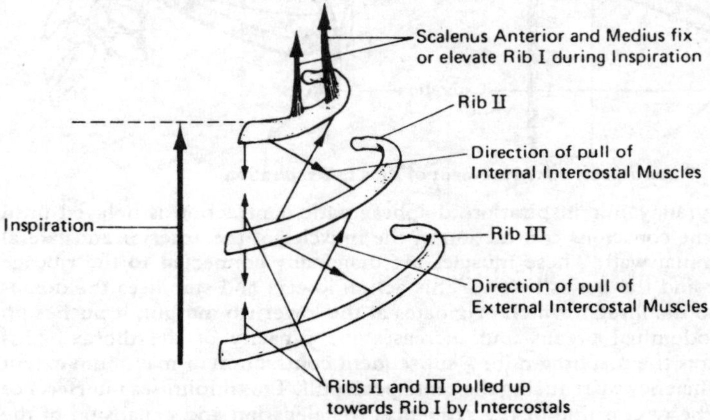

Fig. 12 **Downward Movement of Lower Thoracic Wall during Forced Exhalation**

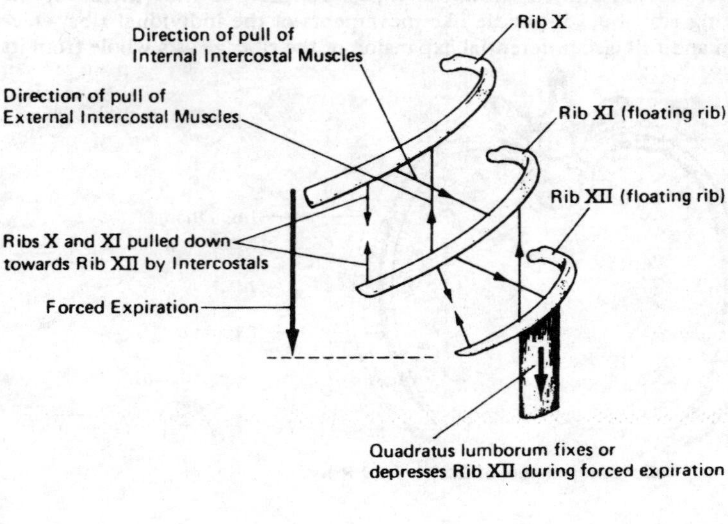

Fig. 13 **Structure of the thoracic wall**

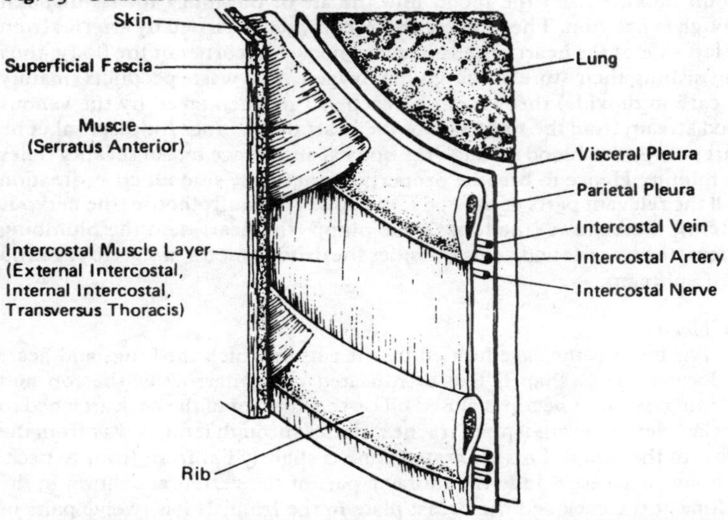

19. This series of movements of the abdomen, chestwall and neck, in which each step of the sequence prepares the ground for the next, results in a maximum filling of the lungs, to create space for the incoming air to reach every corner of each lung.

20. The sādhaka must first direct his body-conscious awareness specifically and intelligently at the lower anterior abdominal wall just above the pelvis. To accomplish this, he has to move the lower abdominal wall towards the spine and against the diaphragm as if massaging from the skin to the muscles and muscles to the inner organs. This sense of active conscious contraction is associated with visible movements of the abdominal wall from the surface skin to its deepest layers, and can be directed at will. After that, direct your attention to expand the lateral and posterior regions of the chest. Elevate the lower chest wall simultaneously expanding the top chest wall with its skin and muscles. The diaphragm gradually and smoothly resumes its domed shape as it starts to relax towards the end of inspiration. During exhalation the dome moves up again. It is active at the start of expiration to encourage a smooth slow start to the elastic recoil of the lungs.

21. The fresh oxygen which is sucked in percolates the minute sacs (the alveolar sacs) which form the basic unit of the lungs. The membranes round these alveoli convey this oxygen into the blood stream and then the

carbon dioxide from the blood into the air of the lungs for its disposal through exhalation. The blood with fresh oxygen is carried by arteries from the left side of the heart to cells in every nook and corner of the body, thus replenishing their store of life-giving oxygen. The waste products (mainly the carbon dioxide) thrown out by each sac are then taken by the venous blood stream from the right side of the heart to the lungs for disposal. The heart pumps this blood through the body at an average rate of seventy times per minute. Hence to breathe properly we need the smooth co-ordination of all the relevant parts of the body, the power or controlhouse (the nervous system), the bellows (the lungs), the pump (the heart) and the plumbing system (the arteries and veins), besides the driving motor of the rib cage and the diaphragm.

The Chest

22. The chest is the cage formed by the ribs in which the lungs and heart are located. It is shaped like a truncated cone, narrow at the top and widening below. The top is closed off by the muscles of the neck attached to the clavicles. The wind-pipe (trachea) passes through it on its way from the throat to the lungs. This truncated cone is slightly flat from front to back. Its bony surfaces include the thoracic part of the vertebral column in the midline at the back and the breast plate in the front. It has twelve pairs of flattened ribs which curve across the gap between the spine at the back and the breastbone in front to form semicircular bridges on each side. The spaces between the ribs are filled by internal and external intercostal muscles. There are, in addition, muscles joining the twelfth rib to the pelvis

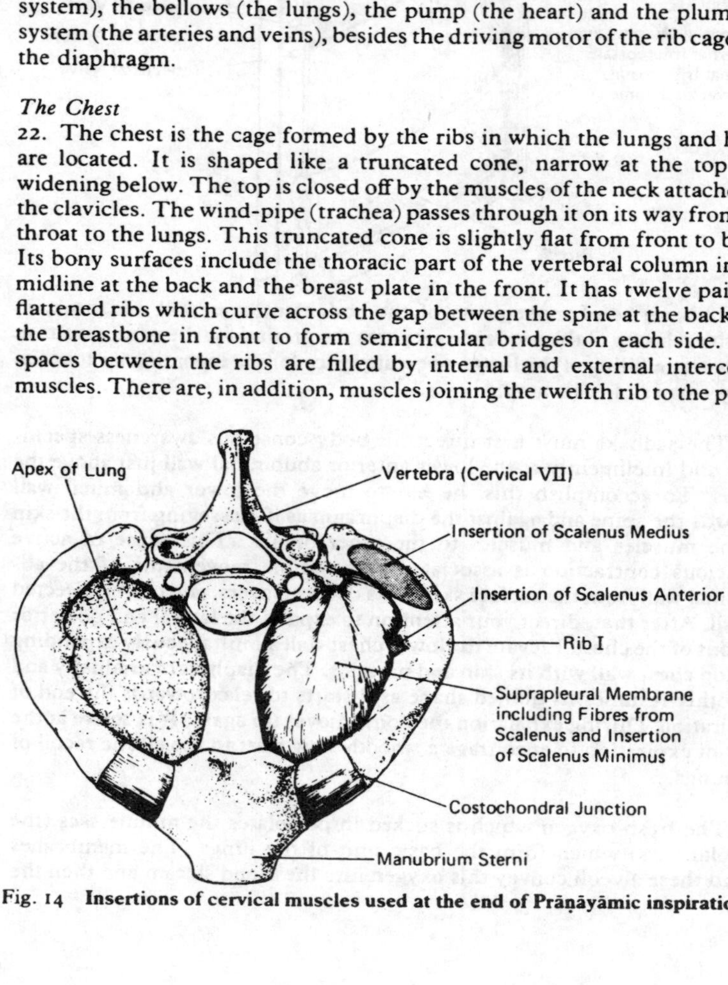

Fig. 14 **Insertions of cervical muscles used at the end of Prāṇāyāmic inspiration**

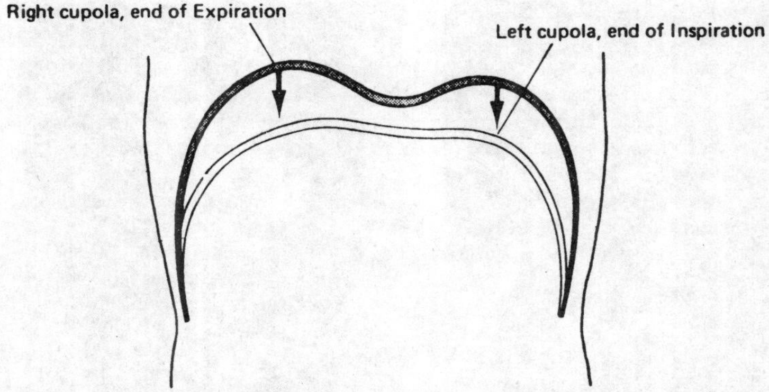

Fig. 15 Movements of diaphragm during Prāṇāyāma

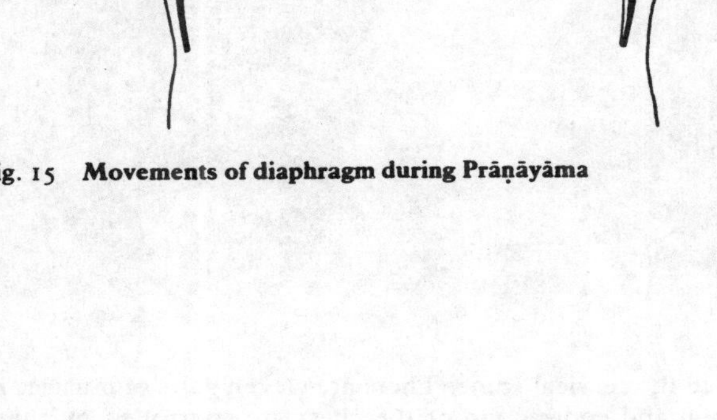

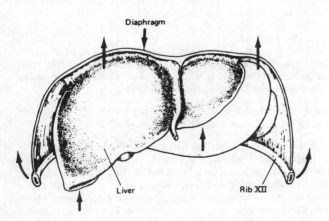

Fig. 16 Diaphragm elevating the floating ribs in inspiration

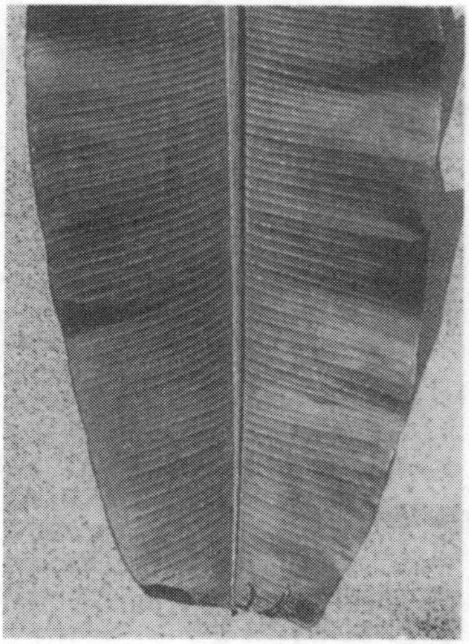

Pl. 1

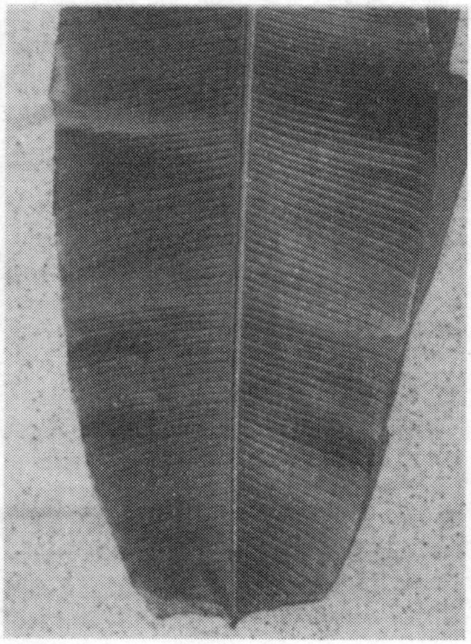

Pl. 2

and the first one to the cervical spine. There are eleven pairs of muscles in all. The expansion and contraction of the chest are controlled by these muscles and the diaphragm. The thoracic dorsal area is like the broad mid-section of a banana leaf, the spine being the stem, the evenly spaced ribs being the veins and the tail bone the thin end of the leaf (Pls 1 & 2).

The Lungs and the Bronchial Tree

23. The right and left lungs differ in shape and capacity. In most of us the bulk of the heart, which is about the size of a fist, is on the left side. Consequently, that lung is smaller. It is divided into two lobes, one above the other, whereas the right lung has three lobes. (Fig. 5)

24. The lungs are covered with a membrane called the pleura and due to their shape expand rather like the bladder of a football.

25. The dome of the right diaphragm is higher than the left. Beneath it is the liver, the largest solid abdominal organ, less compressible and depressible than the stomach and spleen lying below the left diaphragm. In full inhalation, when attempting to fill the lungs, most people can feel a sense of increased resistance below the right side of the diaphragm, where the liver is, when their attention is drawn to the area. In order to equalise the filling of both lungs from base and side, special effort and attention must be directed to diaphragmatic and chest wall movements on the right side.

26. The bronchial system, connecting the windpipe and the alveoli, is in the thoracic cage. It resembles an inverted tree with its roots in the gullet, while the branches spread out downwards towards the diaphragm and the side walls of the chest cavity.

27. The windpipe in the throat is a tube about four inches long and less than an inch wide, which branches out into two primary bronchi, one leading into each lung. Both then branch out into numerous tiny air-passages called the bronchioles. At the end cf each of these bronchioles are the alveoli, the tiny air sacs clustered like bunches of grapes, some 300 million linıng each lung, their surface covers about eighty to one hundred square yards – forty to fifty times that of the human skin.

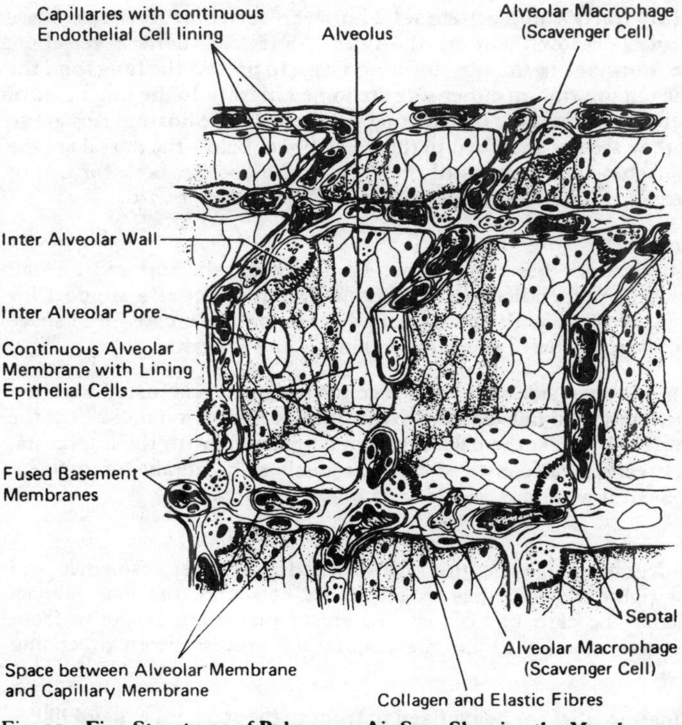

Fig. 17 **Fine Structures of Pulmonary Air Sacs Showing the Membranes across which Gases Exchange between Air and Blood**

28. These alveoli are small, multiple sac-like chambers with an incomplete lining of cells. The gap between the cells (the interstitial space) is filled with fluid. Around the outer wall of the alveoli lie minute blood vessels (the capillaries). Exchange of gases takes place between the alveoli and the red blood cells and plasma of the blood via the fluid in the alveoli or interstitial space.

29. The air in the alveoli contains more oxygen and less carbon dioxide than the blood passing through the capillaries in the lungs. During the exchange of oxygen and carbon dioxide, the molecules of oxygen diffuse into, and carbon dioxide out of, the blood.

The Spine

30. The spine should be kept firm like the trunk of a tree. The spinal cord is protected by thirty-three vertebrae. The seven vertebrae in the neck are called cervical. Below them are the twelve dorsal or thoracic vertebrae which are connected to the ribs, forming a cage to protect the lungs and the heart. The ten top ribs on either side are joined in front to the inner side of the breastbone, but not the two floating ribs below. The floating ribs are so called, as they are not anchored to the breastbone. Below the dorsal are the lumbar vertebrae and lower still the sacrum and coccyx, both formed of fused vertebrae. The lowest coccygeal vertebra curls forward.

The Breastbone

31. The breastbone has three parts. In breathing, the top and bottom should be kept perpendicular to the floor. Use it to act as a support for lifting the side ribs like the handle of a bucket, and so create more space through the expansion of the lungs sideways and upwards.

32. The lungs open sideways and space for expansion is created with the help of the intercostal muscles. Keep the interior intercostal muscles at the back firm. If the skin at the back does not co-ordinate with the intercostal muscles, breathing becomes shallow, reducing the intake of oxygen, causing physical weakness and lack of bodily resistance.

The Skin

33. As a drummer tightens the skin of his drum to get resonance and a violinist tightens his strings to get clarity of sound, the yogi adjusts and stretches the skin of his torso to create maximum response from the intercostal muscles to aid the respiratory process when practising prāṇāyāma.

34. The floating ribs, not being fixed in front to the sternum expand like a pair of calipers to create more space in the chest. Laterally, the thick middle ribs can also expand laterally, thus widening and lifting the rib-cage. This

does not affect the top ribs. To fill the uppermost reaches of the lungs requires training and attention. Learn to use the upper inner intercostal muscles and the top part of the sternum. Expand the rib-cage from the inner frame outwards, as this will stretch the intercostal muscles.

The Diaphragm

35. The diaphragm is a large dome-shaped muscle-like partition which separates the thoracic cavity from the abdominal one. Anchored all around the circumference of the lower thoracic cage, it is attached at the back to the lumbar vertebrae, at the sides to the lower six ribs and in the front to the dagger-shaped cartilage of the breastbone. Above it are the heart and lungs and below it the liver on the right and the stomach and spleen on the left.

Accessory Muscles

36. The respiratory muscles of the throat, torso, spine and abdomen are the accessories used in breathing, which is ordinarily dominated by the diaphragm. Besides the muscles already described, those of the neck, especially the sternomastoids and the scalenus, play their parts. They contribute very little to quiet breathing, but become active when the rate or depth is increased and rigid when the breath is held. The use of accessory respiratory muscles varies from one individual to another. It also varies from time to time in the same person, depending on how powerfully he exerts in his breathing and how efficiently and how tensely.

37. We all breathe, but how many of us do so correctly, with attention? Bad posture, an ill-shaped or caved-in chest, obesity, emotional disorders, various lung troubles, smoking and uneven use of the respiratory muscles, lead to improper breathing, below one's capacity. We are aware of the discomfort and disability which then arises. Many subtle changes take place in our body as a result of poor breathing and bad posture, leading to heavy breathing, inadequate pulmonary function and aggravation of heart disease. Prāṇāyāma can help to prevent these disorders and help to check or cure them, so that one can live fully and well.

38. As light radiates from the disc of the sun, so air is spread through the lungs. Move the chest up and out. If the skin over the centre of the breastbone can move vertically up and down and it can expand from side to side circumferentially, it shows that the lungs are being filled to their maximum capacity.

Chapter 5

Nāḍīs and Chakras

1. The word nāḍī is derived from nād meaning a hollow stalk, sound, vibration and resonance. Nāḍīs are tubes, ducts or channels which carry air, water, blood, nutrients and other substances throughout the body. They are our arteries, veins, capillaries, bronchioles and so on. In our so-called subtle and spiritual bodies, which cannot be weighed or measured, they are channels for cosmic, vital, seminal and other energies as well as for sensations, consciousness and spiritual aura. They are called by different names in accordance with their functions. Nāḍikās are small nāḍīs and nāḍīchakras are ganglia or plexuses in all three bodies – the gross, subtle and causal. The subtle or causal bodies are not yet recognised by scientists or the medical profession.

2. It is said in the *Varāhopaniṣad* (V, 54/5) that the nāḍīs penetrate the body from the soles of the feet to the crown of the head. In them is prāṇa, the breath of life and in that life abides Ātmā, which is the abode of Śakti, creatrix of the animate and inanimate worlds.

3. All nāḍīs originate from one of two centres, the kandasthāna – a little below the navel – and the heart. Though Yoga texts agree about their starting points, they vary about where some of them end.

Nāḍīs Starting from Below the Navel

4. Twelve digits above the anus and the genital organs and just below the navel, there is an egg-shaped bulb called the kanda. From it 72,000 nāḍīs are said to spread throughout the body, each branching off into another 72,000. They move in every direction and have countless outlets and functions.

5. The *Śiva Saṁhitā* mentions 350,000 nāḍīs, of which fourteen are stated to be important. These and a few others are listed with their functions in the given table below. The three that are most vital are the suṣumṇā, iḍā and pingalā.

6. The suṣumṇā, which runs through the centre of the spine, is split at the root and terminates at the crown of the head in the thousand-petalled lotus (sahasrāra), which is the seat of fire (agni). The *Varāhopaniṣad* (V, 29, 30) describes it as blazing and shining (jvalanti), and as being sound incarnate

Table of Nāḍīs Starting from the Kanda Below the Navel

Sl No.	Nāḍī	Place in body	Terminus	Function
1.	Suṣumṇā	Centre of spine	Crown of head	Agni. Fire (sattva), illumination
2.	Iḍā	Left of 1	Left nostril	Chandra Cooling (tamas), inertia
3.	Pingalā	Right of 1	Right nostril	Sūrya Burning (rajas) action
4.	Gāndhāri	Behind 2	Left eye	Seeing
5.	Hastijihvā	In front of 2	Right eye	Seeing
6.	Pūsā	Behind 3	Right ear	Hearing
7.	Yasasvini	Before 3 – Between 4 and 10	Left ear and Left big toe	
8.	Alambusā	Bifurcates mouth and anus.		
9.	Kuhū	In front of 1		Evacuation
10.	Sarasvati	Behind 1	Tongue	Controls speech and keeps all abdominal organs free from disease
11.	Vāruṇi	Between 7 and 9	Flows throughout body	Evacuates urine
12.	Viśvodhari	Between 5 and 9		Absorbs food
13.	Payasvinī	Between 6 and 10	Right big toe	
14.	Śaṁkhinī	Between 4 and 10	Genital organs	Carries the essence of food
15.	Śubhā			
16.	Kauśiki		Big toes	
17.	Śūrā		Between eyebrows	
18.	Rāka			Creates hunger and thirst; collects mucus at sinuses.
19.	Kūrma			Stabilises body and mind
20.	Vijñāna Nāḍīs			Vessels of consciousness

(nādarūpiṇi). It is also called the 'Supporter of the Universe' (Viśvadhāriṇī: viśva = universe, dhāriṇī = supporter), the brahmanāḍī and the aperture of Brahma (Brahmarandhra). It is illumination (sattva). It gives delight to the sādhaka when prāṇa enters it and swallows time.

Nāḍīs Starting from the Heart

7. According to the *Kaṭhopaniṣad* (VI 16, 17) and *Praśnopaniṣad* (III, 6), the Ātmā, which is said to be the size of a thumb, dwells within the heart, from which a hundred and one nāḍīs radiate. In the *Chāndogyopaniṣad* (III, 12,4) it is said that as the outer cover of man is his physical body, his inner core (hṛdayam) is the heart (VIII 3.3), wherein abides the Ātmā. It is also called the antarātma (soul, heart or mind), antaḥkaraṇa (source of thought, feeling and consciousness) and chidātmā (faculty of reasoning and consciousness).

8. Here the heart stands for both the physical and the spiritual one. All the vital breaths or winds (vāyus) are established there and do not go beyond it. It is here that the prāṇa stimulates actions and activates intelligence (prajñā). The intelligence becomes the source of thinking, imagination and will. When the mind is controlled and the intellect and heart are united, the self is revealed. (*Śvetāśvataropaniṣad* IV 17.)

9. From each of these 101 nāḍīs emanate one hundred subtler nāḍīs, each of which branches off into another 72,000. If there is harmony between the five winds (vāyus) (namely, prāṇa, apāna, udāna, vyāna and samāna) and these nāḍīs, then the body becomes a heaven on earth; but if there is disharmony, it becomes a battle ground of diseases.

10. Of the 101 nāḍīs, only the chitrā splits into two parts at the root of the suṣumṇā. One part of the chitrā moves within it, extending upwards to the aperture (randhra) of Brahma at the crown of the head above the sahasrāra chakra. This is the gateway to the Supreme Spirit (Parabrahman). The other part of chitrā moves downwards towards the generative organ for discharge of semen. It is said that at the time of death, yogis and saints consciously leave through the Brahmarandhra. Since the aperture is in the spiritual or causal body (kāraṇa śarīra), it cannot be seen or measured. When prāṇa rises upwards, via the chitrā through the chakras, it takes with it the radiance (ojas), a creative energy latent in semen. The chitrā is transformed into the Brahma nāḍī or parā (supreme) nāḍī. Then the sādhaka becomes one who has sublimated his sexual appetite (an ūrdhva-reta) and is free from all desire.

Dhamanī and Sirā

11. Nāḍīs, dhamanīs and sirās are tubular organs or ducts within the physical and subtle bodies conveying energy in different forms. The word

'dhamanī' is derived from 'dhamana', meaning a pair of bellows. The nearest analogy is an orange. Its rind represents the gross (sthūla), the membranes represent the subtle (sūkṣma), and the segments, containing the juicy buds, the causal (kāraṇa) bodies respectively. The nāḍīs carry air, the dhamanī carry blood, and the sirās distribute the vital seminal energy throughout the subtle body.

12. Āyurveda is the science of life and longevity. According to its texts, which deal with ancient Indian medicine, sirās start from the heart. They carry blood (rakta) and seminal vitality (ojas) from and to the heart. Sirās are thicker at the heart and become thinner as they branch out like the veins of a leaf. Seven hundred of them are considered important. They are divided evenly into four categories, each of which caters for one of the humours: wind (vāta) for proper functioning of the body, bile (pitta) for harmonising the organs, phlegm (kapha) for free movement in the joints, and blood (rakta), which circulates oxygen and its own form of vital energy.

Nāḍīs and Circulation

13. The *Śiva Saṁhitā* (V 52–55) states that when food is digested, the nāḍīs carry the best part to nourish the subtle body (sūkṣma śarīra), the middle part to the gross body (sthūla śarīra), and discharge the inferior part in the form of faeces, urine and sweat.

14. The food that is consumed is turned into chyle, which is carried through certain ducts known in Āyurvedic texts as srotas – a synonym for nāḍīs. Their functions are wide, for they also carry the vital energy or breath known as prāṇa, water, blood and other material to various tissues, marrow and ligaments, as well as discharge semen, urine, faeces and sweat.

15. In breathing, nāḍīs, dhamanīs and sirās perform the dual function of absorbing vital energy from the in-coming air and throwing off the resultant toxins. The in-breath moves through the windpipe to the lungs, on into the bronchioles (dhamanīs) and then to the alveoli (sirās). The blood takes up the energy from the oxygen and percolates it into the dhamanīs with the help of prāṇa in the nāḍīs. The percolation transforms the seminal fluid into vital seminal energy (ojas) and discharges it into the sirās, which distribute it to revitalise the body and the brain. The sirās then discharge used-up energy and gathered toxins such as carbon dioxide into the dhamanīs and through them into the windpipe, to be breathed out.

16. The *Varāhopaniṣad* (V 30) calls the body a 'jewel' filled with essential ingredients (ratna pūrita-dhātu). In Prāṇāyāma the essential ingredient (dhātu), called blood, is enriched and refined like a jewel as it absorbs the various energies. The nāḍīs, dhamanīs and sirās also convey smells,

flavours (essence of food), forms, sounds and intelligence (jñāna). Yoga helps them to function properly by keeping all these channels pure, the body immune from diseases and the intelligence keen, so that the sādhaka can get to know his body, mind and soul (*Varāhopaniṣad*, V 46–9).

17. Some nāḍīs, dhamanīs and sirās may correspond to arteries, veins and capillaries of the respiratory and circulatory systems. They may also be nerves, channels and ducts of the nervous, lymphatic, glandular, digestive and genito-urinary systems of the physical and physiological body. Others carry vital energy (prāṇa) to the mental body, intellectual energy (vijñāna) to the intellectual body, and spiritual energy to the causal or spiritual body (soul). The terminating point of each nāḍī is to be found in follicle, cell or hair. They function as inlets and outlets of various energies. In all, 5.9 billion of them flow in the gross, subtle and causal bodies. No wonder it is said that the body is full of nāḍīs.

Kuṇḍalinī

18. Kuṇḍalinī is divine cosmic energy. The word is derived from 'kuṇḍala', meaning a ring or coil. The latent energy is symbolised as a sleeping serpent with three and a half coils; it has its tail in its mouth, which faces downwards. It lies at the hollow base of the suṣumṇā, two digits below the genital area and two above the anus.

19. The three coils represent the three states of mind (avasthā), namely awake (jāgṛt), dreaming (Svapna) and in deep sleep (suṣupti). There is a fourth state, turīya, combining and transcending the others, which is represented by the last half-coil. It is attained in samādhi.

20. The *Haṭha Yoga Pradīpikā* (III.1) states that as Ādi Śeṣa, the Lord of Serpents, supports the universe, so kuṇḍalini upholds all the disciplines of Yoga.

21. The energy which passes through the iḍā, pingalā and suṣumṇā is called bindu, literally a point having no parts or no magnitude. These three nāḍīs represent respectively the nāḍīs of the moon, the sun and fire. Before the word 'kuṇḍalini' came into vogue, 'agni' (fire) was used to represent the divine power which purifies and rises upwards like fire. Through the discipline of Yoga the direction of the mouth of the coiled serpentine energy is made to turn upwards. It rises like steam through the suṣumṇā via the chitrā (emanating from the heart) till it reaches the sahasrāra. When the creative energy (śakti) of kuṇḍalinī is awakened, iḍā and piṅgala merge within the suṣumṇā. (*Śiva Saṁhitā*, V 13.)

22. Metal is refined by burning out of the dross. By the fire of yogic discipline, the sādhaka burns up within himself the impurities of desire,

anger, greed, infatuation, pride and envy. Then his intellect becomes refined. The cosmic energy latent within him is then awakened by the grace of God and the guru. (*Haṭha Yoga Pradīpikā*, III.2.). As this rises, the sādhaka gets more and more in tune with the Divine. He becomes free from attachment towards fruits of action (karma mukta) and unattached to life (jīvana mukta).

23. According to Tāntric texts, the object of Prāṇāyāma is to arouse the latent power (śakti) called kuṇḍalinī, the divine cosmic energy in our bodies, lying at the base of the spinal column in mūlādhāra chakrā, the nervous plexus situated in the pelvis above the anus at the root of the spine. This energy has to be aroused and made to ascend through the suṣumṇā from the mūlādhāra chakra to the thousand-petalled lotus (sahasrāra) in the head, the net-work of nerves in the brain. After piercing the intervening chakras, it finally unites with the Supreme Soul. This is an allegorical way of describing the tremendous seminal vitality which is obtained by the practice of uḍḍīyāna, mūla bandhās (Ch. 13) and self-restraint. It is a symbolic way of describing the sublimation of sexual energy.

24. When the kuṇḍalinī reaches the sahasrāra, the sādhaka has no feeling of his own separate identity and nothing exists for him. He has crossed the barriers of time and space, and becomes one with the universe.

Chakras

25. 'Chakra' means a wheel, a ring. Chakras are flying wheels, radiating energy, located at vital centres along the spine, connecting the nāḍīs to the various sheaths (kośas).

26. As antennae pick up radio waves and transform them into sound through receiving sets, chakras pick up cosmic vibrations and distribute them throughout the body in the nāḍīs, dhamanīs and sirās. The body is a counterpart of the universe, a microcosm within the macrocosm on the gross, subtle and spiritual levels.

27. According to Yoga texts, two other important types of energy pervade the body, that from the sun radiating through the pingalā nāḍī, and from the moon through the iḍā nāḍī. Both these currents criss-cross at the chakras, the vital centres along the suṣumṇā, the nāḍī of fire in the spinal cord.

28. To conserve the energies generated within the body and to prevent their dissipation, āsanas and mudrās (seals), Prāṇāyāmas and bandhās (locks) were prescribed. The heat so generated causes the kuṇḍalinī to uncoil. The serpent lifts its head, enters the suṣumnā and is forced up through the chakras one by one to the sahasrāra.

29. The generation and distribution of prāṇa in the human system may be compared to that of electrical energy. The energy of falling water or rising steam is made to rotate turbines within a magnetic field to generate electricity. The electricity is then stored in accumulators and the power is stepped up or down by transformers which regulate the voltage or current. It is then transmitted along cables to light cities and run machinery. Prāṇa is like the falling water or rising steam. The thoracic area is the magnetic field. The breathing processes of inhalation, exhalation and retention of breath act like the turbines, while the chakras represent the accumulators and transformers. The energy (ojas) generated by prāṇa is like electricity. It is stepped up or down by the chakras and distributed throughout the system along the nāḍīs, dhamanīs and sirās, which are the transmission lines. If the power generated is not properly regulated it will destroy the machinery and the equipment. It is the same with prāṇa and ojas, for they can destroy the body and the mind of the sādhaka.

30. The main chakras are: (1) mūlādhāra (mūla = source, ādhāra = support, vital part), situated in the pelvis above the anus; (2) svādhiṣṭhāna (seat of a vital force), situated above the organs of generation; (3) maṇipūraka, situated in the navel; (4) sūrya, the sun; and (5) manas (mind), between the navel and the heart; (6) anāhata (heart), in the cardiac area; (7) viśuddhi (pure), in the pharyngeal region; (8) ājñā (command), between the eyebrows; (9) Soma, the moon in the centre of the brain; (10) lalāṭa, at the top of the forehead; and (11) sahasrāra, which is called the thousand-petalled lotus in the brain. The most important of them are mūlādhāra, svādhiṣṭhāna, maṇipūraka, anāhata, viśuddhi, ājñā and sahasrāra.

31. The mūlādhāra chakra is the seat of the element of earth (pṛthvi tattva) and of smell. It is the base of the annamaya kośa, the body of nourishment, connected with the absorption of food and the evacuation of faeces. When this chakra is activated, the sādhaka becomes firm in vitality and ready to sublimate his sexual energy (ūrdhvarētas)

32. The svādhiṣṭhāna chakra is the seat of the element of water (ap) and of taste. When it is activated, the sādhaka becomes free from disease and acquires vibrant health. Feeling no fatigue, he becomes friendly and compassionate.

33. The maṇipūraka chakra is the seat of the element of fire (agni), and when it is activated the sādhaka obtains calmness even in adverse circumstances.

34. The svādhiṣṭhāna and the maṇipūraka chakras are the foundations of the Prāṇamaya kośa, the physiological body. Both have to move together,

co-ordinating their functions during inhalation and exhalation in Prāṇāyāma.

35. The sūrya chakra, commonly known as the solar plexus, lies between the navel and the diaphragm. It keeps the abdominal organs healthy and increases the lifespan.

36. The manas chakra lies between the sūrya and the anāhata. It is the seat of emotion, igniting imagination and creativity, and can be stabilised by Prāṇāyāmas involving retention of the breath.

37. The anāhata chakra lies in the region of the physical and the spiritual heart. It is the element of air (vāyu) and of touch.

38. The manas and the anāhata chakras represent the psychological body (manomaya kośa). When activated, they strengthen the heart, develop adoration (bhakti) and knowledge (jñāna). They free the sādhaka from sensual pleasures and make him follow the path of spirituality.

39. The viśuddhi chakra, in the region of the throat above the chest, and at the base of the neck, is the element of ether (ākāśa). It represents the intellectual body (vijñānamaya kośa). When it is activated, the sādhaka's power of understanding increases. He becomes intellectually alert. His speech becomes distinct, clear and fluent.

40. The ājñā chakra represents the abode of joy (ānandamaya kośa). When it is activated, the sādhaka gains perfect control over his body and develops a spiritual aura.

41. Soma chakra regulates the temperature of the body.

42. When the lalāṭa chakra is activated, the sādhaka becomes the master of his destiny.

43. The sahasrāra chakra, also called sahasrāra dala (dala = a body of troops, a large number) is the seat of the Supreme Spirit (Parabrahman) at the end of the Brahma nāḍī or suṣumṇā.

44. When the kuṇḍalinī energy reaches the sahasrāra, the sādhaka has crossed all barriers and becomes an emancipated soul (siddha). This state is referred to in the *Ṣaṭ Chakra Nirūpaṇa* (Verse 40) as the State of Void (Śūnya Deśa).

Chapter 6

Guru and Śiṣya

1. The guru (teacher) and his pupil (śiṣya) are together concerned with spiritual knowledge (Brahma-vidyā). The guru first studies his pupil and discusses what the pupil knows, while the pupil studies the guru and the subject he is being taught. The next step for the pupil is prolonged ascetic practice (tapas) until the knowledge has been fully absorbed. In time wisdom (prajñā), the fruit of first-hand experience, matures and the guru and śiṣya explore it together.

2. The Sanskrit word guru is derived from the two roots 'gu' meaning darkness and 'ru' light. As a teacher of sacred knowledge he removes the darkness of ignorance and leads his pupil towards enlightenment and truth. He is also one from whom we learn right conduct or under whom one studies how to lead a good life. Free from hatred, he has searched widely for truth. He puts his spiritual knowledge into practice. He is not content with the theoretical level only. He shows by example what he has experienced and lives up to what he preaches. A guru should be (a) clear in his perception and knowledge, (b) regular in spiritual practice (anuṣṭhāna), (c) constant and determined in study (abhyāsa), (d) free from desire for the fruits of his actions (karma phala thyāgi or vairāgya), and (e) pure in what he does to guide his pupils in the true essence of knowledge (paratattva). He shows them how to turn their senses and intelligence inwards, so that they learn to explore themselves and to reach the source of their own being (Ātmā). The guru is the bridge between the individual (jīvātmā) and God (Paramātmā).

3. The classical examples of the guru-śiṣya relationship are those mentioned in the *Kaṭhopaniṣad* and in the *Bhagavad Gītā*. In the former, Yama, the God of Death gives spiritual knowledge to the earnest seeker Nachiketā, who with unhesitating courage faces death. In the latter, Śri Kṛṣṇa removes the doubts and dejection of the mighty bowman Arjuna, whose unerring aim and spirit of humility led him to the highest goal of life.

4. The strength and energy of a robber named Ratnākara were diverted by the sage Nārada towards God. The robber ultimately became the sage Vālmīki, the author of the epic *Rāmāyaṇa*. By way of parable the *Rāmāyaṇa* compares the human body to Laṅkā, the island kingdom of Rāvaṇa,

the ten-headed demon king with an inflated ego. The ten heads are the organs of knowledge and action, whose desires have no bounds; like the ocean around the island, Sītā, the individual soul or prakṛti, is kept confined in Aśokavana, Rāvaṇa's pleasure garden. Sītā is dejected and full of sorrow at the forced separation from her Lord, Rāma, and thinks of him constantly. Rāma sends his messenger Hanumān, son of Vāyu (the vital wind), to console Sītā and raise her flagging spirit. Hanumān helps to destroy Rāvaṇa, the ego, and to reunite Sītā and Rāma (prakṛti and puruṣa; jīvātmā and Paramātmā). As Hanumān brought about the reunion of Sītā and Rāma, prāṇāyāma brings about the reunion of the sādhaka with his Ātmā.

5. Initially the guru brings himself down to the level of his pupil, whom he encourages and gradually lifts up by precept and example. This is followed by teaching adjusted to the pupil's fitness and maturity until the latter becomes as fearless and independent as his guru. Like a mother cat holding a blind and helpless kitten in her mouth, he first checks the movements of his pupil, leaving him with little initiative. In the next stage, he allows him the same freedom that a mother monkey does when her baby first releases its grip on her fur, for she keeps it close to her. In the first stage, the pupil is under the unquestionable discipline of the guru; in the second stage he surrenders his will completely. In the third stage, like the fish with unwinking eyes he becomes both skilful and clean in thought, word and deed.

6. Pupils are of three categories – dull, average and intense or superior. The dull pupil has little enthusiasm, being sensual, unstable and cowardly. He is unwilling to shed his negative qualities or to work hard for self-realisation. The second type of pupil is a waverer, equally attracted towards worldly matters as by the spiritual, sometimes giving weight to the one and sometimes to the other. He knows what is the highest good, but lacks courage and determination to hold on steadfastly. He needs strong treatment to correct his fickle nature of which the guru is aware. The intense or superior pupil has vision, enthusiasm and courage. He resists temptations and has no hesitation in casting off qualities which take him away from his goal. He therefore becomes stable, skilful and steady. The guru is always alert to find a way to guide his intense pupil to realise his highest potential until he becomes a realised soul (siddha). The guru is always happy with his pupil, who may eventually surpass him.

7. A worthy pupil finds his guru by the grace of God. Satyakāma-Jābāli, who confessed that he was not aware of his parentage, was accepted as a pupil by the sage Gautama, who was impressed by his innocence and truthfulness. Śvetaketu proudly returned home after years of study, but

failed to answer when his father Uddālaka asked him what had made a huge tree grow from a tiny seed. When with due humility Śvetaketu confessed his ignorance, his father accepted him as a pupil and gave him spiritual knowledge. A disciple should hunger after spiritual knowledge and self-control. He should practise constantly with attention and possess great endurance.

8. Spiritual training (sādhana) has nothing to do with theoretical study, but it leads to a new way of life. Just as sesame seeds are crushed to yield oil and wood ignited to bring out its latent heat, so must the pupil be unswerving in his practice to bring out the knowledge latent within him and find his own identity. When he realises that he is a spark of the Divine Flame burning throughout the universe, then all his past impressions (saṁskāras) are burnt out, and he becomes enlightened. He is then a guru in his own right.

Chapter 7

Food

1. The *Mahānārāyaṇopaniṣad* (79–15) describes food (anna) as the primary requisite without which man cannot develop his anatomical body to the spiritual level. It is stated that the sun radiates heat which evaporates water. The vapour becomes clouds from which rain falls to the earth. Man tills the earth and produces food which, when consumed, creates the energy that maintains vigour. Vigour engenders discipline, which develops the faith that gives knowledge; knowledge bestows learning, which brings composure that creates calmness; calmness establishes equanimity, which develops memory that induces recognition; recognition brings judgement, which leads to the realisation of the 'Self'.

2. The body needs food containing the right balance of carbohydrates, proteins, fats, vitamins and mineral salts. Water is needed to help digestion and assimilation. Food in the form of nourishment is finally assimilated in various forms throughout the body.

3. Food should be wholesome, palatable and congenial to the body, and should not be eaten merely to gratify the senses. It is broadly divided into three kinds – sāttvic, rājasic and tamasic. The first promotes longevity, health and happiness; the second produces excitement, and the third creates disease. Rājasic and tāmasic food make the consciousness dull and impede spiritual progress. It is the duty of the sādhaka to find out by trial and experience which is suitable for him.

4. Whereas it is true that character is influenced by food, it is equally true that the practice of Prāṇāyāma changes the eating habits of the sādhaka. Man's temperament is influenced by his diet because what he eats affects the functioning of the mind. Sāttvic vegetarian food, however, may be taken by tyrants with disturbed minds, full of hatred, yet they remain rājasic or tāmasic. In the same way noble characters (like the Buddha or Jesus) may not be affected by the type of food offered to them or by those persons who give it, though they would normally be regarded as tāmasic. It is the state of mind of the eater that is important. Yet a diet consisting of sāttvic food only will help the practitioner to maintain a clear and unwavering mind.

5. The body is the abode of the individual self (jīvātmā). If it were to perish from lack of food the 'Self' would leave it just like a tenant who refuses to reside any longer in a dilapidated house. The body therefore, has to be protected to house the 'Self'. To neglect this body leads to death and destruction of the 'Self'.

6. According to the *Chāndogyopaniṣad* (VI 7.2) solid food, fluids and fats which fuel the body are each split up into sixteen parts on consumption. Food is divided into three of these; the grossest becomes faeces, the medium becomes flesh, and the subtlest becomes the mind, in the ratio of 10/16, 5/16 and 1/16 respectively. With fluids, the grossest becomes urine, the medium becomes blood and the subtlest becomes energy (prāṇa). Similarly with fats, the grossest ingredient becomes bone, the medium becomes marrow and the subtlest speech (vāc). Śvetaketu lived on fluid for fifteen days and lost his power of thinking, but regained it as soon as he ate solid food again; his power of speech diminished when he went without fats. This experience revealed to him that the mind is the product of food, energy of fluids and speech of fats.

7. The *Haṭha Yoga Pradīpikā* (II.14) says that during his practice of prāṇāyāma the sādhaka has to eat pounded rice cooked in milk and clarified butter. When well established in prāṇāyāma, he may choose the food congenial to him and his practice.

8. Do not eat when saliva does not flow, for this indicates that the body does not need more food. Both the quantity and quality of food should be moderated. Chosen food might appear to be dainty and delicious, but it may not be good for the sādhaka. It may have high nutritive value and yet it may develop toxins affecting progress in prāṇāyāma. When one is really hungry or thirsty, food is immediately absorbed into the system and becomes nourishing. Water by itself can always quench thirst. Real thirst chooses no other drink but water. Restrain artificial hunger and thirst. Yoga texts prescribe that the sādhaka should fill half his stomach with solid food, one-fourth with fluids and keep one-fourth empty for the free flow of breath.

9. Do not eat when emotionally disturbed. While dining, talk well and eat wisely. When a noble frame of mind prevails while eating, all but poisonous food is sāttvic.

10. The fire of digestion is lit by the energy that arises from respiration. Moderate and nourishing food is essential to maintain vigour, strength and alertness. Avoid fasting.

11. According to *Taittirīya Upaniṣad*, food is Brahman. It is to be respected, not derided or abused.

Chapter 8

Obstacles and Aids

1. The sādhaka must be aware of the obstacles which disturb his prāṇāyāma practice consciously or unconsciously. He should avoid distractions and lead a disciplined life to prepare his body and mind.

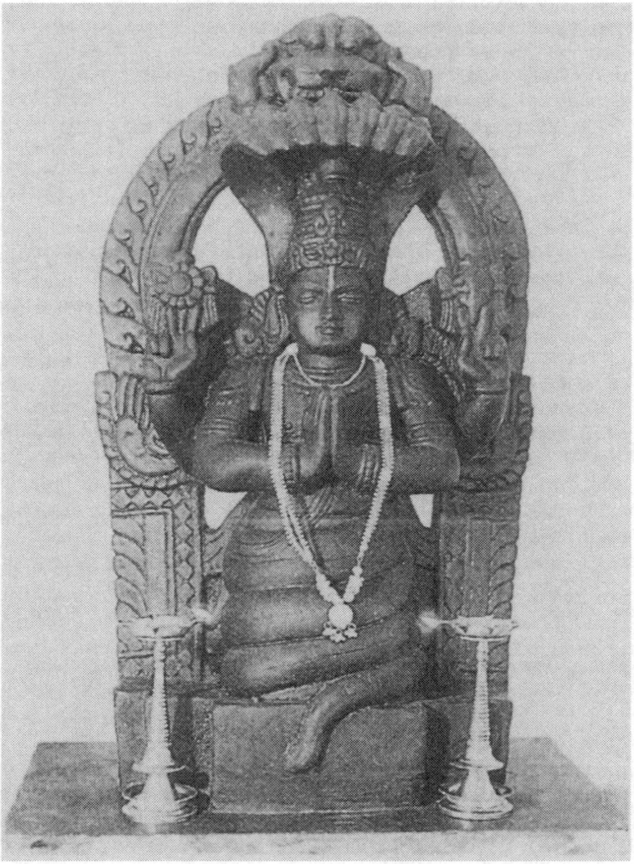

Sage Patanjali

2. Patanjali gives a list of obstacles to yogic practices. They are: sickness (vyādhi), lack of mental disposition (styāna), doubt about one's practices (saṁśaya), insensibility (pramāda), laziness (ālaysa), sensuality or rousing of desire when sensory objects possess the mind (avirati), false or invalid knowledge (bhrānti-darśana), failure to attain continuity of thought or concentration (alabhdha-bhūmikatva), inability to continue the practice due to slackness and failure (anavasthitattva), pain (duḥkha), despair (daurmansya), unsteadiness of the body (angamejayatva) and breathing (śvāsa-praśvāsa). (*Yoga Sūtra*, I 30/31). These either originate in man or are due to natural calamities and accidents. Man-made afflictions, brought about by over-indulgence and lack of discipline, affect the sādhaka's body and mind. Their cures are laid down in Yoga texts.

3. It may be noted that out of thirteen obstacles to yogic practices mentioned by Patanjali, only four deal with the physical body, namely, sickness, laziness, unsteadiness of the body and respiration. The remaining nine obstacles deal with the mind. The sage mentioned the stage of āsanas to enable the sādhaka to get rid of the obstacles affecting the pḥysical body, before he was ready to tackle the mental obstacles by the practice of prānāyāma.

4. The *Haṭha Yoga Pradīpikā* (I 16) mentions the six destroyers of yoga practices; over-eating, over-exertion, useless talk, undisciplined conduct, bad company and restless inconstancy. According to the *Bhagavad Gītā* (VI 16) Yoga is not for those who gorge themselves, starve or sleep or stay awake too much. The *Yoga Upaniṣads* include bad physical posture and self-destroying emotion, like lust, anger, fear, greed, hatred and jealousy.

5. To continue and maintain his training, the pupil needs faith, virility, memory, meditation (samādhi) and acute insight (prajñā). (*Yoga Sūtras*, I 20.)

6. To overcome these obstacles, Patanjali offered the four-fold remedy of friendliness and feeling at one with all that is good, compassion with devoted action to relieve the misery of the afflicted; delight at the good work done by others and avoidance of disdain for or feeling superior to the victims of vice. The *Haṭha Yoga Pradīpikā* prescribes enthusiasm, daring, fortitude, true knowledge, determination and a feeling of detachment, of being in the world but not of it, as the means to overcome the obstacles in the path of Yoga.

7. By moderation in eating and resting, by regular working hours and by the right balance between sleeping and waking, Yoga destroys all pain and sorrow, says the *Bhagavad Gītā* (VI 17). Yoga is working wisely and living a skilful, active life in harmony and moderation. What the sādhaka needs most is single-minded, devoted practice (*Yoga Sūtra*, I 32).

Chapter 9

The Effects of Prāṇāyāma

1. Āsanas improve the blood circulation throughout the body, including the head, trunk and limbs.

2. Those appropriate for legs and arms keep the circulatory system active. The arterial, capillary, venous and lymphatic circulation is stimulated by the rhythmic contraction and relaxation of the muscles which act as pumps by the opening up of new and unused vascular beds. This allows efficient supply and utilisation of energy and promotes a remarkable resistance to disease.

3. Although āsanas produce similar effects in the trunk, prāṇāyāma affects rhythmic expansion of the lungs, creating the proper circulation of the bodily fluids within the kidneys, stomach, liver, spleen, intestines, skin and other organs, as well as the surface of the torso.

4. The lungs are directly concerned with the disposal of carbon dioxide in the venous blood and preventing ammonia, ketones and aromatic amines from building up to toxic levels. The lungs need to be kept clean and free from bacterial diseases by an efficient circulation of blood and lymph. Prāṇāyāma helps here by keeping the lungs pure and by increasing the flow of fresh blood.

5. The functions of the liver depend on hepatic arterial current bringing in waste substances to be chemically altered so that they can be excreted in the bile and urine. It also depends on portal venous circulation to bring in blood from the stomach and small intestine to be filtered and processed to remove toxins and bacterial products. The liver also has an active lymphatic circulation and supplies scavenger cells (macrophages) which wander in the blood lymph, picking up solid wastes, foreign cells and their products for breakdown or storage. All these activities are stimulated by prāṇāyāma.

6. In the kidneys, production of urine is dependent upon the continuous filtration of large volumes of arterial blood through the renal cortex. This flow is susceptible to conflicting demands and is often too low. Tendencies to shunt blood away from the renal cortex are countered by auto-regulation

of flow by the local small arteries. This process depends on proper intra-renal pressures and hence will be aided by Prāṇāyāma in achieving the correct position, shape and state of tension in the kidneys. Internal massage by phasic activity in the abdominal and back muscles will stimulate renal lymph flow, so essential to keeping the organ healthy.

7. The rhythmic use of the diaphragm and abdominal muscles in prāṇāyāma directly stimulates the peristaltic and segmenting movements of the intestines, as well as promoting intestinal circulation. Thus, it helps the intestine in its functions of absorbing food materials and disposing of solid wastes, mainly unabsorbed food and the products of our friendly bacteria, the colonic flora, as well as those containing the residue of secretions from the liver (bile), pancreas and intestines.

8. The spleen, just under the left diaphragm, acts as a filter to purify the circulating blood of worn-out oxygen-carrying red cells. Much of the splenic blood circulation is within lymphatic structures and is stimulated by prāṇāyāma.

9. Prāṇāyāma helps to maintain the flow of pure blood, which tones the nerves, brain, spinal cord and cardiac muscles, thus maintaining their efficiency.

10. The sweat glands act as accessory micro-kidneys, especially when stimulated by prāṇāyāma.

11. According to yogic texts, regular practice of Prāṇāyāma prevents and cures diseases. Improper practice, however, may cause asthma, cough, hyper-tension, pain in the heart, ears and eyes, dryness of the tongue and hardness of the bronchioles. (*Haṭha Yoga Pradīpikā*, II 16–17.)

12. Prāṇāyāma purifies the nāḍīs, protects the internal organs and cells, and neutralises lactic acid, which causes fatigue, so that recovery is quick.

13. Prāṇāyāma increases digestion, vigour, vitality, perception and memory. It frees the mind from the grasp of the body, sharpens the intellect and illumines the self.

14. An erect spine can be compared to a cobra which has lifted its hood. The brain is the hood and the organs of perception are the fangs, while bad thoughts and desires are the poison glands. Practice of prāṇāyāma quietens the upsurge of the senses and desires. Thus the mind becomes sacrosanct or free of thoughts (nirviṣaya). The sādhaka's words, thoughts and deeds become clean and pure. He maintains firmness (achalatā) in the body and steadiness (sthiratā) in his intellect.

15. Practice alone brings strength and knowledge. Daily practice ensures success and perfect consciousness, which purge the sādhaka from the fear of death. (*Śiva Saṁhita*, IV 17/18.)

16. The sādhaka experiences a state of serenity. He no longer thinks of the past, nor fears the future, but remains ever in the present. When he has mastered prāṇāyāma while sitting in padmāsana, he is ready to become a liberated soul says the *Haṭha Yoga Pradīpikā* (1 49).

17. As wind drives away smoke and impurities from the atmosphere and its inherent quality is to burn and purify the area, prāṇāyāma is a divine fire which cleanses the organs, senses, mind, intellect and ego.

18. As the rising sun slowly disperses the darkness of night, prāṇāyāma removes the impurities and refines the sādhaka and prepares his body and mind to become fit for concentration (dhāraṇā) and meditation (dhyāna)—*Patanjali Yoga Sūtra*, II 52, 53.

19. Prāṇāyāma is the window of the 'Self'. That is why it is called the great austerity (mahā tapas) and the true knowledge of the Self (Brahma-vidyā).

Section II

The Art of Prāṇāyāma

Chapter 10

Hints and Cautions

1. As Ādi Śeṣa, the Lord of the serpents, is the supporter of Yoga (*Haṭha Yoga Pradīpikā*, III 1), so Prāṇāyāma is the heart of Yoga. Yoga is lifeless without Prāṇāyāma.

2. The normal rate of breathing is fifteen times a minute and 21,600 times in every twenty-four hours. However, the number varies according to one's way of life, health and emotional state. Since prāṇāyāma lengthens the time taken by each in and out breath, thereby slowing down the process of ageing, its practice leads to a longer life.

3. In old age, the respiratory function decreases, due to the contraction of the air cells of the lungs, which take in less oxygen. Prāṇāyāma will help to normalise their size and make the red corpuscles circulate in all parts of the body, infusing life and vigour throughout. By its practice even old people can delay the ageing process.

4. The body is the field (kṣetra) of righteousness (dharma) and also of tribulation (kuru). It is the former when used for good and the latter when for bad. It is the field and the Self is the knower (kṣetrajña) thereof. Prāṇāyāma is the bond between the two.

5. Breathing in prāṇāyāma should always be through the nose, except where otherwise stated as in Ch. 24.

Qualifications for Fitness

6. Mastery of the alphabet leads to mastery of the language. Prāṇāyāma is the root of spiritual knowledge, knowledge of the Self (Ātma jñāna).

7. Mastery in prāṇāyāma is the next step after āsanas have been mastered. There is no short-cut.

8. Āsanas bring elasticity to the fibres of the lungs for better performance of prāṇāyāma.

9. The overall length of the nerves in the body is about 6000 miles. Their functions being supremely delicate, extra care and attention are needed to

keep them clean and clear. Repeated performance, with greater duration of each āsana in many varieties, keeps the nervous system clean and clear, thus aiding an uninterrupted flow of energy (prāṇa) while doing prāṇāyāma.

10. Bad and poorly performed postures lead to shallow breathing and low endurance.

11. If the body is neglected or pampered, it becomes a treacherous ally. Discipline the body by āsanas and the mind by prāṇāyāma. This is a sure step to self-realisation, which frees you from the dichotomy of pleasure and pain.

12. As food is essential to sustain the body, the proper intake of air must be provided for the lungs to maintain the life force (prāṇa).

13. Before attempting prāṇāyāma, learn how to move the intercostal muscles correctly, also the pelvic and thoracic diaphragm, by practising the relevant āsanas.

14. Empty the bladder and bowels before starting prāṇāyāma. Constipated persons can practice prāṇāyāma, as the bowels cannot be damaged in the same way as the bladder.

15. A trainer of tigers, lions or elephants studies their habits and moods and then puts them through their paces slowly and steadily. He treats them with kindness and consideration lest they turn on him and maim him. It is the same with the sādhaka. A pneumatic tool can cut through the hardest rock. If not used properly, it may destroy both the tool and the user. Study your breathing carefully and proceed step by step, for if you practise prāṇāyāma hastily or too forcibly, you may well harm yourself.

16. Practise at a fixed time each day and in the same posture. Occasionally, the same set of prāṇāyāma creates uneasiness. Be quick to switch over to a breathing pattern more conducive to the body and mind, and soothing to the nerves and brain, so that they are rejuvenated and refreshed. Prāṇāyāma should not become a blind routine.

17. Analyse and mould the breath with thorough understanding, clarity and wisdom.

Place

18. Choose a secluded, clean, airy place, free from insects, and practise during quiet hours.

19. Noise creates restlessness, disturbance and anger. Avoid prāṇāyāma at such times.

Cleanliness

20. One does not enter a temple with a dirty body or mind. Before entering the temple of his own body, the yogi observes the rules of cleanliness.

Time

21. Yoga texts insist that one should complete eighty cycles of prāṇāyāma four times a day in the early morning, noon, evening and at midnight, which not everyone can do. However, a minimum of fifteen minutes per day is essential, but this is not long enough for a devoted sādhaka. (One cycle of prāṇāyāma consists of inhalation, internal retention, exhalation and external retention.)

22. The best time for practice is the early morning, preferably before sunrise, when industrial pollution is at its lowest, and the body and brain are still fresh. If mornings are unsuitable, prāṇāyāma may be practised after sunset, when the air is cool and pleasant.

Posture

23. Prāṇāyāma is best practised while sitting on the floor on a folded blanket. Study Ch. 11 on the art of sitting. The postures suitable are siddhāsana, swastikāsana, bhadrāsana, vīrāsana, baddhakoṇāsana and padmāsana (Pls 3 to 14). However, any other posture will do provided the back is kept erect from the base of the spine to the neck and perpendicular to the floor.

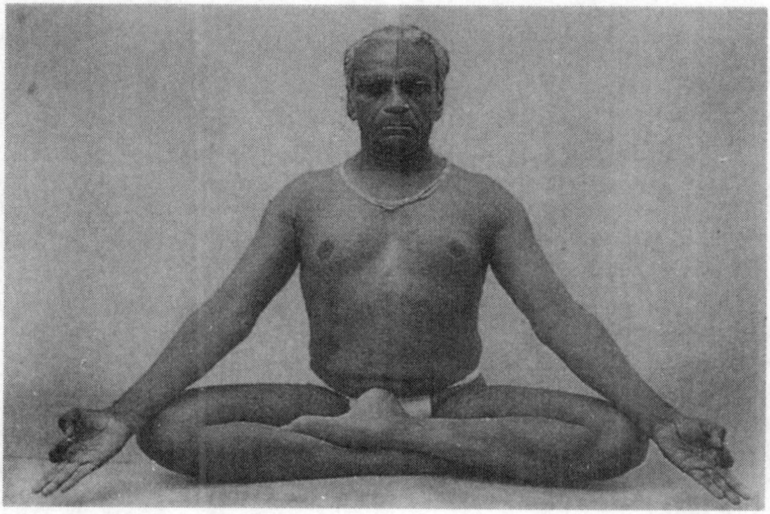

Pl. 3 **Siddhāsana (front view)**

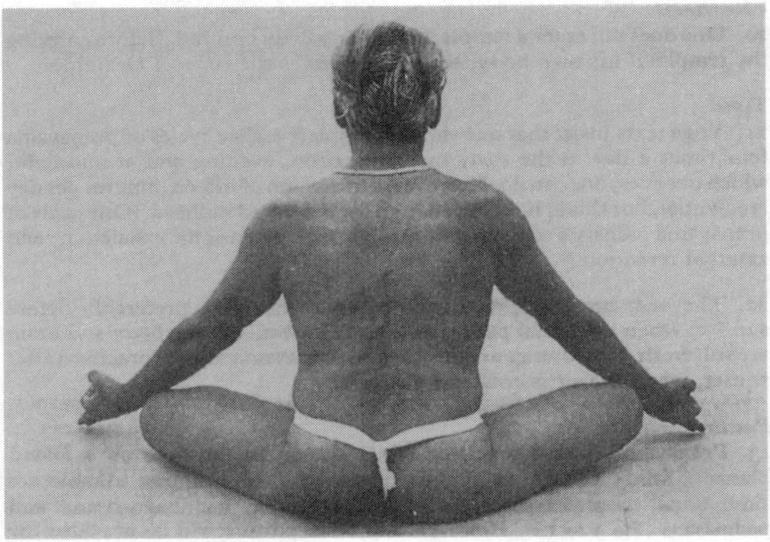

Pl. 4 **Siddhāsana (back view)**

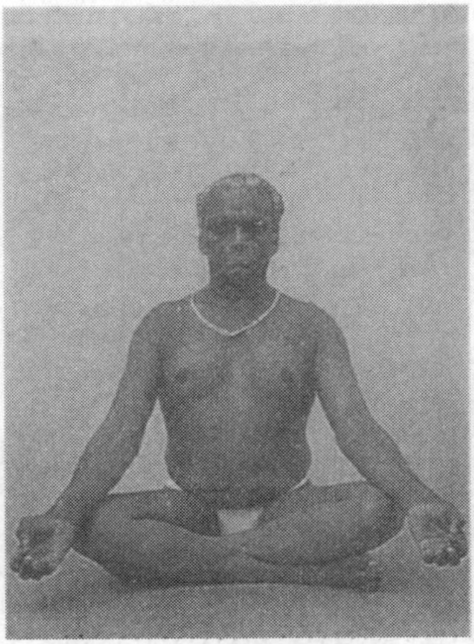

Pl. 5 **Swastikāsana (front view)**

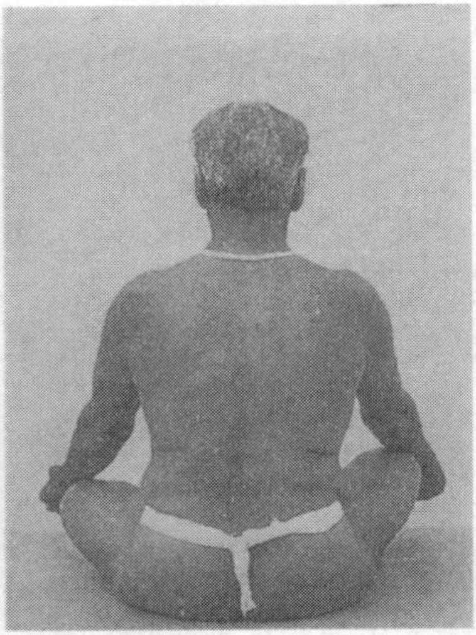

Pl. 6 **(back view)**

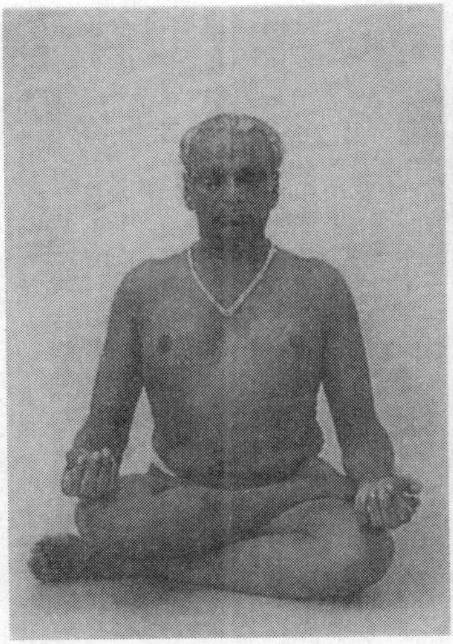

Pl. 7 **Bhadrāsana (front view)**

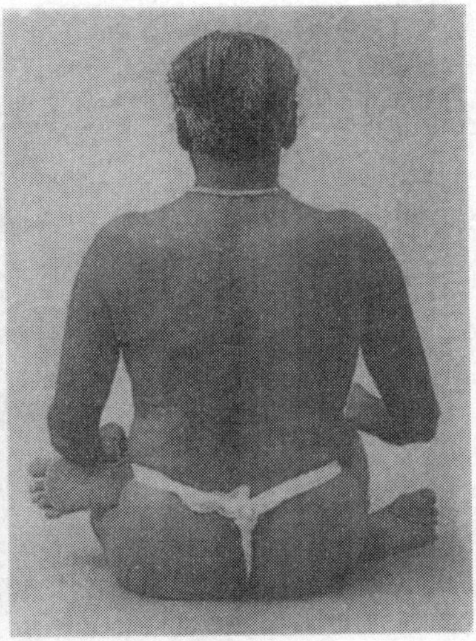

Pl. 8 **(back view)**

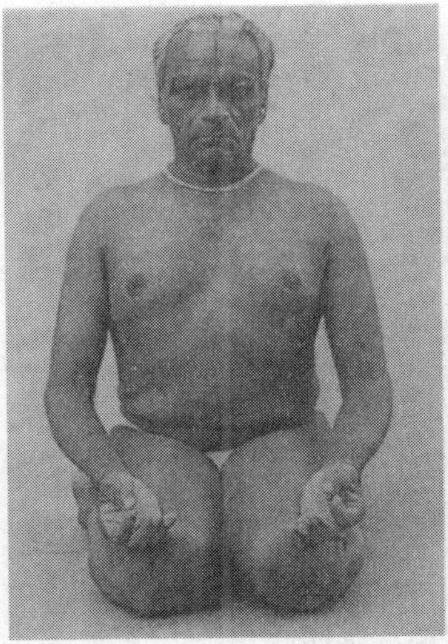

Pl. 9 **Vīrāsana (front view)**

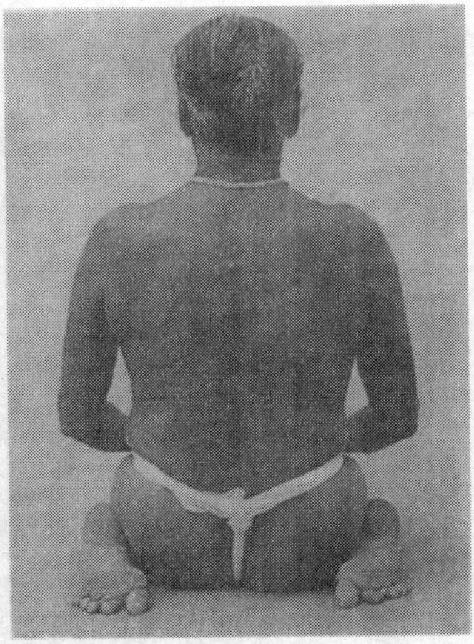

Pl. 10 **(back view)**

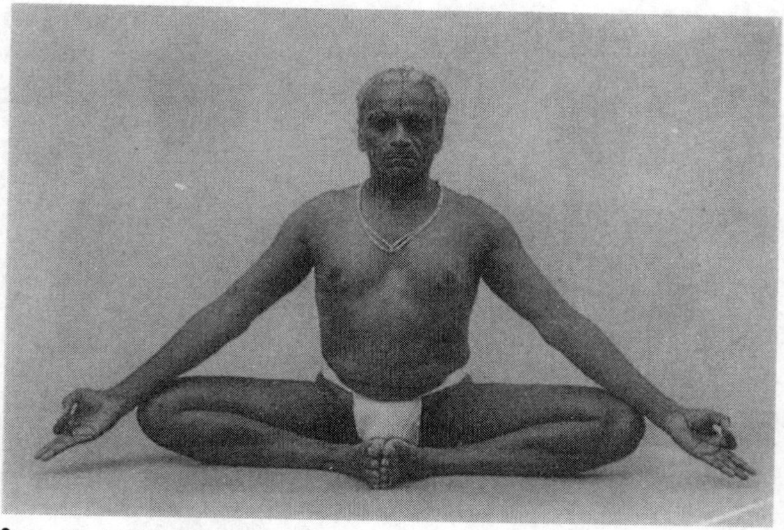

Pl. 11 **Baddhakoṇāsana (front view)**

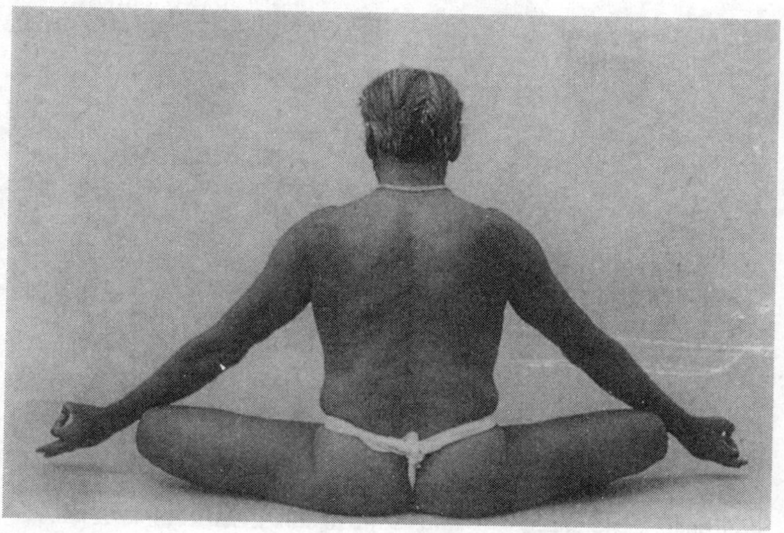

Pl. 12 **(back view)**

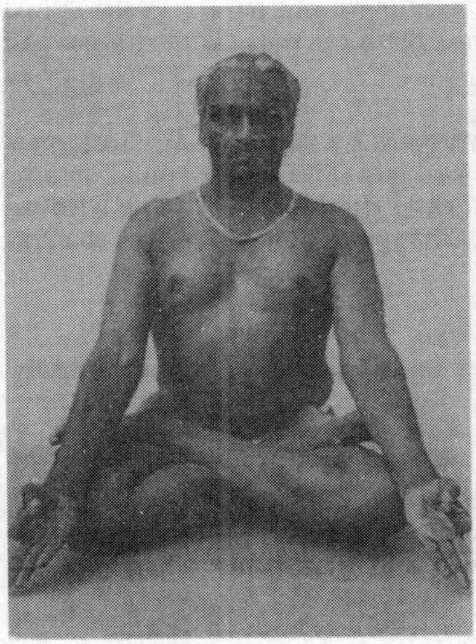

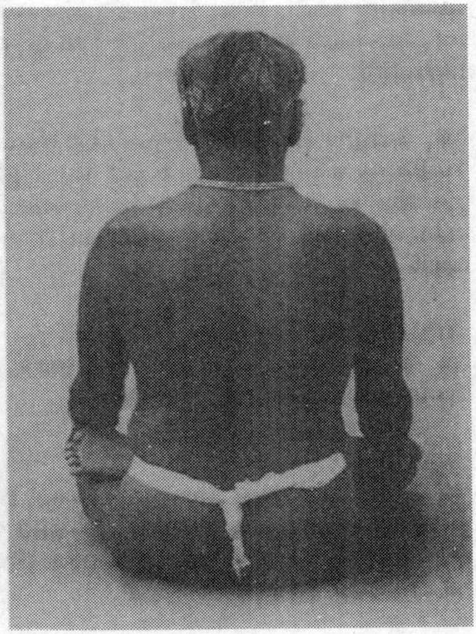

Pl. 13 **Padmāsana (front view)** Pl. 14 **(back view)**

Body

24. As an earthen pot must be baked in a furnace before it is used to store water, so should the body be baked by the fire of āsanas to experience the true effulgence of prāṇāyāma.

25. The body is tāmasic, the mind rājasic and the Self sāttvic. Develop body intelligence to the level of the mind through āsanas. Then raise both body and mind to the level of the Self through prāṇāyāma for the prāṇa to move throughout the body. This in turn keeps the body agile, the mind steady and the Self attentive.

26. The body is like a pit in which breath snakes in and out of the body. The chitta is the snake-charmer who entices the breath and acquires control over it.

Spine

27. The spine in man can be compared to an Indian lute (vīṇa). The gourd is the head from which sound is produced. The nose is the bridge which controls the sound vibrations caused by inhalation and exhalation. The resonance depends upon the tautness of the strings. If they are loose no sound is produced; if they are too tight there is no vibration and they may even snap. String tension is adjusted to produce the required resonance,

intensity and pitch. In the same way, the nāḍīs and nerves in the spinal column have to be positioned so that the breath can move with rhythm and harmony.

28. Adjust the spine from the base, vertebra by vertebra, as if you were building a brick wall. Keep the right and left sides of the spinal column parallel by moving them independently and rhythmically in line with the central spine. In prāṇāyāmā the front of the spine is more dynamic than the back.

Ribs

29. Move simultaneously the back ribs in, the side ones forward and the front ones upwards together.

Legs and Shoulders

30. Keep the arms passive. Do not tighten or lift them up or backwards. If they are tight, pins and needles and numbness result. This also happens at the start in any unaccustomed posture and disappears when you get established in it.

Nails

31. Pare the nails so that they do not hurt the delicate nasal skin while doing digital Prāṇāyāma.

Saliva

32. Saliva flows at the beginning of Prāṇāyāma. Swallow it after breathing out, but before breathing in, and never while holding the breath. Do not stiffen or press the tongue against the teeth and palate, but keep it and the throat passive.

Eyes and Ears

33. Prāṇāyāma should be practised with closed eyes and āsanas with open eyes.

34. Close the eyes gently and look down within at the heart without hardening the eye-balls. This inner observation or feeling is most revealing.

35. If the eyes are kept open, a burning sensation results, you feel irritable and restless and the mind is distracted.

36. Open your eyes for a split second once in a while to check your posture and correct any unevenness.

37. Keep the inner ears alert but passive. They are the windows of the mind. Tune them to the vibrations of inhalation and exhalation and to the soundless state of retention.

Skin

38. The skin performs two important functions, absorption and elimination. It absorbs and gives out heat, acting as a thermostat to keep the body temperature even. It also helps to eliminate organic and inorganic salts.

39. Skin is a source of perception. Maintain a constant and coherent communication between its movement with the inner awareness throughout your practices.

40. Keep the skin of the trunk active and dynamic and that of the skull, face, legs and arms soft and passive.

41. Perspiration appears at the start but disappears in due course.

Brain

42. Keep the brain receptive and observant. Use it to induce the lungs to act without becoming involved in the action; for if it does it cannot at the same time watch the process of breathing.

43. Prāṇāyāma is tāmasic when the trunk and spine are dull and rājasic when the brain is involved. Only when the torso is firm, the brain receptive and the self attentive, is prāṇāyāma sāttvic.

44. Memory is a friend if you use it for progress and refinement in your practice. It is a hindrance when you brood over and repeat past experiences. See new light each time in your practice.

45. Practice and surrender of desire are the wings of prāṇāyāma which take the sādhaka to higher spheres of knowledge and to the realisation of the Self (Ātmā).

46. Master samavṛtti prāṇāyāma (equal duration of inhalation, exhalation and retention) before attempting viṣama vṛtti (breathing with different ratios and duration of the three types). See Ch. 18 for details.

47. Never do āsanas immediately after prāṇāyāma. There is no harm in practising prāṇāyāma after āsanas. Prāṇāyāma, however, cannot be performed well after strenuous āsanas. It is advisable to practice both at different times. Mornings for the former and evenings for the latter are ideal.

48. Do not practise when the mind or body are dull or depressed. For mental distress or disturbances perform āsanas described in *Light on Yoga* and śavāsana for physical exhaustion (see Ch. 30). Then resume prāṇāyāma.

49. Do not perform internal retention (antara kumbhaka) when the brain is highly sensitised, as it may suffer injury from sudden disturbances, nor before you go to sleep, as it keeps you awake. Instead, perform prāṇāyāma without retention of breath or pensive external retention (bāhya kumbhaka), for both induce sleep, the latter being a cure for insomnia (see Chs 19, 20: Stage II in lying positions, and 21).

50. Do not perform prāṇāyāma in haste nor when the lungs are congested.

51. Do not talk or walk immediately after prāṇāyāma, but relax in śavāsana for a time before attending to other activities.

52. Do not practise just after meals or when hungry, in which case a cup of tea or milk will do. An interval of four to six hours is necessary between meals and prāṇāyāma, but you can eat half an hour after practice.

53. Do not allow mistakes to take deep root, but watch for and eradicate them by training and experience.

54. Do not attempt retention (kumbhaka) at a tender age, but start at sixteen or eighteen years, otherwise your face will become prematurely old.

55. Stop prāṇāyāma for the day the moment heaviness and tightness are felt in the lungs or when the sound of your breathing becomes harsh or rough.

56. Faulty practice tenses the facial muscles, shakes the mind and invites disease. Irritability, heaviness and restlessness are the symptoms.

57. Prāṇāyāma helps to regulate one's conduct and energy perfectly.

58. When prāṇāyāma is performed properly diseases disappear and a radiant state of well-being, enlightenment and serenity is experienced.

59. Correct practice reduces the craving for worldly pleasures and leads towards the realisation of the Self, freeing the sādhaka from domination by the senses.

Prāṇāyāma for Women

60. During pregnancy, women can do all prāṇāyāma except kapāla-bhāti, bhastrikā, viṣamavṛtti prāṇāyāma, antara kumbhaka with long duration,

and bāhya kumbhaka with uḍḍīyāna. The following prāṇāyāmas are, however, very beneficial: ujjāyī, viloma, sūrya bhedana, chandra bhedana and nāḍī śodhana.

61. One month after delivery start both āsanas and prāṇāyāma as for a beginner and gradually increase the timings and variations.

62. The practice of prāṇāyāma is safe during the menstrual period. But uḍḍīyāna must be avoided.

Note

63. When heat is generated in the body due to practising āsanas and prāṇāyāma, stop for the day. Apply oil to the body, head, heels and soles and rub it in. After a while, take a hot bath and then do śavāsana for about fifteen minutes. The body will then be cool and fit for practice the next day.

Chapter 11

The Art of Sitting in Prāṇāyāma

How to Sit

1. In the *Bhagavad Gītā* (VI 10–15) Kṛṣṇa explains to Arjuna how a yogi should practise to purify himself:

> '10. In a secret place, in solitude, let the yogi be constantly in harmony with his soul, master of himself, free from hope and worldly possessions.
>
> '11. Let him find a spot which is clean and pure and sit on a seat that is firm, neither too high nor too low, covered with layers of cloth, deer-skin and with sacred (kuśa) grass.
>
> '12. Seated there, let him practise Yoga for self-purification, with a concentrated mind, and with his organs of perception and action under control.
>
> '13. With his body, neck and head erect, immovable and still, with his vision indrawn, his sight fixed as if at the tip of his nose.
>
> '14. With soul at peace and fearless, firm in the vow of Brahmacharya, let him rest, with a vigilant controlled mind absorbed in Me as the Supreme.
>
> '15. The yogi, whose mind is ever under his control, always striving to unite with the Self, attains the peace of Nirvāna – the Peace Supreme that rests in Me.'

2. Without giving anatomical details, the above quotation describes the traditional method of sitting for meditation (dhyāna). The Self (Ātmā) is no doubt beyond purity and impurity, but it gets caught by the desires and by the mind. Lord Kṛṣṇa says, 'As fire is covered by smoke and a mirror by dust, as an embryo is enveloped by the womb, so is the Self (Ātmā) engulfed in desires generated by the senses and by the mind'. (*Bhagavad Gītā*, III 38.) So keep the body firm as a mountain peak, and the mind still and steady as an ocean, for meditation (dhyāna). The moment the body loses its own intelligence or firmness, the intelligence of the brain loses its power of clarity, both in action and receptivity. When the body and the brain are well balanced, pure intellectual illumination (sāttvic prajñā) is experienced.

3. In meditation, the head and neck are held erect and perpendicular to the floor, whereas in prāṇāyāma chin-lock (jālandhara bandha) is performed. This prevents strain on the heart, keeps the brain passive and enables the mind to experience inner silence (see Ch. 13).

4. In the art of sitting for meditation (dhyāna) the aim is to sit straight, with the spine upright and the back ribs and muscles firm and alert. Therefore, position the body so that if a vertical line is drawn from the centre of the head to the floor, then the centre of the crown, the bridge of the nose, the chin, the hollow between the collar-bones, the breastbone, navel and pubic symphysis are in alignment (Pl. 15).

5. On the other hand, the eye-brows, ears, tops of the shoulders, collar-bones, nipples, floating ribs and pelvic bones at the hip joints should be kept parallel to each other (Pl. 16). Finally keep the mid-point between tops of the shoulder-blades in perpendicular with the sacrum to avoid body tilt.

6. In prāṇāyāma the first essentials are to learn how to sit correctly with the head down, so that the body remains straight and steady, and how the maximum amount of air can be taken into the lungs to oxygenate the blood. Keep the height of the spinal column the same throughout the practice.

Pl. 15 and Pl. 16 **Vertical and horizontal alignment in sitting position**

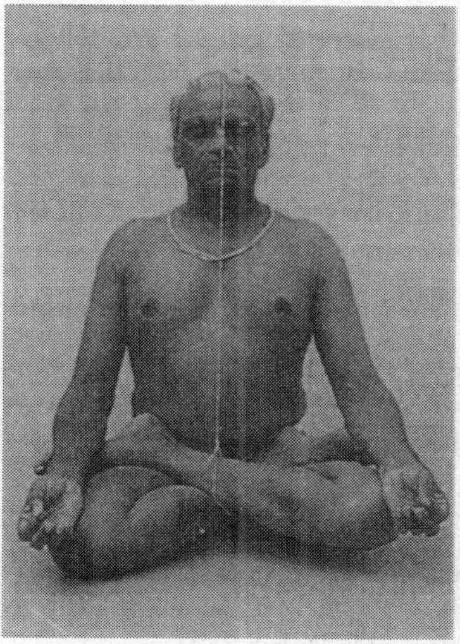

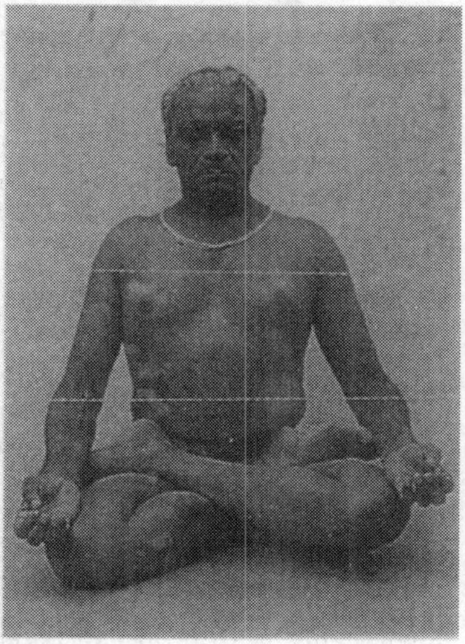

7. Be continuously alert and adjust the body to a correct alignment throughout the practice, whether it be inhalation (pūraka), exhalatior (rechaka) or retention of the breath (kumbhaka).

8. Just as an interior decorator arranges a room to make it spacious, so does the sādhaka create maximum space in his torso to enable his lungs to expand fully in prāṇāyāma. His capacity to do so increases with practice.

9. According to the *Bhagavad Gītā* the body is called the field (kṣetra) or abode of the Self (Ātmā) and the Self is the Knower of the Field (kṣetrajña), who watches what takes place when the body has been cultivated by Prāṇāyāma. Prāṇāyāma is the bridge between the body and the Self.

10. In order to cultivate the requisite field of activity in the torso, the first thing to bear in mind is how to sit. Unless the seat is firm, the spine will sink and give way, the diaphragm will not function properly and the chest will cave in, making it difficult to fill the lungs with life-giving air.

11. Here an attempt is made to describe in detail the technique of sitting for prāṇāyāma by dividing the body into four areas, namely: (a) the lower limbs, that is the buttocks and pelvis, hips, thighs, knees, shins, ankles and feet; (b) the torso; (c) the arms, hands, wrists and fingers; (d) the neck, throat and head. Be firm in the areas of buttocks and pelvis, which are the foundation for correct sitting.

12. When practising prāṇāyāma, one normally sits on the ground in a posture, such as siddhāsana, swastikāsana, bhadrāsana, vīrāsana, baddhakoṇāsana or padmāsana (Pls 3 to 14). In all of them see that the spine and the ribs resemble the broad middle portion of a banana leaf (see Pl. 2), the spine being the stem and the evenly-spaced ribs the veins. The tailbone is like the end of the leaf. These postures have been described in *Light on Yoga*.

13. Although a number of postures are in use, in my experience padmāsana is the king of them all for the practice of prāṇāyāma or meditation (dhyāna). It is the key to success in both cases. In it, all the four areas of the body mentioned above are evenly balanced (as in Para. 11) and the brain rests correctly and evenly on the spinal column, giving psychosomatic equilibrium.

14. The spinal cord passes through the spinal column. In padmāsana, the adjustment and alignment of the spinal column and the ridges on either side move uniformly, rhythmically and simultaneously. The prāṇic energy flows evenly, with proper distribution throughout the body.

15. In siddhāsana the top part of the spine is more stretched than its other parts, while in vīrāsana it is the lumbar area that is more stretched. Some of these postures may be more comfortable, but for accuracy and efficacy padmāsana is the best of them all. In padmāsana the thighs are lower than the groin, the lower abdomen is kept stretched, with maximum space between the pubis and the diaphragm, enabling the lungs to expand fully. For those using padmāsana, particular attention should be paid to the three important joints of the lower body – the hips, knees and ankles – which have to move effortlessly.

PADMĀSANA (Plates 15–43)

16. Sit on the base of the pelvis after doing padmāsana. Rest both buttocks evenly on the floor. If you sit more on one than the other, the spine will be uneven. Press the thighs down to the floor, bringing the thigh bones deeper into the hip sockets. Stretch the skin of the quadriceps towards the knees. This creates freedom round the knees to move diagonally and circularly from the top of the outer to the bottom of the inner knees. Bring the hamstring muscles closer in order to lessen the distance between the thighs. Then the anus and the genitals will not rest on the floor (Pl. 13). The line of gravity here is a very small area of the perineum between the anus and the genitals. The upward stretch of the spine begins from here and the body is simultaneously lifted upwards and sideways from the inner frame of the pelvis. Try and keep the top and bottom of the pubic areas perpendicular. If this is difficult, sit with the buttocks resting on a rolled blanket (Pls 17–18). In padmāsana both knees will not rest evenly on the floor (Pl. 13).

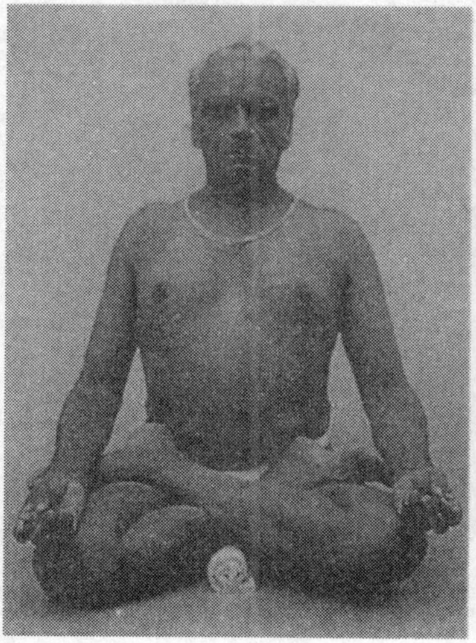

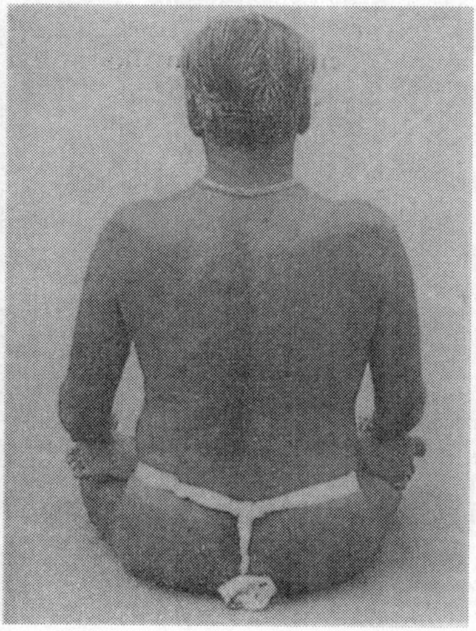

17. Do not turn the soles of the feet up to the ceiling, but keep them facing the side walls (Pl. incorrect 19 and correct 20). Stretch the metatarsals (the insteps), by turning the big toes towards the little ones, then the arches of the feet remain firm. If either arch drops, then the buttocks and the anus lose their grip, the trunk inclines and the spine sags in the middle, disturbing the whole balance of the torso. Do not spread out the knees or deliberately press them to touch the floor (Pl. 21 and 22). Any such attempt will only disturb the centre of gravity. Later, due to regular practice, though the knee remains above the ground one does not feel it. In order to get evenness in balance on the hips, it is advisable to rest the knee which is above the ground on a rolled towel (Pl. 23). Change the crossing of the legs on alternate days to get evenness in balance (Pl. 24).

The Torso

18. The torso or the trunk plays the most important part in the practice of prāṇāyāma. Keep the torso vigorously active, legs and arms dormant as if asleep, and the area from the neck to the crown of the head in a pure state of alert calmness. The trunk acts like a bridge between the static legs and arms and the alert but calm mind.

19. The torso will collapse if the spinal and intercostal muscles lose their grip, or if the vertebrae are not fully stretched. The muscles from the armpits to the hips, in front, in the back and on either side, are the keys. They

Pl. 19

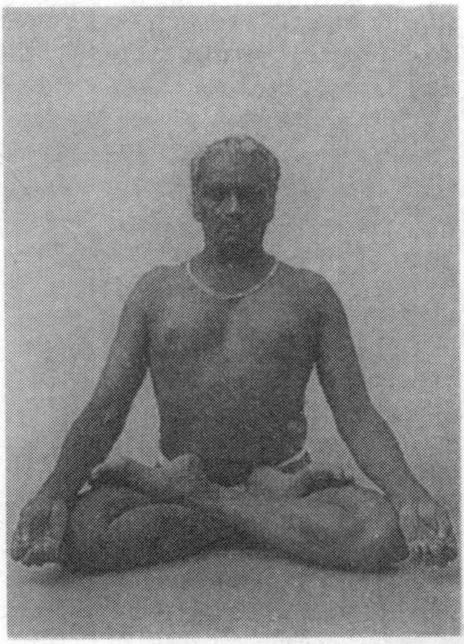

Pl. 20

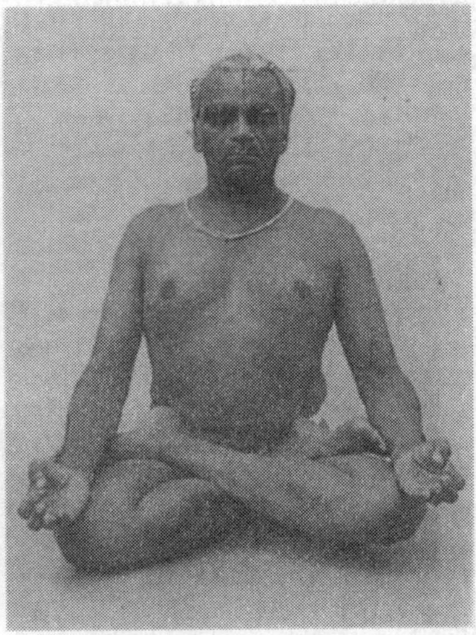

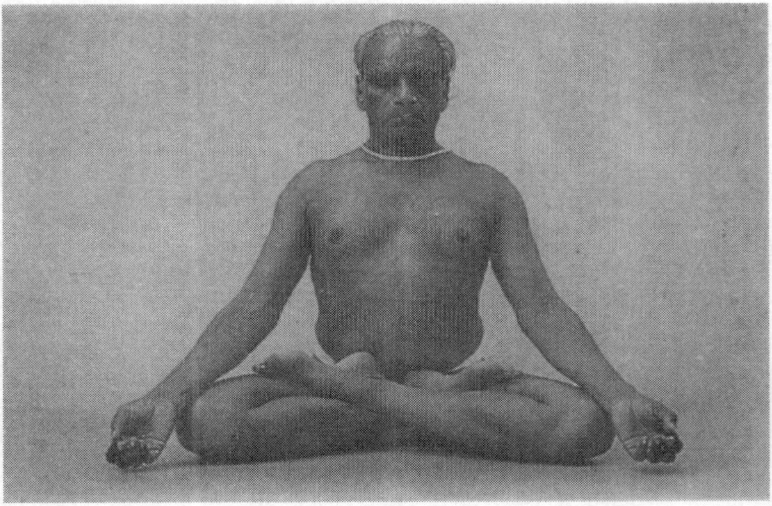

Pl.21

Pl.22

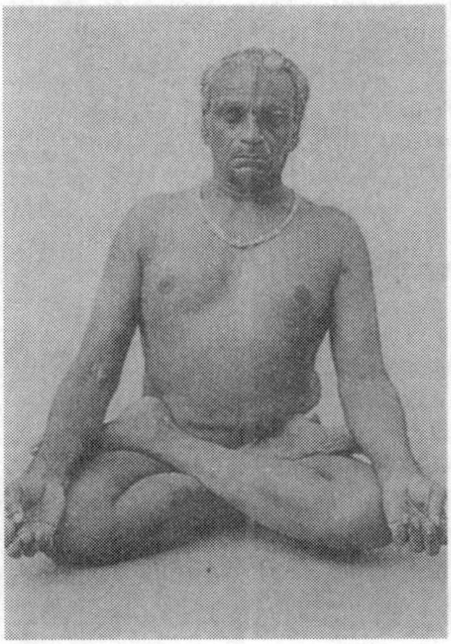

Pl.23

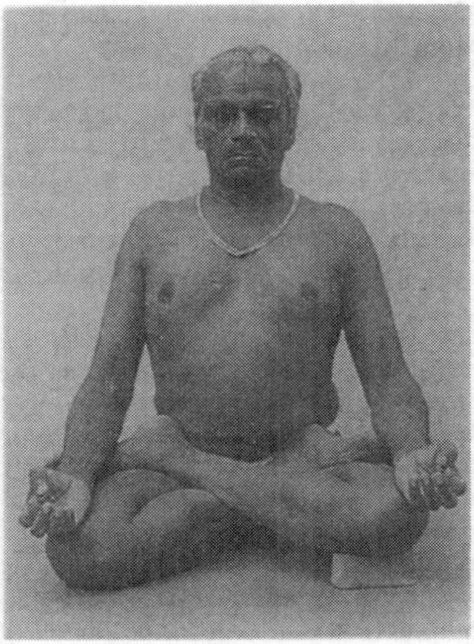

Pl.24

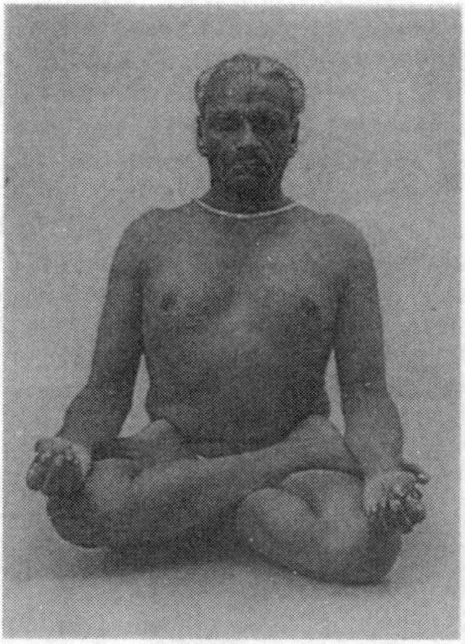

Pl.25

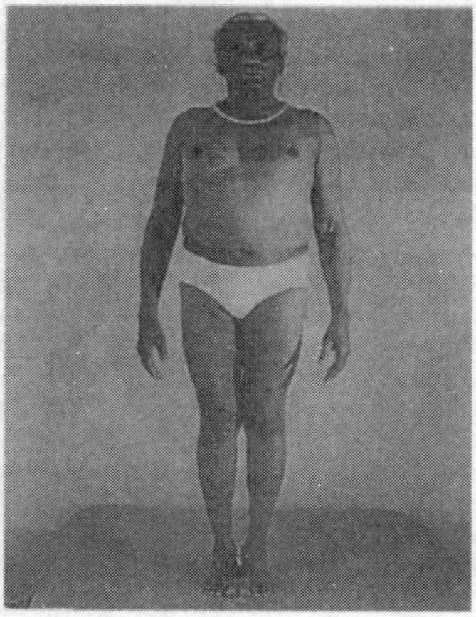

are anchored at the top to the collar-bones and shoulders, and at the bottom to the pelvis and the hip bone. Keep the back firm. Adjust the spine from the base to the top, that is, from the coccyx to the cervical vertebrae. Stretch the spinal column not only from the centre, but also from the left and right sides as well.

20. Keep the area of the navel passive and perpendicular to the floor. Narrow the area of the waist by lifting it up on either side. When lifting it up take care not to tighten it. Emotions, particularly fear, cause this area to become hard or tight, which affects the diaphragm and consequently breathing. When this area is passive the mind and the intellect stay serene. Then the body, mind and intellect are united with the Self.

21. In tāḍāsana (Pl. 25) (see *Light on Yoga*) space is created from the base of the pubis to the navel and the area there is kept flat. In sitting positions simulate the tāḍāsana stretch. Always stretch from the frontal spine. Stretch all the way up from the anus to the pubis, to the navel, to the diaphragm, to the sternum and finally to the hollow of the collar-bones. If the pubis collapses, the purity of the sitting posture vanishes and the practice loses precision. When the chest is stretched correctly the lungs function efficiently and more oxygen flows into the system. Any blockages in the subtle channels (nāḍīs) of prāṇic energy are removed and the energy which is drawn in through inhalation flows freely through the system. As

the disc of the sun emits rays of light uniformly in all directions, so the Self radiates the vital energy of the inhaled breath in all the corners of the lungs when the sternum is well lifted and stretched.

22. Remember that extension cultivates the field which brings freedom, freedom brings precision, which in turn creates purity and this leads to divine perfection.

23. To find out whether you are sitting correctly or not, slightly bend the tips of the thumbs and separated fingers and press them lightly, gently and evenly on the floor beside the buttocks. Place the nails perpendicularly to the floor (Pls, side view 26, front view 27, back view 28). If the forefingers press down too hard, the head tilts forwards; if the little fingers, then the body tilts backwards. If the fingers of one hand press the floor more than the fingers of the other, the body tilts to the side where the pressure is more (Pl. 29). An even but steady pressure on the thumbs, middle and little fingers, and light pressure on the other fingers keeps the body upright. Do not jerk the shoulders or lift them up while pressing the fingers. Without lifting the knees, raise the buttocks slightly from the floor (Pl. 30), tighten the buttock muscles, tuck in the tail-bone and then place the buttocks on the floor. Those who cannot raise the buttocks with the tips of the fingers can do so by placing the palms on the floor as in Pl. 31.

Pl.26

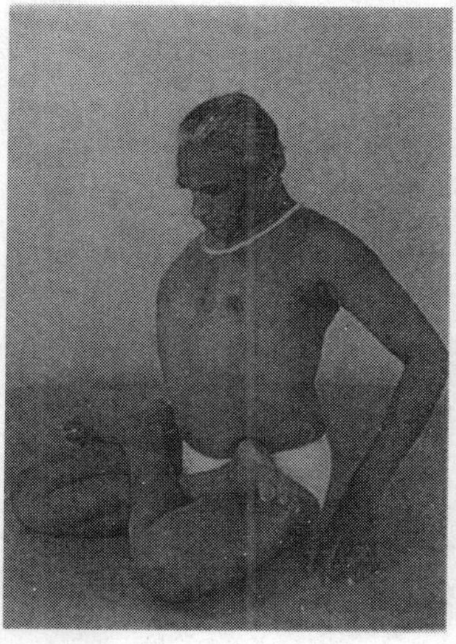

Pl.27

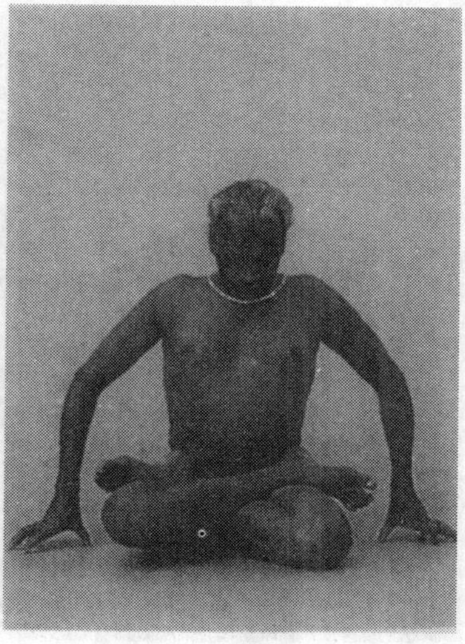

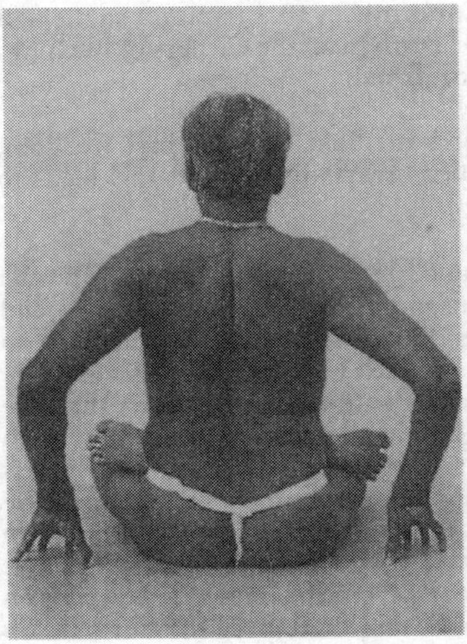

Pl.28

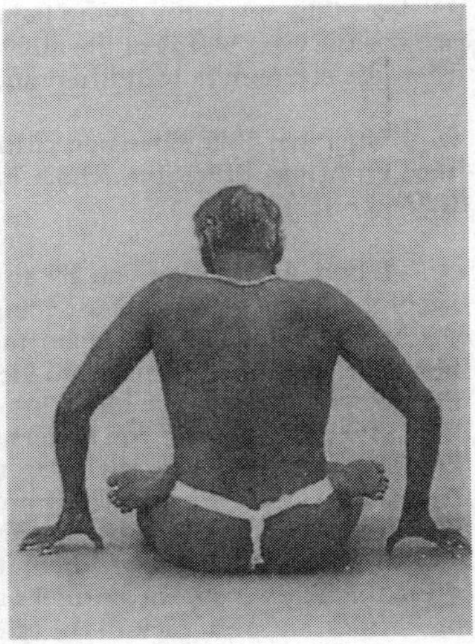

Pl.29

Pl.30

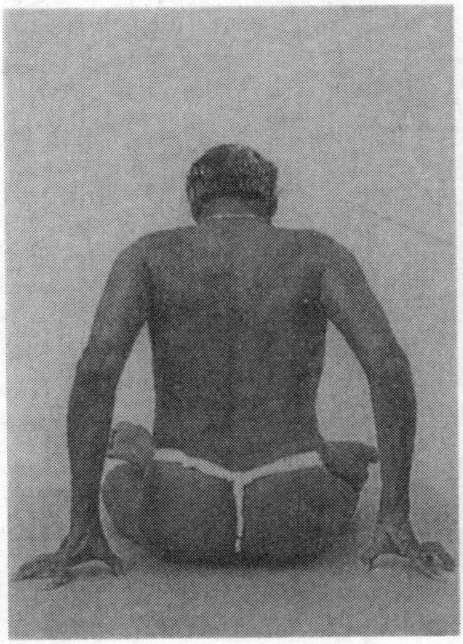

Pl.31

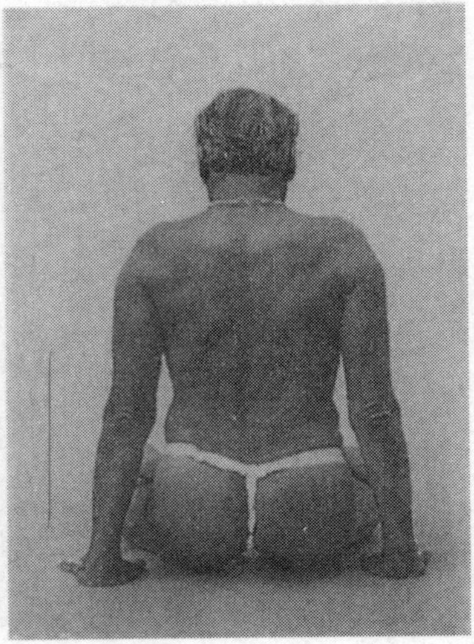

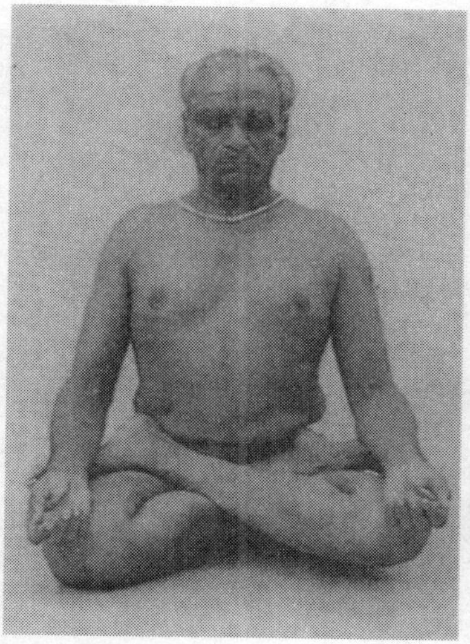

Pl.32

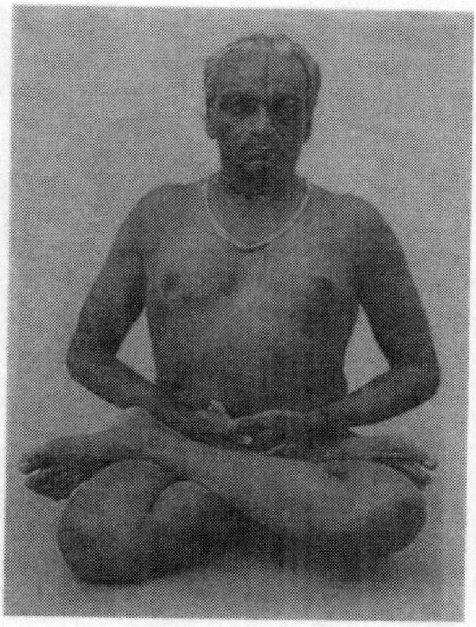

Pl.33

24. Lift the hands from the floor and rest the back of the wrists on the knees (Pl. 32) or left palm over the right on the lap and vice-versa (Pl. 33). This change of hands helps the back muscles to get a harmonious stretch. Do not straighten the arms at the elbows as this makes you lean forward (Pl. 34).

Three Crucial Spots

25. Remember the following three crucial spots in the body:

(i) the perineum between the anus and the genitals;
(ii) the sacrum and the first lumbar vertebra;
(iii) ninth thoracic vertebra at the back, and the centre of the breastbone in front (Pl. 35 and Fig. 18).

When the posture is correct, the skin from the back of the neck and shoulders moves down towards the base and that from the buttocks and hips stretches upwards. The maximum tension is felt at the first lumbar vertebra where these two opposing movements meet. The thoracic vertebra at the back and the centre of the breastbone in the front are lifted towards the chin, while the chin is bent downwards as in jālandhara bandha. The upward stretch of the skin at the centre of the breastbone helps the chin to bend down so that it rests in the notch between the collar-bones. The first lumbar is used as a fulcrum for stretching the spine vertically and opening the chest sideways to maintain the strength of the four pillars of the body

Pl.34

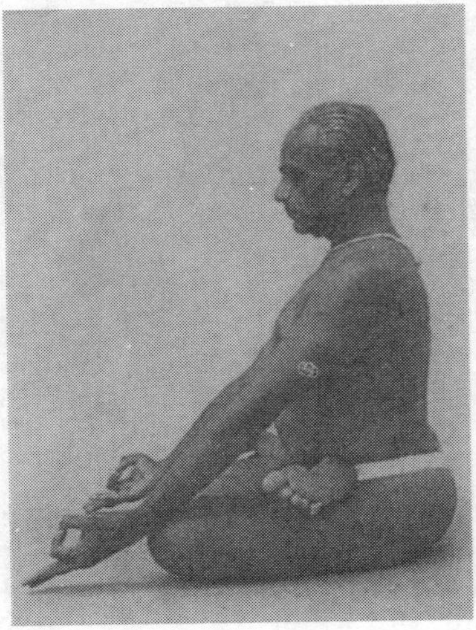

Pl.35

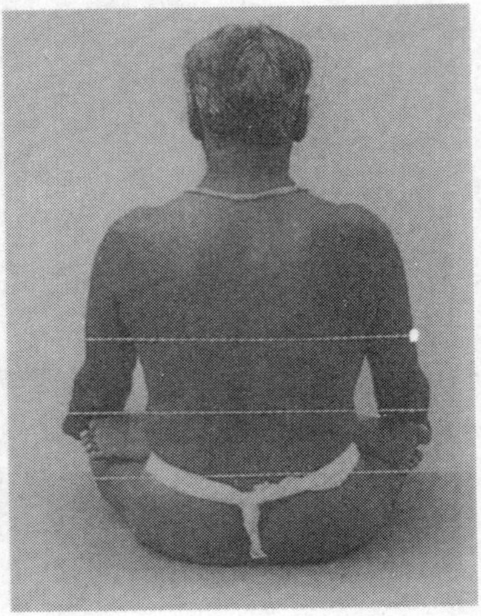

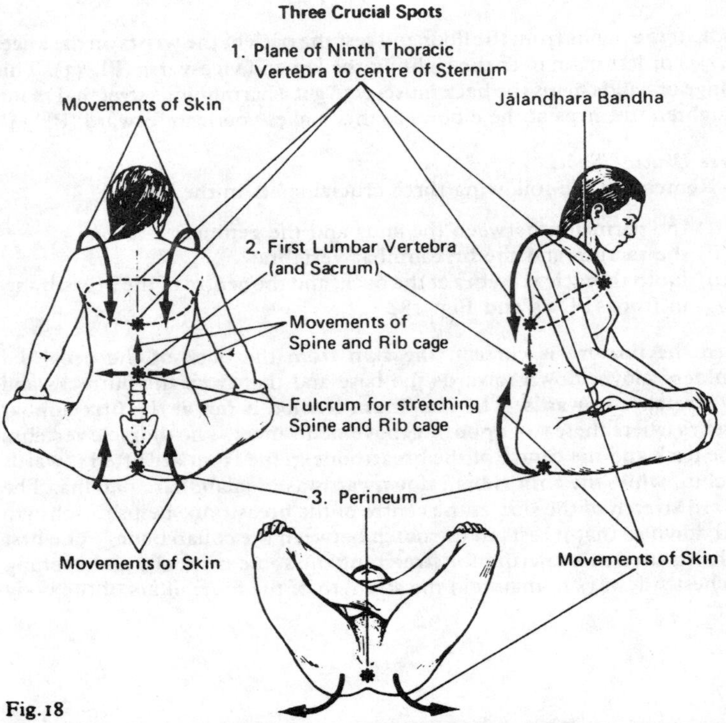

Fig. 18

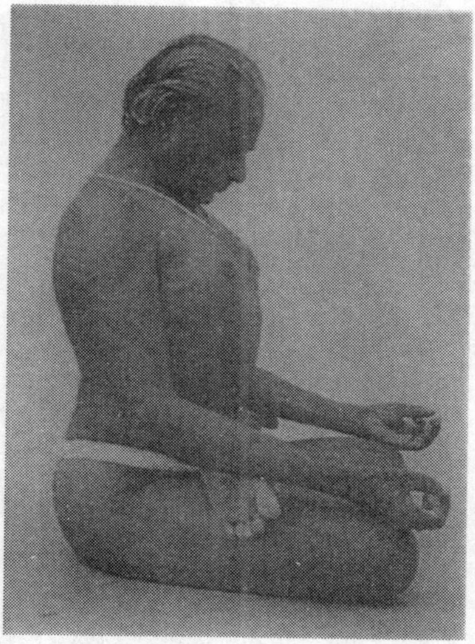

Pl.36

(corners of the torso) on either side. If the dorsal or the lumbar spine sags, the lungs do not expand properly. Only the correct movement and stretch of the skin at the back, the sides and the front of the torso enables the top lobes of the lungs to be filled.

Skin of the Torso

26. Like a bird spreading its wings in flight, keep the shoulder-blades down and open them away from the spine. Then the skin there moves down and the back of the armpits are slightly lower than the front ones. This prevents the back from drooping. The skin of the front is stretched sideways on each side as the breasts are lifted away from the armpits (Pl. 36).

27. The inner and the outer intercostal muscles inter-connect the whole rib cage and control diagonal cross-stretches. It is commonly understood that the action of the inner intercostal muscles is expiratory and the action of the outer intercostal muscles is inspiratory. Normal deep breathing techniques differ from that of prāṇāyāma techniques. In prāṇāyāma, the inner-intercostal muscles at the back initiate inspiration and the outer intercostal muscles at the front initiate expiration. In internal retention (see Ch. 15) the sādhaka has to balance evenly and fully the muscles of the chest wall throughout to release tension in the brain. The muscles and skin at the back must act in unison, as if interwoven, both in prāṇāyāma as well as in meditation (dhyāna).

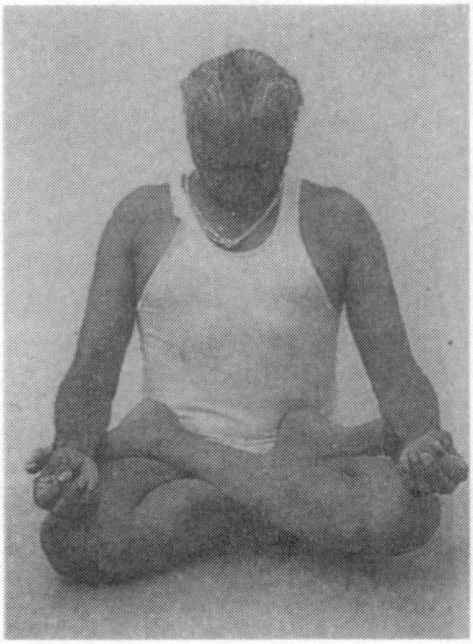

Pl.37

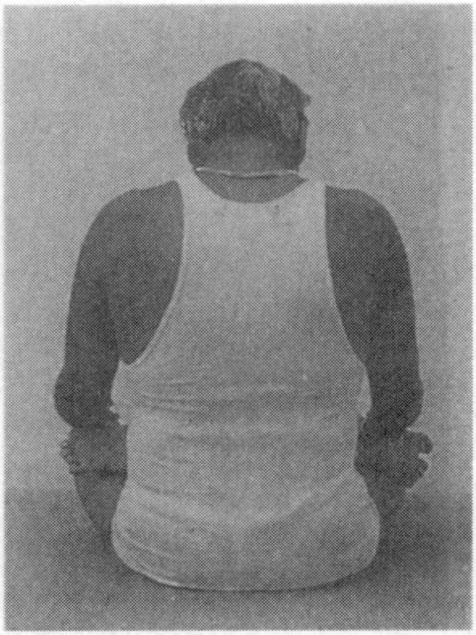

Pl.38

Pl.39

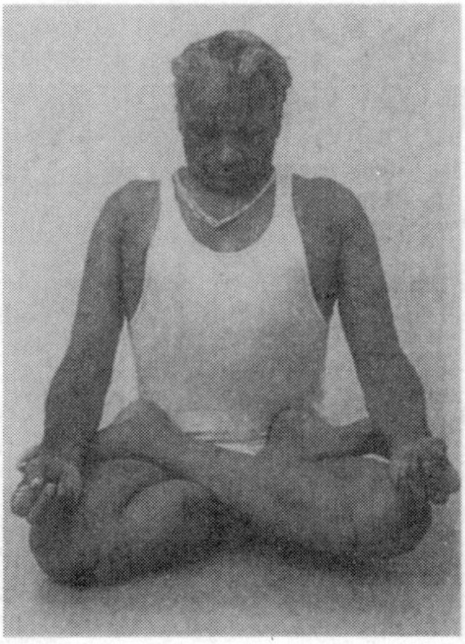

Pl.40

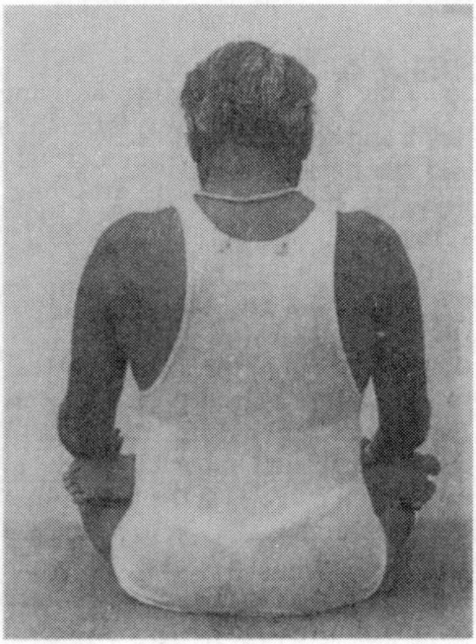

28. The tautness or the slackness of the skin of the trunk indicates emotional stability or the lack of it, and shows whether a person has achieved serenity and tranquillity of mind. If the skin at the top of the chest near the collar-bones caves in and sags, the person is a victim of his emotions. A firm chest is a sign of stability. If the chest and diaphragm are not kept steady and the activity of the skin is not co-ordinated with the movements of the back muscles, no serenity in breathing will be felt. If they are activated in co-ordination, courage comes to inspire the mind.

29. In the art of sitting, the back moves forward to meet the chest. Watch your clothing, for if your back touches the cloth, the movement is wrong, whereas if the front touches it is correct (faulty, Pls 37 and 38; correct, Pls 39 and 40).

30. Beginners may sit near a wall, tucking the buttocks close to it. Keep the base of the sacrum and the top of the shoulder-blades touching the wall. When the shoulders touch the wall the base of the sacrum tends to move away from the wall (Pl. 41). If this occurs, readjust the position (Pl. 42). Stretch the shoulder-blades outwards. To get the correct position, place between them, just behind the breastbone, a cake of soap, a piece of wood of a similar size, or a small rolled towel (Pl. 43).

Pl.41

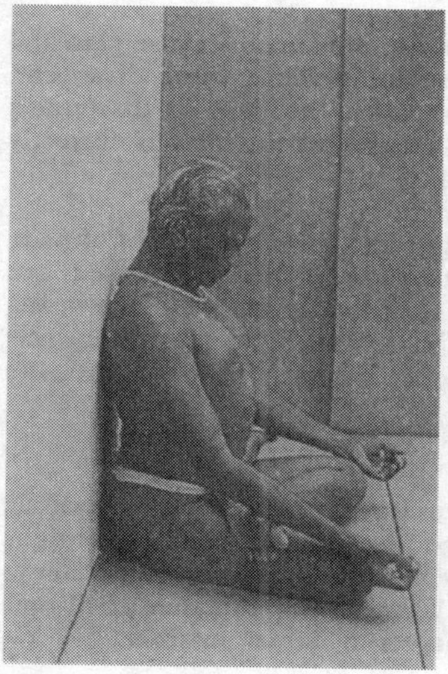

Pl.42

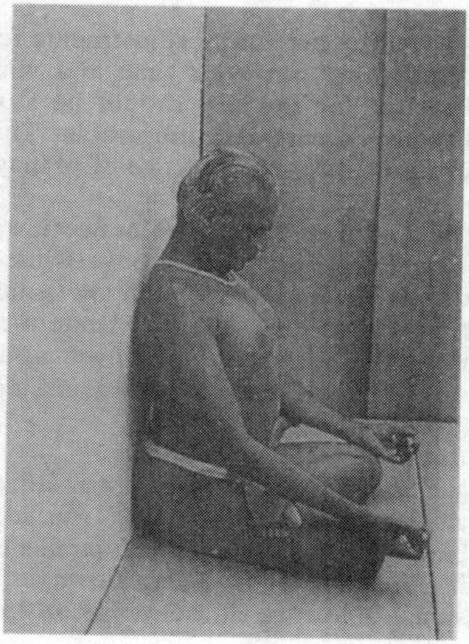

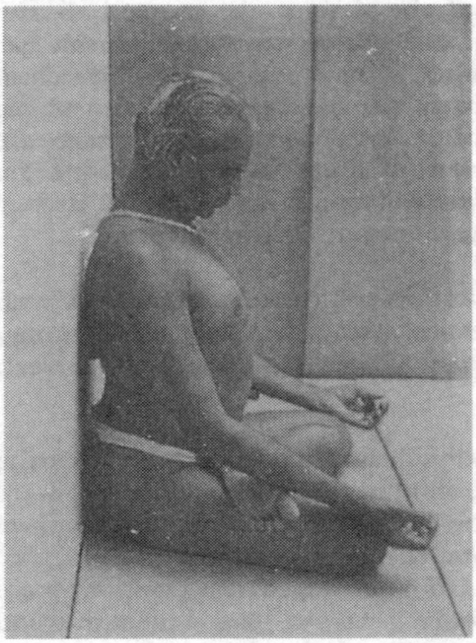

Pl.43

31. Jerky movements are a sign of fatigue, loss of attention or want of confidence. If they occur, do not waste time on prāṇāyāma, but practise āsanas, which develop the lungs and quieten the nerves.

32. At the beginning adjustments for correct movements cause pain and discomfort, but with time and with regular practice these disappear. Practice for the day should be stopped when the pain or discomfort becomes severe and unbearable. This is a sign that the torso is correctly positioned for the practice of prāṇāyāma.

33. Learn to distinguish between the right and the wrong types of pain. The right pain occurs only while prāṇāyāma is being practised and disappears immediately after śavāsana. If the pain persists it is of the wrong type and will continue to irritate the sādhaka, whereas the right type acts like a real friend, teaching fresh adjustments and adaptations, continually moulding the brain as well as the body.

Inability to Sit on the Floor

34. If through age, weakness or infirmity, sitting on the floor is impossible, a chair or stool may be used. But keep the feet flat on the floor, the thighs parallel with each other and parallel to the floor, and shins perpendicular to it (Pls 44 and 45). Keep the arms and legs relaxed, and free of all tensions, following all the points of this chapter as far as possible.

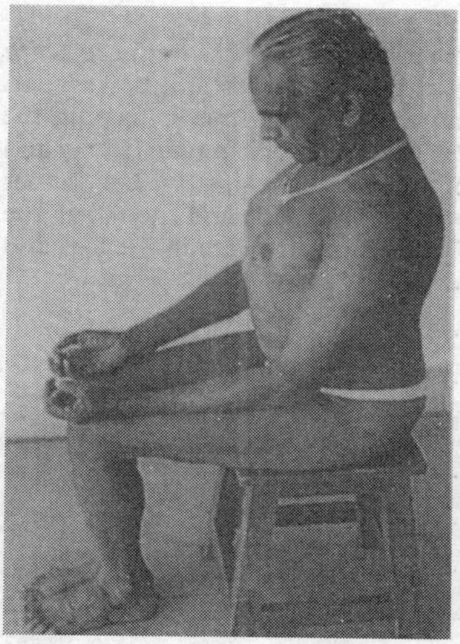

Pl.44

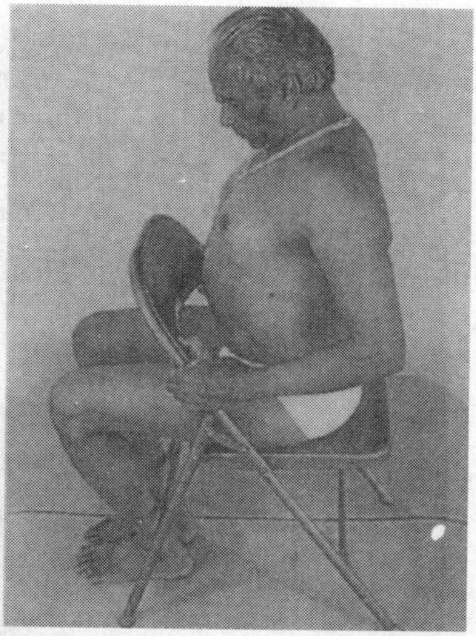

Pl.45

Pl.46

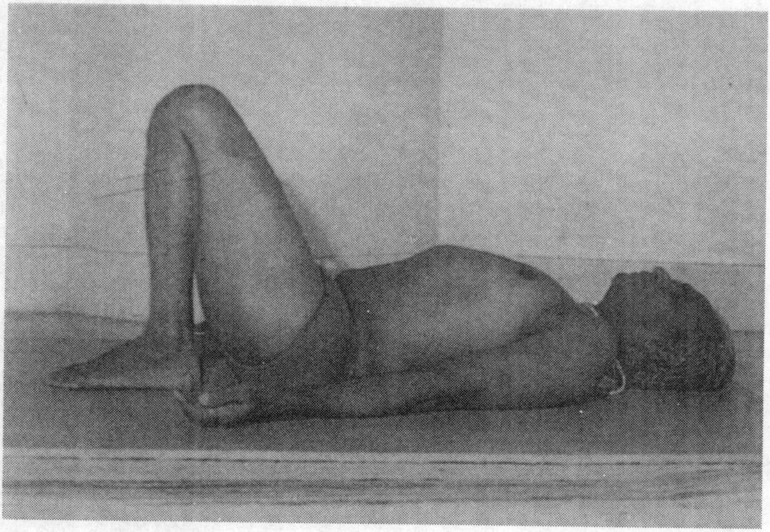

Pls. 46–50 **Śavāsana**

Numbness in the Feet

35. Sitting in any posture for prāṇāyāma causes numbness in the feet, for sitting in one position restricts the flow of blood. Correction, however, is easy. Do śavāsana for two or three minutes with bent knees, keeping the heels near the buttocks (Pl. 46). Then straighten the legs in turn (Pl. 47 and 48). Stretch the calf muscles, the back of the knees, heels, arches, with toes pointing to the ceiling (Pl. 49). Remain there for a while and then drop the feet to the sides (Pl. 50). This will make the blood circulate in the legs and the numbness of the feet will disappear.

Pl.47

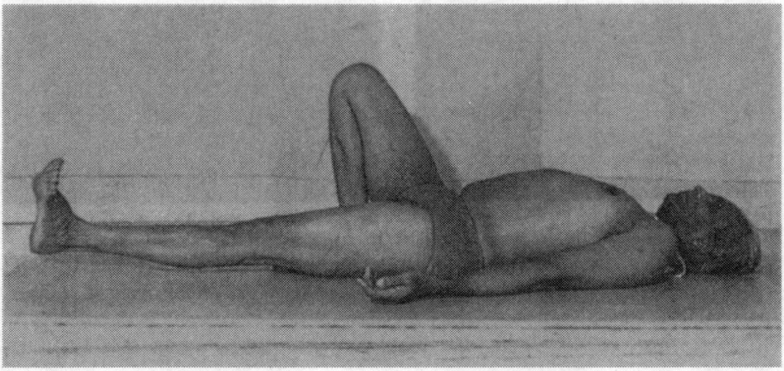

Pl.48

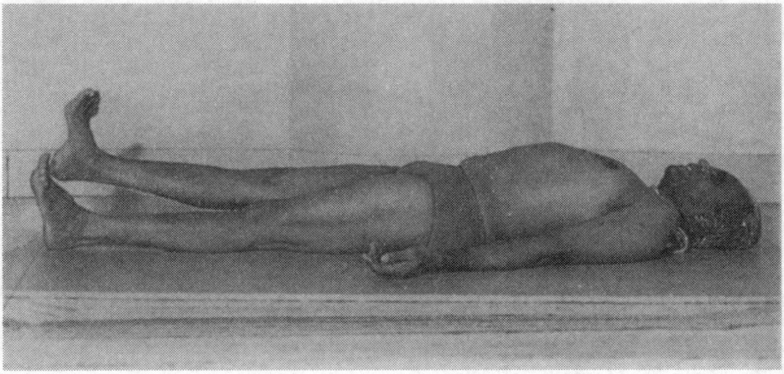

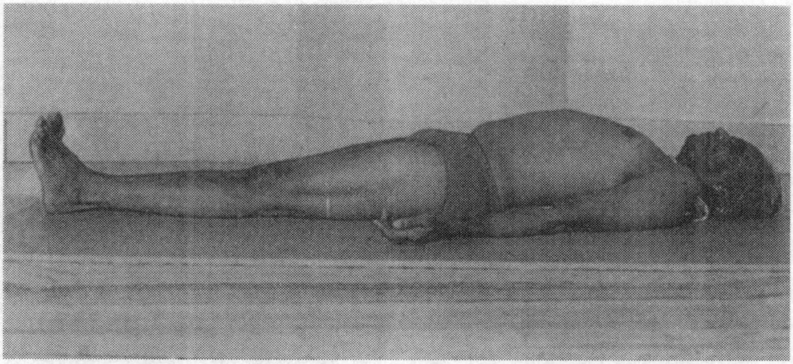

Pl.49

Pl.50

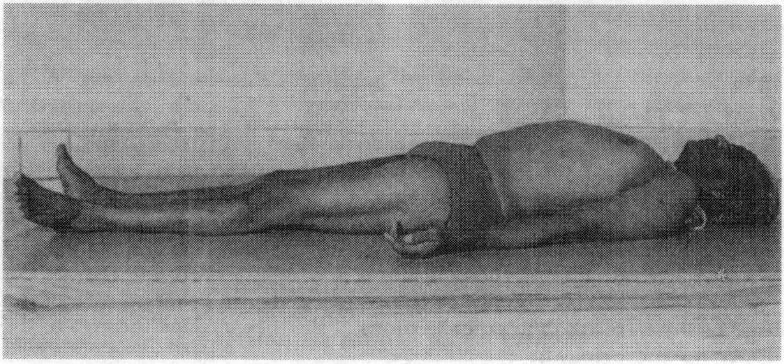

Arms and Shoulders

36. Spread the shoulders away from the neck on either side. Take them down as low as possible away from the lobes of the ears, and keep them parallel to the floor. The skin at the front of the armpits faces upwards, that at the back downwards. The shoulders tend to move up towards the ears during the practice of prāṇāyāma. Consciously and continually adjust them. This brings the elbows closer to the ground and ensures that the stretch and length of the upper arms at the front and back is even. Do not spread the elbows or move them up towards the shoulders (Pls 51 and 52).

37. The adjustment of the lower arms and placement of the fingers on the nostrils for certain types of prāṇāyāma are discussed in detail in Ch. 22.

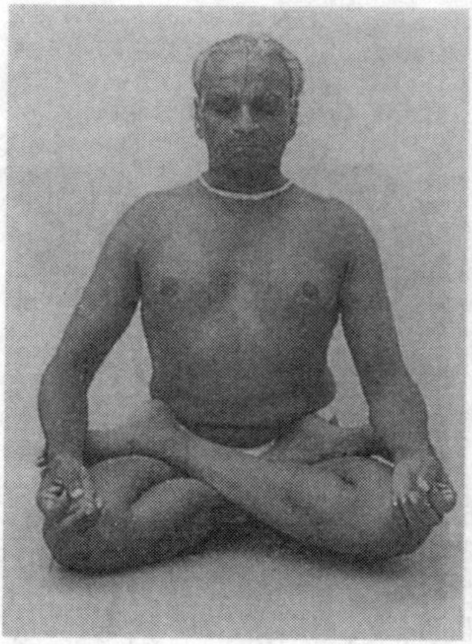

Pl.51

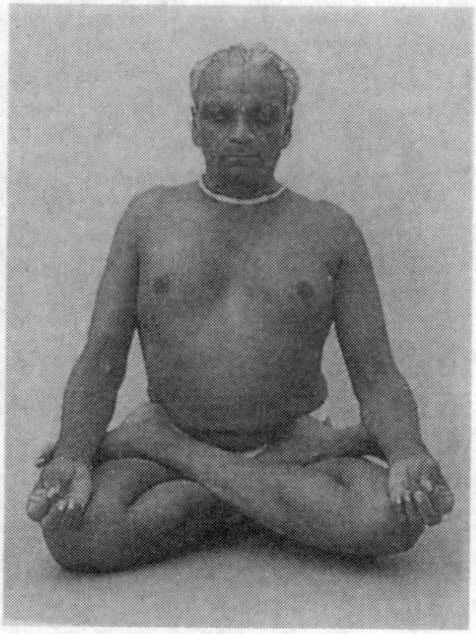

Pl.52

Head and Throat

38. Except when lying down, never keep the head erect; form a chinlock, so that the crown of the head does not go up, but remains undisturbed throughout the practice of prāṇāyāma. This clears the subtle passages of the two nāḍīs at the sides of the bridge of the nose. Constriction at the bridge of the nose, stiffness of the throat and tightness around the back of the neck indicate that the head position is wrong. In order to correct the head position, release the inner tensions of the throat, relax the area of the upper lip and bring the eye-balls down.

39. Relax the skin of the skull and keep the nerves passive, so that the brain remains quiet and stable. Never tighten or raise the skin over the temples. Do not compress the lips, but keep them relaxed and passive with the corners soft.

Tongue

40. Keep the tongue passive and relaxed, resting on the lower palate. See that its tip does not touch the upper palate or the teeth. Do not clench the jaws nor move the tongue while inhaling, exhaling or holding the breath. If the tongue moves, saliva will flow. However, when you begin practising Prāṇāyāma saliva will flow and accumulate. Do not worry, but swallow it before taking a fresh breath. If you keep the tongue passive, the flow will stop gradually.

Nose

41. The nose regulates the flow and sound of breath. Keep the tip of the nose and the bridge between the eye-brows pointing to the sternum without tilting the head to the side. The tip of the nose tends to rise during inhalation, so be attentive and keep the bridge down deliberately. If the bridge or the tip of the nose moves up, the sound of breathing will be rough.

Eyes and Ears

42. The eyes control the fluctuations of the brain; the ears of the mind. They are the rivers that take the brain and the mind to the sea of the soul. Prāṇāyāma should be practised with eyes closed and motionless and ears receptive to the sound of breathing. Close the eyes gently, applying slight pressure on the pupils with the upper eye-lids, while keeping the lower lids passive. The eyes will then be soft. Do not let them harden and dry. Move the upper eye-lids towards the outer corners of the sockets, thus easing any tension of the skin at the inner corners near the bridge of the nose. Keep the pupils steady and equidistant from the bridge. Release the tension of the skin from the centre of the forehead, as this relieves the creases between the eye-brows and keeps the area passive.

43. At first it is difficult to master the art of sitting, for the body tilts unconsciously. Therefore, periodically open the eyes for a fraction of a second and check whether the body has sagged, the head is up or down or tilted to one side. Next, check tension in the throat and tautness of the facial skin, particularly around the temples. Lastly, find out whether the eyes are flickering or steady. Then adjust the body and head to correct positions, relax the throat and keep the eyes passive. When the muscles there relax so does the skin. The upper lips and the nostrils influence the working of the senses and organs. Relax the area of the upper lip, for this helps the facial muscles to relax and the brain too. While practising prāṇāyāma in a sitting position, if the skin around the temples moves towards the ears, it means that the brain is under pressure; if it moves towards the eyes, then the brain is at rest. In recumbent positions, the skin around the temples moves towards the ears and not towards the eyes.

44. Direct the vision inwards as if looking with closed eyes at something behind. It will seem as if the eyes are wide open, though the vision is directed inwards (Pls. 53 and 54). The pupils tend to move up and down as you breathe in and out. Try to stop this as their movement tends to create activity in the brain.

45. Dullness sets in once the eye-lids are loose; the moment the pupils start to flicker distraction arises. If the upper eye-lids contract, thoughts flicker like a flame in the wind. None of this takes place when completely relaxed.

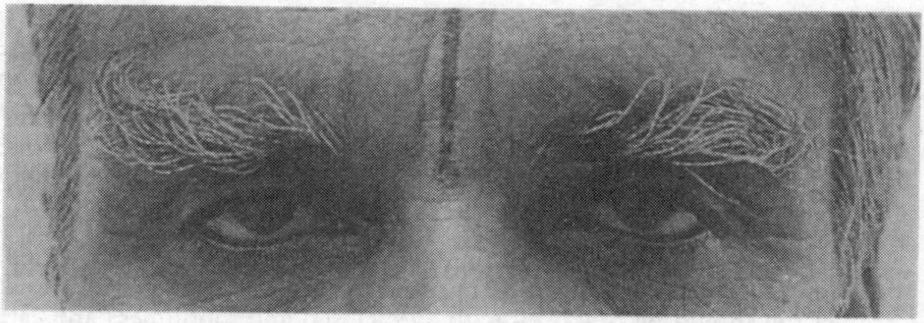

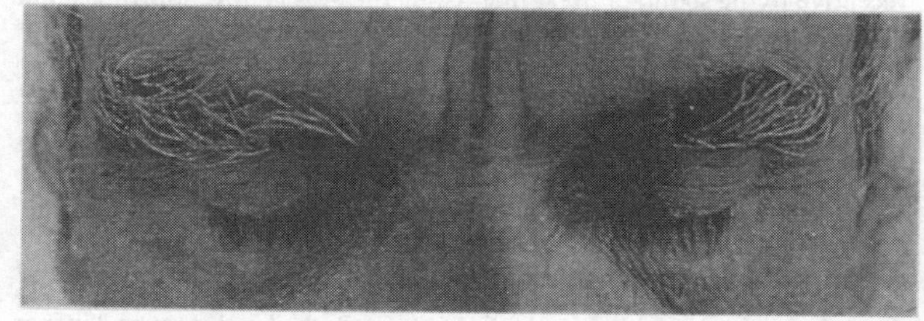

Pls. 53–54 **Inward vision**

46. If the eye-lashes do not meet, the brain is active and does not relax. If there is tension at the arch of the brows, the hair at this point will bristle as when angry; but if the brows are flat, the brain is at rest.

47. Keep the ear apertures level to each other and equidistant from the top of the shoulders. The ears must listen to the sound of breathing and feel light throughout practice. Do not clench the jaws as this will harden the area around the ears and block them, giving a sense of heaviness and itching inside.

48. Pay particular attention to the spot where the subtle energy channels (nāḍīs) from the eyes, ears and lungs criss-cross in the centre of the brain behind and between the eyes. This is the centre from which these energies are controlled. (See Ch. 5). This is where breath control starts.

Brain

49. The brain is a computer and an instrument of thinking. The mind has feeling, but not the brain. Since the brain controls the functions of the body and the organs of sense, it should be kept motionless. In Prāṇāyāma, it is the

inducer, not the actor but a witness. The lungs are the actors, the brain is the director.

50. If the sitting posture is correct, firm, steady and evenly balanced, the emotions are held in check. The brain feels light as if floating. Then no tension is felt there and hence no waste of energy. If there is an upward lift of the frontal brain, irritability and tensions are felt; if tilted to one side, the other side feels heavy, disturbing its equilibrium.

51. Intellectuals tend to be arrogant. Intelligence, like money, is a good servant but a bad master. When practising prāṇāyāma, the yogi bows his head low, adjusting the position of the front in relation to the back of the skull in order to make himself humble and without pride in his intellectual attainments.

52. The yogis know that the brain is the seat of acquiring objective knowledge (vidyā), while the mind (manas) is where subjective knowledge (buddhi) is experienced. Manas is the outer envelope, buddhi its content. Manas is located at the heart centre, where the emotional upheavals take place.

53. While both emotions and the intellect are silent and do not fluctuate, the yogi first experiences tranquillity of the senses followed by that of the mind. This is followed by the rarer and maturer experience of spiritual tranquillity, which frees him from worldly thoughts and cares. He becomes aware of the rare, pure state of being, a total awareness, the divine state in man. In it the finite merges in the infinite. This is samādhi, the endless goal of the yogi.

Chapter 12

The Art of Preparing the Mind for Prāṇāyāma

When the breath is steady or unsteady, so is the mind, and with it the yogi. Hence, the breath should be controlled.
Haṭha Yoga Pradīpikā Ch. II.2.

1. The tree of life is said to have its roots above and its branches below, and so it is with man, for his nervous system has its roots in his brain. The spinal cord is the trunk descending through the spinal column, while the nerves run down from the brain into the spinal cord and branch off throughout the body.

2. The art of sitting for prāṇāyāma is explained in detail in Ch. 11, while this chapter is concerned with the mental preparation.

3. The arteries, veins and nerves are channels (nāḍīs) for circulating and distributing energy throughout the body. The body is trained by practice of āsanas, which keep the channels free from obstruction for the flow of the prāṇa. Energy does not radiate throughout the body if the nāḍīs are choked with impurities. If the nerves are entangled, it is impossible to remain steady, and if steadiness cannot be achieved the practice of prāṇāyāma is not possible. If the nāḍīs are disturbed, one's true nature and the essence of things cannot be discovered.

4. The practice of āsanas strengthens the nervous system, and the practice of savāsana soothes ruffled nerves. If the nerves collapse so does the mind. If the nerves are tense, so is the mind. Unless the mind is relaxed, silent and receptive, prāṇāyāma cannot be practised.

5. In its search for peace the modern world has become interested in the benefit of meditation and the ancient art of prāṇāyāma. Both disciplines are fascinating at first, but as time passes it is apparent that they are not only very difficult to learn but that they are very tedious and repetitive, because progress is very slow. On the other hand, the practice of āsanas is fascinating and absorbing throughout, as the intelligence is focused and recharged in various parts of the body. This creates a feeling of exhilar-

ation. In prāṇāyāma attention is initially on the two nostrils, sinus passages, thorax, spine and diaphragm. Thus the intelligence cannot be diverted to the other parts of the body. Thus prāṇāyāma cannot become absorbing until body and mind are trained to receive the flow of breath; months or years may pass without much progress, yet by sincere and unwavering efforts, and by perseverance, the sādhaka's mind becomes receptive to the regulated flow of breath. Then he starts to experience the beauty and fragrance of prāṇāyāmas, and after years of practice he will appreciate its subtlety.

6. For the practice of prāṇāyāma there are two essentials, a stable (achala) spine, and a still (sthira) but alert mind. Bear in mind, however, that those who practice excessive backward bends may have an elastic spine, but it does not remain stable for long; others, who practice excessive forward stretches, may have a stable spine but not a still and alert mind. In backward bends, the lungs are stretched, whereas they do not expand in forward bends. The sādhaka has to strike a balance between the two, so that the spine remains stable and the mind stays alert and unwavering.

7. The practice of prāṇāyāma should not be mechanical. The brain and the mind should be kept alert, to correct and adjust the body position and the flow of breath from moment to moment. One cannot practise prāṇāyāma by force of will; hence, there should be no regimentation. Complete receptivity of the mind and intellect are essential.

8. In prāṇāyāma the relationship between chitta (mind, intellect and ego) and breath is like that between a mother and her child. Chitta is the mother and prāṇa is the child. As a mother cherishes her child with love, care and sacrifice, chitta should cherish prāṇa.

9. Breath is like a turbulent river, which, when harnessed by dams and canals, will provide abundant energy. Prāṇāyāma will teach the sādhaka how to harness the energy of breath to provide vitality and vigour.

10. However, the *Haṭha Yoga Pradīpikā* (Ch. 2, 16–17) gives warning: as a trainer tames a lion, an elephant or a tiger slowly, so should the sādhaka acquire control over his breath gradually, otherwise it will destroy him. By the proper practice of Prāṇāyāma, all diseases are cured or controlled. Improper practice, however, gives rise to all sorts of respiratory ailments, like cough, asthma, pains in the head, eyes and ears.

11. Steadiness of mind and breath interact and makes the intellect steady too. When it does not waver, the body becomes strong and the sādhaka is filled with courage.

12. The mind (manas) is the lord of the sense organs (indriyas), as the breath is of the mind. The sound of the breath is its lord and when that sound is maintained uniformly the nervous system quietens down. Then the breath flows smoothly, preparing the sādhaka for meditation.

13. The eyes play a predominant part in the practice of āsanas, and the ears in prāṇāyāma. By being fully attentive and using one's eyes, one learns āsanas and proper balance in the poses. They can be mastered by the will, to which the limbs can be made subservient. Prāṇāyāma, however, cannot be performed in this way. During its practice the eyes are kept closed and the mind concentrated on the sound of breathing; while the ears listen to the rhythm, the flow and nuances of the breath are regulated, slowed and smoothened.

14. In āsanas there is endless variety, because of the number of different postures and movements, and attention changes while performing them. In prāṇāyāma there is monotony. The reasons are: first, the sādhaka has to practise in one position only; second, he has to maintain a continuous and unwavering sound in breathing. It is like practising scales in music before learning melody and harmony.

15. While practising āsanas, the movement is from the known gross body to the unknown subtle one. In prāṇāyāma, the movement is from the subtle breath within to the gross body without.

16. As ashes and smoke obscure a burning, smouldering piece of wood, impurities of the body and the mind cover the soul of the sādhaka. Just as the breeze clears the ashes and smoke, and the wood blazes forth, so the divine spark in the sādhaka shines out when by the practice of prāṇāyāma his mind becomes free of impurities and fit for meditation.

Chapter 13

Mudrās and Bandhās

1. In order to follow the techniques of Prāṇāyāma, it is necessary to know something about mudrās and bandhās. The Sanskrit word mudrā means a seal or a lock. It denotes positions which close the body apertures, and where the fingers are held, together with special hand gestures.

2. Bandhā means bondage, joining together, fettering or catching hold. It also refers to a posture in which certain organs or parts of the body are gripped, contracted and controlled.

3. When electricity is generated, it is necessary to have transformers, conductors, fuses, switches and insulated wires to carry the power to its destination; otherwise the current would be lethal. When prāṇa is made to flow in the yogi's body by the practice of prāṇāyāma, it is equally necessary for him to employ bandhās to prevent the dissipation of energy and to carry it to the right places without damage. Without the bandhās, prāṇāyāma practice disturbs the flow of prāṇa and injures the nervous system.

4. Out of the several mudrās mentioned in Haṭha-yoga texts, jālandhara, uḍḍīyāna and mūla bandhā are essential to prāṇāyāma. They help to distribute energy and prevent its waste through hyper-ventilation of the body. They are practised to arouse the sleeping kuṇḍalinī and direct its energy up through the suṣumṇā channel during prāṇāyāmas. Their use is essential for experiencing the state of samādhi.

JĀLANDHARA BAṆDHA (Plates 55–65)

5. The first bandha the sādhaka should master is jālandhara bandha, jāla meaning a net, a web or a mesh. It is mastered while performing sarvāṅgāsana and its cycle, during which the sternum is kept pressed against the chin.

Technique

(a) Sit in a comfortable position like siddhāsana, swastikāsana, bhadrāsana, vīrāsana, baddhakōṇāsana or padmāsana (see Pls 3 to 14).

(b) Keep the back erect. Lift the sternum and the front part of the rib cage.

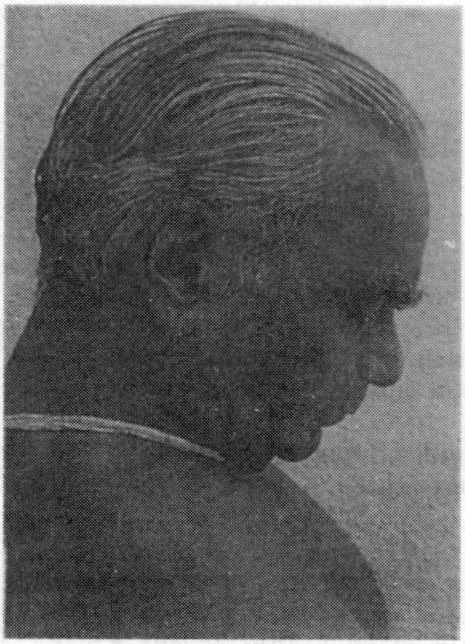

Pl.55

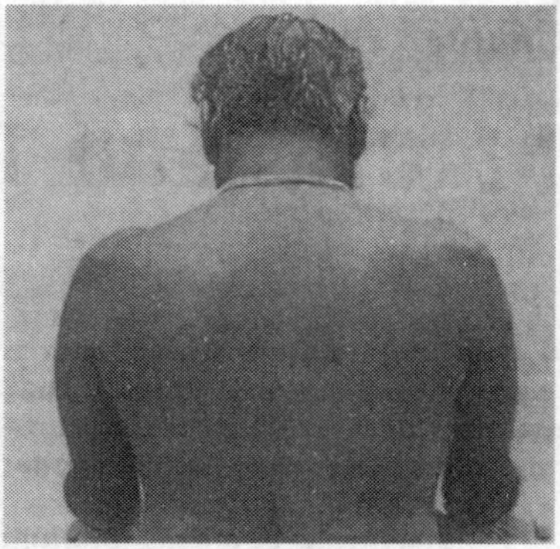

Pl.56

(c) Without tensing, stretch the sides of the neck and move the shoulder-blades into the body; keep the thoracic and cervical spine concave and bend the head forwards and downwards from the back of the neck towards the chest.

(d) Do not constrict the throat or strain the neck muscles. It should not be forced forward, downward or tensed back (Pls 55 and 56). Keep the neck and throat muscles soft.

(e) Bring the head down so that the point and both sides of the jaw-bone rest evenly in the notch between the collar-bones on the front wall of the chest (Pls 57 and 58).

(f) Do not stretch the chin more to one side or the other (Pl. 59). Also do not tilt the neck to one side (Pl. 60), which may cause pain and strain that continue for a long time. As elasticity is gained, the neck bends down increasingly.

(g) Do not force the chin to the chest as in Pl. 55, but lift the chest to meet the descending chin as in Pl. 58.

(h) Keep the centre of the head and chin in alignment with the middle of the sternum, the navel and the perineum (Pl. 61).

(i) Do not cave in the ribs, while resting the chin on the chest (Pl. 62).

(j) Relax the temples and keep the eyes and ears passive (Pl. 57).

(k) This is jālandhara bandha.

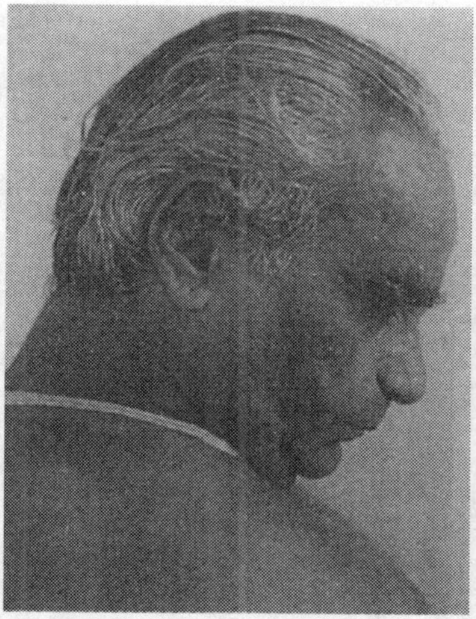

Pl.57

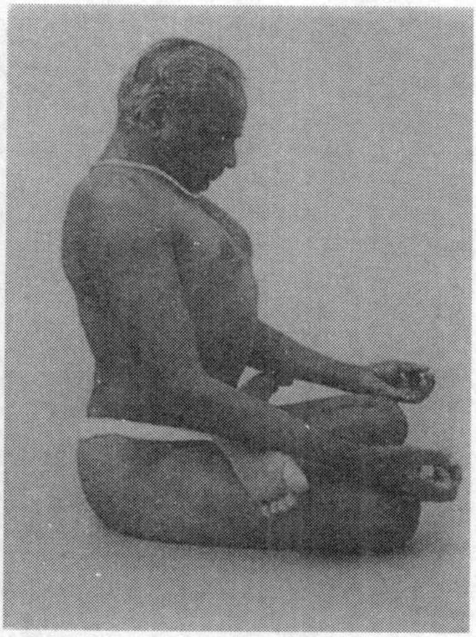

Pl.58

Pl.59

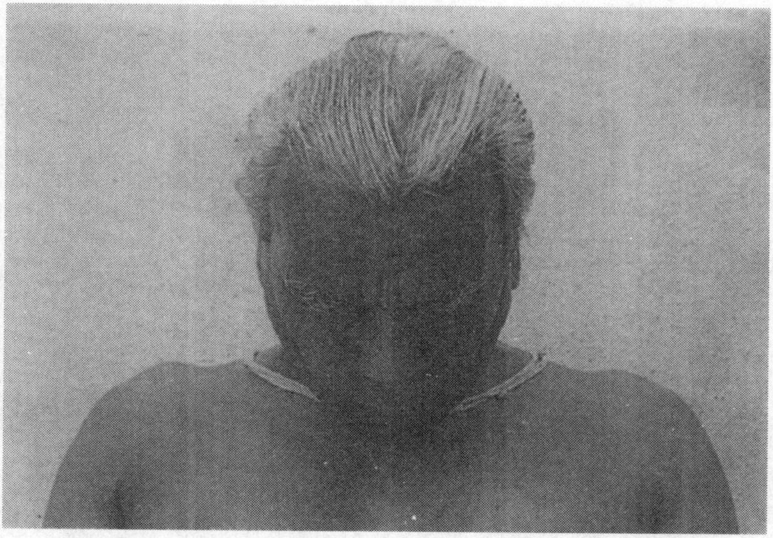

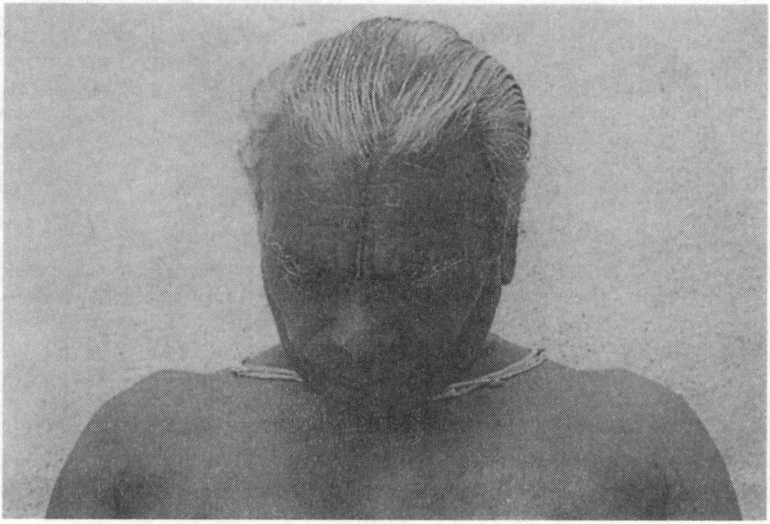

Pl.60

Pl.61

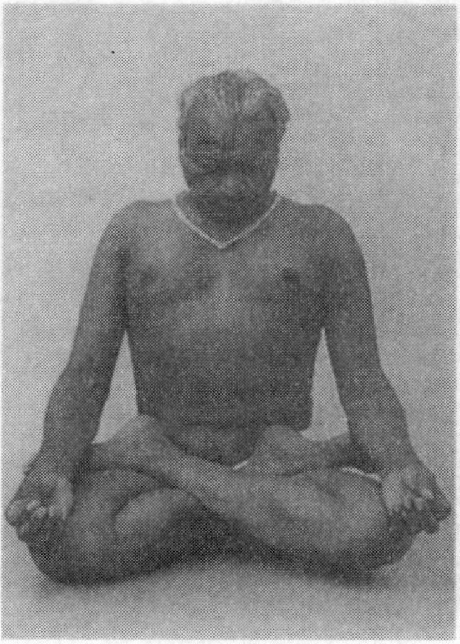

Pl.62

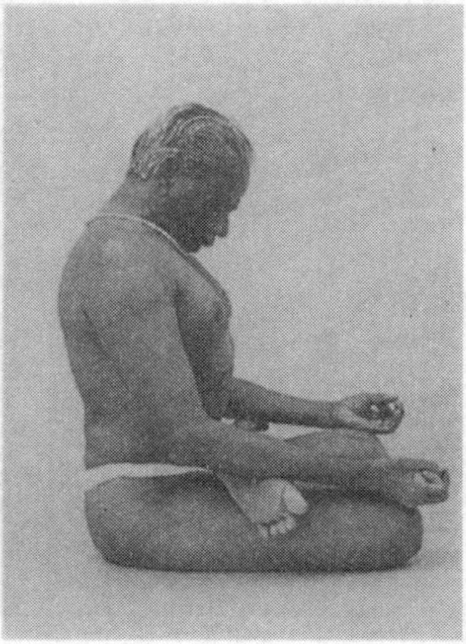

Effects

The solar plexus is situated at the centre of the trunk. According to Yoga, it is the seat of the digestive fire (jāṭharāgni), which burns food and creates heat. The lunar plexus is in the centre of the brain and creates coolness. By performing jālandhara bandha, due to the lock of the nāḍīs around the neck, the cool energy of the lunar plexus is not allowed to flow down or to be dissipated by the hot energy of the solar plexus. In this way the elixir of life is stored and life itself is prolonged. The bandha also presses the iḍā and piṅgalā channels and allows the prāṇa to pass through suṣumṇā.

The jālandhara bandha clears the nasal passages and regulates the flow of blood and prāṇa (energy) to the heart, head and the endocrine glands in the neck (thyroid and para-thyroid). If prāṇāyāma is performed without jālandhara bandha, pressure is immediately felt in the heart, brain, eye-balls and in the inner ear. This may lead to dizziness.

It relaxes the brain and also humbles the intellect (manas, buddhi and ahaṁkāra).

Note

Those with stiff necks should keep the head as far down as possible without undue discomfort (Pl. 63), or roll a piece of cloth and place it on the top of the collar-bones (Pls 64 and 65). Hold it by lifting the chest rather than by pressing down with the chin (see Pl. 57). This releases tension in the throat and breathing becomes comfortable.

Pl.63

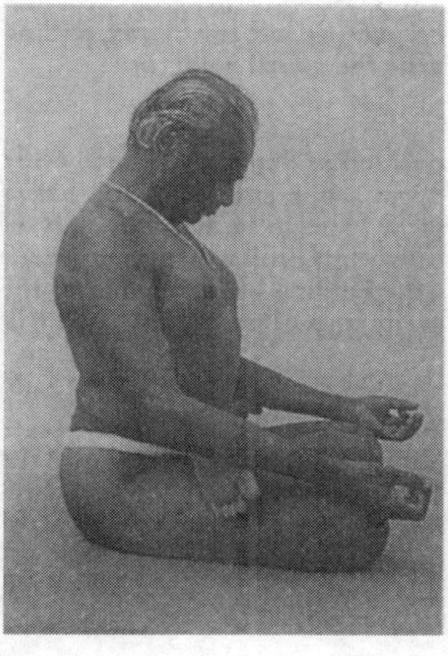

Pl.64

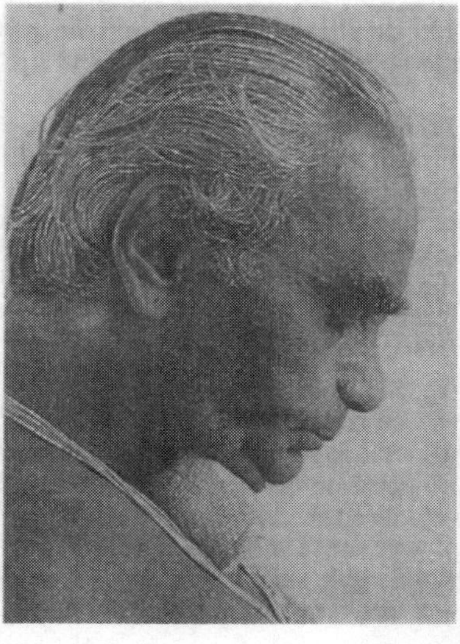

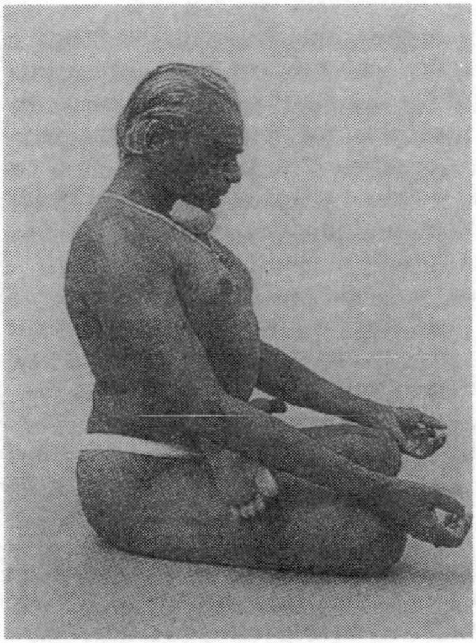

Pl.65

UḌḌĪYĀNA BANDHA

6. Uḍḍīyāna, which means flying up, is an abdominal grip. In it the prāṇa or energy is made to flow up from the lower abdomen towards the head. The diaphragm is lifted from the lower abdomen up into the thorax, pulling the abdominal organs back and up towards the spinal column.

Technique

First master uḍḍīyāna in the standing position as explained below. Only then introduce it into Prāṇāyāma practices while sitting during bāhya kumbhaka (the interval between complete exhalation and the start of inhalation). Never do uḍḍīyāna during Prāṇāyāma until you have mastered the latter, nor during antara kumbhaka (the holding of breath during the interval between complete inhalation and the start of exhalation), as it will strain the heart.

(a) Stand in tāḍāsana (Pl. 25).
(b) Spread the legs about a foot apart.
(c) Stoop slightly forward with bent knees, spread the fingers and grip the middle of the thighs with the hands.
(d) Bend the arms slightly at the elbows and lower the chin as far down as possible into jālandhara bandha.
(e) Inhale deeply and then exhale quickly so that the air is expelled from the lungs in a rush.

(f) Hold the breath without inhalation. Pull the whole abdominal region back towards the spine and lift it upwards (Pl. 66). Never hollow the chest during uḍḍīyāna practice.
(g) Raise the lumbar and dorsal spine forwards and upwards. Squeeze the abdominal organs towards the spine and press them against it.
(h) Maintain the abdominal grip, lift the hands from the thighs and rest them a little higher on the pelvic rim for a still firmer contraction.
(i) Straighten the back without loosening the abdominal grip or raising the chin up (Pl. 67).
(j) Hold the grip as long as you can, from ten to fifteen seconds. Do not try to hold it beyond your endurance, but gradually increase the time as it becomes comfortable.
(k) First relax the abdominal muscles without moving the chin and the head. If they move, strain is at once felt in the region of the heart and temples.
(l) Allow the abdomen to return to its normal position. Then inhale slowly (Pl. 68).
(m) Do not inhale during the processes described in Paras (f) to (k).
(n) Take a few breaths, then repeat the cycle in Paras (a) to (k) not more than six to eight times at a stretch. Increase the duration of the grip or the number of cycles as your capacity increases, or do so under the personal supervision of an experienced teacher or a guru.
(o) The cycles should be performed once a day only.
(p) When firmness is achieved in practice of uḍḍīyāna, gradually introduce it in various types of prāṇāyāma, but only while holding your breath after exhalation (bāhya kumbhaka).

Note:
(i) Practise on an empty stomach only.
(ii) Do not squeeze the abdomen until the breath has been expelled.
(iii) If strain is felt on the temples or if the intake of breath is laboured, this means that the uḍḍīyāna has been done beyond capacity.
(iv) Never inhale until the grip of uḍḍīyāna is released and the abdominal organs are brought to their original relaxed state.
(v) Do not constrict the lungs while the abdominal organs are compressed.

Effects
It is said that through uḍḍīyāna bandha the great bird prāṇa is forced to fly up through the suṣumṇā nāḍī, the main channel for the flow of nervous energy, which is situated inside the spinal column (mĕrudaṇḍa). It is the best of bandhās, and he who constantly practises it, as taught by his guru, becomes young again. It is said to be the lion that kills the elephant named death. It should be performed only during the interval between a complete exhalation and a fresh inhalation. It exercises the diaphragm and

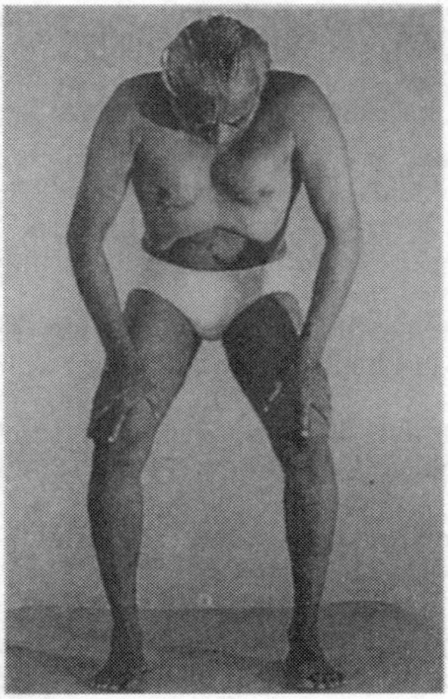

Pl.66

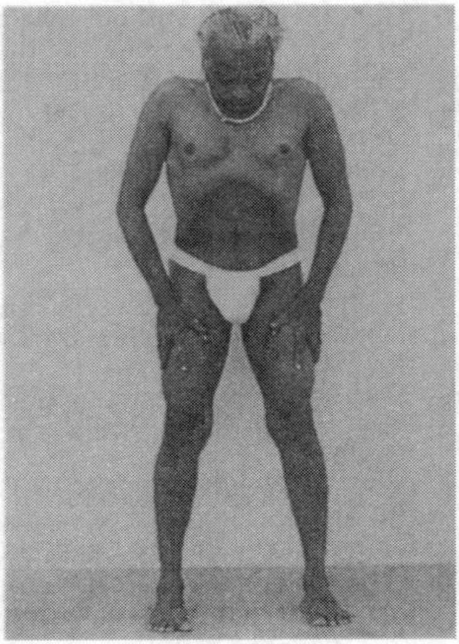

Pl.67

Pl.68

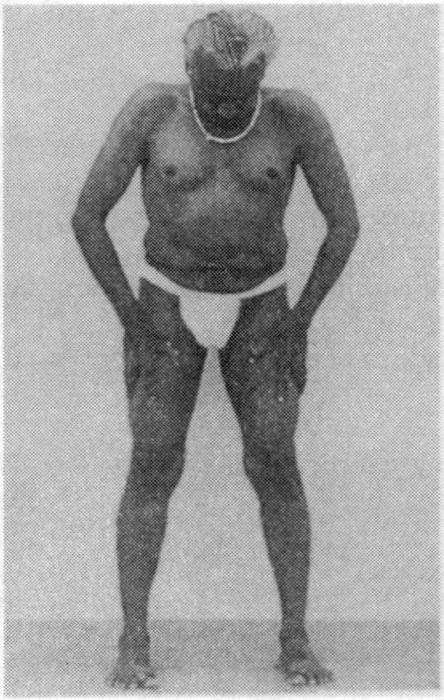

Pl.69

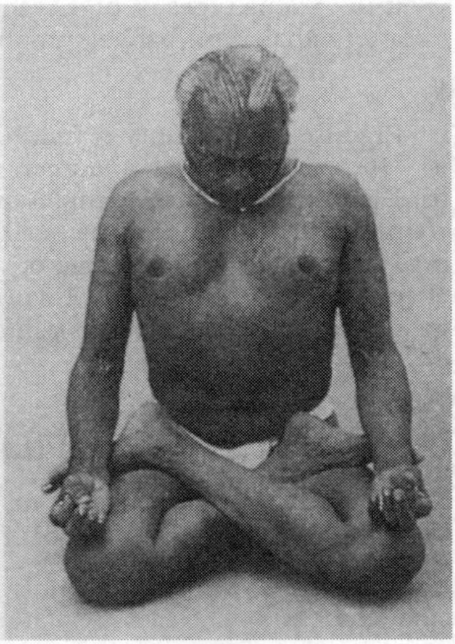

Pls. 66–8 **Uḍḍīyāna Bandha**

Pl. 69 **Mūla Bandha**

abdominal organs. The lift of the diaphragm gently massages the muscles of the heart, thereby toning them. It tones the abdominal organs, increases the gastric fire and eliminates toxins in the digestive tract. As such it is also called śakti chālana prāṇāyāma.

MŪLA BANDHA

7. Mūla means root, source, origin, or cause and basis, or foundation. It refers to the principal region between the anus and the genitals. Contract the muscles of this area, and lift them vertically towards the navel. Simultaneously, the lower anterior abdomen below the navel is pressed backwards and upwards towards the spine. The downward course of apāna vāyu is changed and then made to flow up to unite with the prāṇa vāyu, which has its seat in the region of the chest.

Mūla bandha should be attempted first in internal retention after inhalation (antara kumbhaka). There is a difference between the abdominal grips in uḍḍīyāna and in mūla bandha. In the former the entire region from the anus to the diaphragm is pulled back towards the spine and lifted up. But in the latter only the perineal and lower abdominal area between the anus and navel is contracted, pulled back to the spine and lifted up towards the diaphragm (Pl. 69).

The practice of contracting the anal sphincter muscles (aśvini mudrā) helps one to master mūla bandha. Aśva means a horse. This mudrā is so called because it suggests the staling of a horse. It should be learnt while doing various āsanas, especially tāḍāsana, śīrṣāsana, sarvāngāsana, ūrdhva dhanurāsana, uṣṭrāsana and paśchimottānāsana. (See *Light on Yoga*).

There is a grave danger in attempting to learn the uḍḍīyāna and mūla bandhās by oneself. Improper performance of the former will cause involuntary discharge of semen and loss of vitality, while that of the latter will seriously weaken the practitioner, who will lack virility. Even the correct performance of mūla bandha has its own dangers. It increases sexual retentive power, which the practitioner is tempted to abuse. If he succumbs to this temptation, all his dormant desires may be aroused and become lethal like a sleeping serpent stirred by a stick. With the mastery of the three bandhās, the yogi is at the cross-roads of his destiny, one road leading to bhoga (the enjoyment of worldly pleasures) and the other to Yoga or union with the Supreme Soul. The yogi, however, feels greater attraction for his creator. Normally, the senses open outwards and are attracted to objects and follow the path of bhoga. If this direction is changed, so that they turn inwards, then they follow the path of Yoga. The yogi's senses are turned inwards to meet the Source of all Creation. It is when the aspirant has mastered the three bandhās, that the guidance of a guru is most essential, for under proper guidance this increased power is sublimated to higher and nobler pursuits. The practitioner is then known as a celibate (ūrdhvareta). Having mastered the sexual urge naturally but not by force, he stops dissipating his virility. He is fully potent yet a master of himself (bhava vairagī). He then acquires moral and spiritual power, which will shine forth like the sun.

While practising mūla bandha, the yogi attempts to reach the true source or mūla of all creation. His goal is the complete restraint or bandha of the chitta which includes the mind (manas), the intellect (buddhi) and the ego (ahaṁkāra).

Chapter 14

The art of Inhalation (Pūraka) and Exhalation (Rechaka)

1. Inhalation (pūraka) is the intake of cosmic energy by the individual for his growth and progress. It is the path of action (pravṛtti mārga). It is the Infinite uniting with the finite. It draws in the breath of life as carefully and as gently as the fragrance of a flower might be indrawn and distributes it evenly throughout the body.

2. While performing āsanas, the mind and breath of the sādhaka are like those of an enthusiastic child, ever ready to invent, create and show its skill, whereas in practising prāṇāyāma the breath is like an infant child demanding special attention and care from its mother. As the mother loves her child and devotes her life to its well-being, so the consciousness has to foster the breath.

3. To understand this art, it is essential to know its methodology, what is right and wrong and what is gross and subtle. Then one can experience the essence of prāṇāyāma. It is helpful to note that the relationship between consciousness (chitta) and breath (prāṇa) should be like that between a mother and her child. But before this can happen the lungs, the diaphragm and the intercostal muscles must be trained and disciplined by āsanas so that the breath moves rhythmically.

4. The action of the consciousness in respiration is like that of a mother absorbed in watching her child at play. Though outwardly passive, she is mentally alert, observing him minutely while remaining completely relaxed.

5. When the mother first sends her child to school, she accompanies him, holding his hand to guide his way, emphasising the importance of being friendly with his future school-mates and of studying his lessons. She submerges her own identity in attending to her child until he gets accustomed to school life. So also has the consciousness to transform itself

into the same condition as the flow of breath, following it like a mother and guiding it to rhythmic flow.

6. The mother trains the child to walk and cross the streets cautiously. In the same way, the consciousness has to guide the flow of breath through the respiratory passages for absorption into the living cells. As the child gains confidence and becomes adjusted to school, the mother then leaves him when he reaches the gate. Similarly, when the breath moves with rhythmic precision, chitta observes its movements and unites it with the body and the Self.

7. In inhalation, the sādhaka attempts to transform his brain into a receiving and distributing centre for the flow of energy (prāṇa).

8. Do not inflate the abdomen while inhaling as this prevents the lungs from expanding fully. Breathing in or out must be neither forcible nor quick, for strain of the heart or damage to the brain may result.

9. Exhalation (rechaka) is the breath that goes out after inhalation. It is the expiration of impure air or the expulsion of carbon-dioxide. The outgoing breath feels warm and dry and the sādhaka senses no fragrance.

10. Exhalation is the outflow of the individual energy (jīvātmā) to unite with the cosmic energy (Paramātmā). It quietens and silences the brain. It is the surrender of the sādhaka's ego to and immersion in the Self.

11. Exhalation is the process by which the energy of the body gradually unites with that of the mind, merges into the soul of the sādhaka and dissolves into cosmic energy. It is the path of return from the peripheries of the body towards the source of consciousness known as the path of renunciation (nivṛtti mārga).

12. Hold the chest high with consiousness and lead the outgoing breath steadily and smoothly.

13. Inhale and exhale systematically with close attention to the rhythmic pattern of breath, as a spider symmetrically weaves its web and moves to and fro along it.

14. For some persons inhalation is longer than exhalation, whereas for others it is exhalation that is longer. This is due to the challenges we have to face in life and our responses to them, which change the flow of breath and the pressure of the blood. Prāṇāyāma aims to eradicate these disparities and disturbances in the flow of breath as well as in blood pressure, and to make one unperturbed and unattached to one's own personality.

Technique for Inhalation (Pūraka).

(a) Sit in any comfortable posture.
(b) Raise the spine along with the chest, floating ribs and navel and keep it erect.
(c) Now bring the head down as far as you can. (Pls 63 or 64). When elasticity is achieved at the back of the neck, perform jālandhara bandha (Pl. 57).
(d) According to Yoga, the mind (manas), which is the source of the emotions, is located in the region between the navel and the heart. Keep the back in constant contact with the emotional centre. Stretch the front of the body up and out without losing contact with the centre of consciousness.
(e) During inhalation, expand the chest up and out, without tilting forwards, backwards or sideways.
(f) Do not tense or jerk the dome of the diaphragm, but keep it relaxed. Start inhalation from the base of the diaphragm. The key point for starting deep inhalation is from the navel band, down below the floating ribs on either side (Pl. 70).
(g) Keep the lungs passive and non-resistant during inhalation in order to receive and absorb the incoming energy. While inhaling, fill the lungs fully with complete attention. Synchronise the movement of the breath evenly with the interior expansion of the lungs.

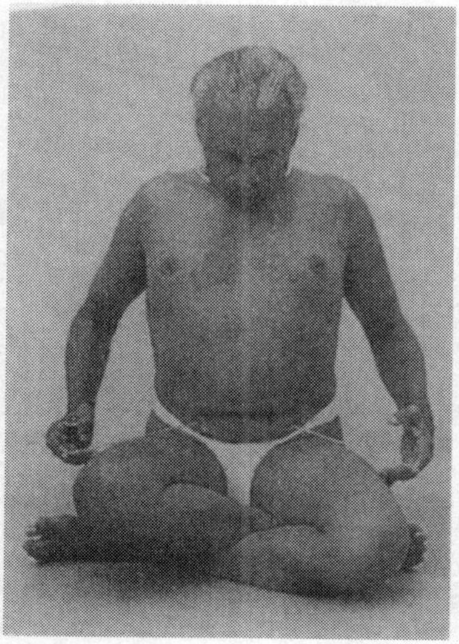

Pl. 70

(h) As a jug is filled from bottom to top, so fill the lungs from their base to the brim. Fill them to the top of the collar-bones and inner armpits.

(i) As special care and attention are needed to train an underdeveloped person, similarly careful training is required for the lungs to receive the full intake of breath. So explore carefully by stretching the nerve fibres of the lungs during soft deep inhalation.

(j) The bronchial tubes reach from the trachea to the periphery of the lungs, where they branch off into numerous bronchioles. See that each inhalation reaches to the very tip of the bronchioles.

(k) The in-breath is absorbed by the living cells in the body, as water is absorbed into the soil. Feel this absorption and the exhilarating sensation of percolation of the cosmic energy (prāṇa) that follows.

(l) The energy of inhalation enters from the nose and is received by the causal frame or the spiritual body. In inhalation the consciousness (chitta) ascends from the navel (maṇipūraka chakra) to the top of the chest (viśuddhi chakra). The sādhaka has to maintain throughout a single unifying contact between the causal and subtle frames of the body (see Ch. 2) and the consciousness ascending from its source. This contact unifies the body, breath, consciousness and the Self. Then the body (kṣetra) and the Ātmā (kṣetrajña) become one.

(m) Each pore of the skin of the trunk should act as the eye of intelligence (jñāna chakṣu) for absorbing prāṇa.

Pl.71

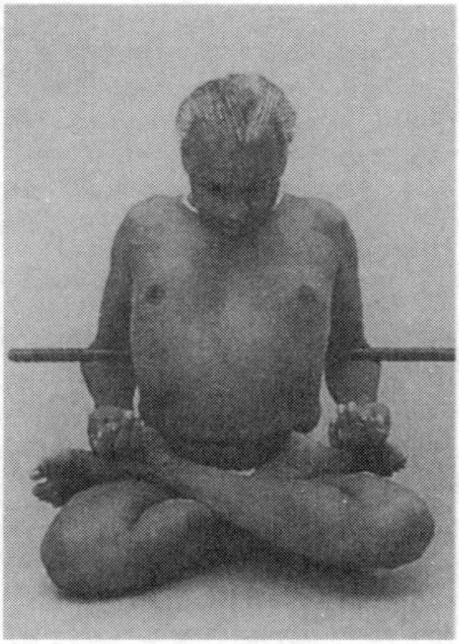

Pl.72

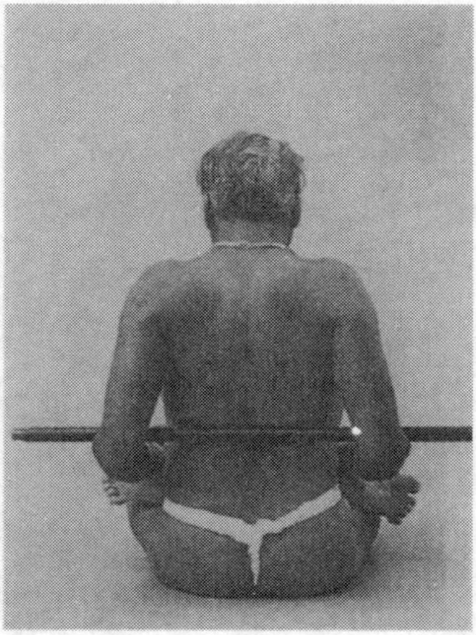

Pl.73

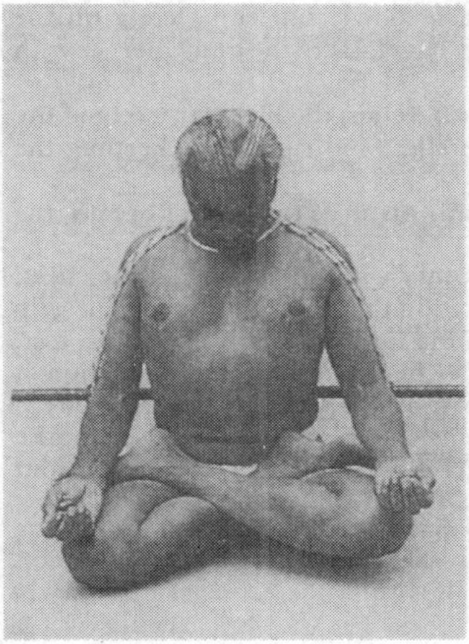

Pl.74

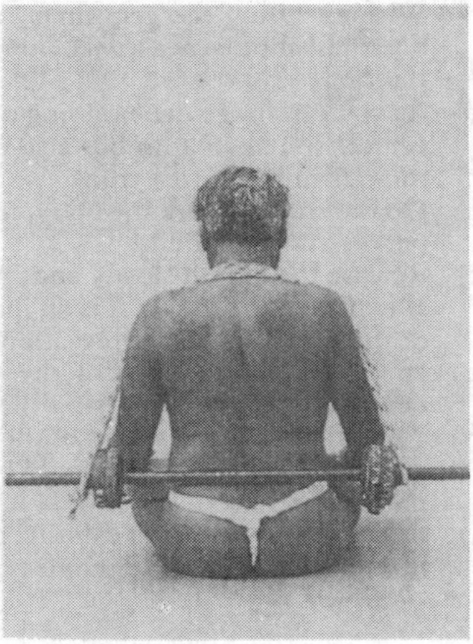

(n) If the inhalation is too pronounced the skin of the palms feels gritty. Regulate the breath so as to keep the skin of the palms soft throughout.

(o) If the shoulders are raised during inhalation, the upper areas of the lungs are not expanded fully and the nape of the neck becomes taut. Watch this tendency of the upward lift (Pl. 52) and bring the shoulders down immediately. In order to keep them down and the chest up, take a rod or weights and use them as shown in Pls 71 to 74.

(p) Relax the throat. Rest the tongue on the floor of the lower jaw without touching the teeth.

(q) Keep the eyes closed and relaxed, but the inner vision active (Pl. 54). When inhaling the eyes tend to turn up (Pl. 95); avoid this.

(r) See that the ears, the facial muscles and the skin on the forehead remain relaxed.

(s) The right method of inhalation removes sluggishness, stimulates and energises the body and the mind.

Technique for Exhalation (Rechaka)

(a) Follow Paras (a) to (d) regarding the techniques for inhalation.

(b) In inhalation the body acts as an instrument for receiving energy in the form of breath. In exhalation it becomes dynamic, acting as an instrument for the slow release of breath. Retain the grip of the intercostal muscles and the floating ribs throughout. Without this grip, steady and smooth exhalation is not possible.

(c) In exhalation, the source or the starting point is the top of the chest. Without losing the grip there, exhale slowly but completely till the breath is emptied at a level below the navel. Here the body merges with the Self.

(d) As you discharge the outgoing breath, retain the lift not merely of the central spinal column but also on its left and right side, keeping the torso firm like a tree trunk.

(e) Do not shake or jerk the body, for this disturbs the flow of breath, the nerves and the mind.

(f) Release the breath slowly and smoothly without collapsing the chest. If exhalation is rough, it is an indication that the attention on the grip of the body and the observation of the flow of breath have been lost.

(g) In inhalation, the skin of the torso becomes taut, in exhalation it becomes soft without losing the grip on the inner structural body.

(h) The skin of the chest and of the arms should not touch closely at the armpits (Pl. 75). There should be freedom and space (Pl. 76) without undue widening of the arms as in Pls 51 and 52.

(i) Exhalation is the art of calming the nerves and the brain. This creates humility and the ego becomes quiet.

Pl.75

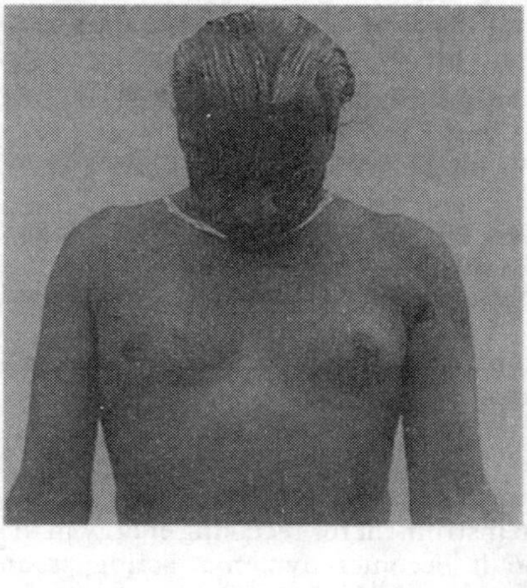

Pl.76

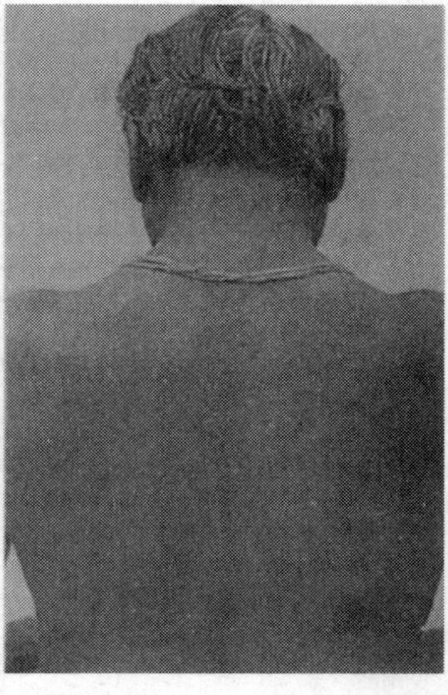

Chapter 15

The Art of Retention (Kumbhaka)

1. Kumbha means a pot which can be full or empty. Kumbhaka is of two types. It is either (a) a pause between an in and an out breath or (b) between an out and an in breath. It is the art of retaining the breath in a state of suspense.

2. It also means the withdrawal of the intellect from the organs of perception and action, to focus on the seat of the Ātmā (puruṣa), the origin of consciousness. Kumbhaka keeps the sādhaka silent at the physical, moral, mental and spiritual levels.

3. Retention of breath in kumbhaka should not be misinterpreted as re-tension of the brain, the nerves and the body to hold the breath. Re-tensioning leads to hyper-tension. Kumbhaka has to be done with the brain relaxed so as to re-vitalise the nervous system.

4. When the breath is stilled in kumbhaka, the senses are stilled and the mind becomes silent. Breath is the bridge between the body, the senses and the mind.

5. Kumbhakas are performed in two ways: sahita and kevala. When the breath is held intentionally and deliberately, this is sahita. Sahita kumbhaka is the pause in breathing (a) after full inhalation before commencing exhalation (antara or pūraka kumbhaka), or (b) after complete exhalation prior to starting inhalation (bāhya or rechaka kumbhaka). Kevala means 'by itself' or 'absolute'. Kevala kumbhaka is the pause in breathing unaccompanied by pūraka or rechaka, as when an artist is totally absorbed in his art or a devotee is breathless with adoration. This state is often preceded by body tremors and fear like that of a man on the point of being overwhelmed by the unexpected. Patience and perseverance will overcome this feeling. Kevala kumbhaka is instinctive and intuitive. In this state one is completely absorbed in the object of one's devotion and isolated from the world, experiencing a feeling of joy and peace which passes understanding. One is in tune with the Infinite. (*Haṭha Yoga Pradīpikā*, II. 71.)

6. Antara kumbhaka is the holding of the Lord in the form of cosmic or universal energy, which is merged into the individual energy. It is a state wherein the Lord (Paramātmā) is united with the individual soul (jīvātmā).

7. Bāhya kumbhaka is the state in which the yogi surrenders his very self, in the form of his breath, to the Lord and merges with the Universal Breath. It is the noblest form of surrender, as the yogi's identity is totally merged with the Lord.

8. In the *Bhagavad Gītā* (IV, 29/30) Kṛṣṇa explains to Arjuna the different kinds of sacrifices (yajñas) and of yogis. Kumbhaka prāṇāyāma is one of these yajñas and has three categories: inhalation-retention, exhalation-retention (both of which are sahita kumbhaka) and absolute retention (kevala kumbhaka). The yogi's body is the sacrificial altar, the in-flow of breath (pūraka) is the oblation and the out-flow (rechaka) is the fire. Kumbhaka is the moment when the oblation of pūraka is consumed in the fire of rechaka, and the oblation and the flame become one. The yogi acquires the knowledge of how to control his breathing (prāṇāyāma vidyā). The upper part of the thorax is the abode of the inflowing breath (prāṇa), and the lower part of the outgoing breath (apāna). When the two unite in the intake of breath, this is the state of pūraka kumbhaka. When apāna comes in contact with the prāṇa and flows out in exhalation, the empty state is the rechaka kumbhaka. Absorbing this knowledge by experience, the yogi makes Prāṇāyāma vidyā a part of his wisdom (buddhi), to which he finally offers his knowledge, his wisdom, his very life breath and his 'Self' as oblation (Ātmāhuti). This is the state of kevala kumbhaka, or absolute surrender, in which the yogi is absorbed in adoration of the Lord.

9. As a mother protects her child from every catastrophe, consciousness (chitta) protects the body and breath. The spine and torso are active and dynamic like a child and the chitta is alert and protective like a mother.

10. In kumbhaka the vibration in the body is like that of a locomotive stationary under steam, its driver alert and ready to start, but relaxed. Similarly, the prāṇa vibrates in the torso, but the chitta is kept relaxed and ready to let go or let in the breath.

11. The sensitivity, the grip and stretch of the skin on the trunk is like that of a disciplined child, who is both bold and cautious.

12. The length of time that the breath is held may be compared with that of traffic signals. If one passes the red light, accidents may occur. So also in kumbhaka, if one goes beyond one's capacity, the nervous system will be damaged. Tension in the body and brain indicates that the chitta cannot hold the prāna in kumbhaka.

13. Do not retain the breath by force of will. The moment the brain becomes tense, the inner ears hard and the eyes red, heavy or irritable, one is exceeding one's capacity. Watch for these warning signs, which indicate that the danger point is near.

14. The aim of kumbhaka is to restrain the breath. While breath is being held, speech, perception and hearing are controlled. The chitta in this state is free from passion and hatred, greed and lust, pride and envy. Prāṇa and chitta become one in kumbhaka.

15. Kumbhaka is the urge to bring out the latent divinity in the body, the abode of Ātman.

The Technique of Antara Kumbhaka

(a) Do not attempt to hold your breath after inhalation (antara kumbhaka) before mastering deep in and out breathing (pūraka and rechaka). Do not attempt to hold it after exhalation (bāhya kumbhaka) before mastering antara kumbhaka.

(b) Mastery means artistic adjustment by disciplined refinement and control of the movement of breath. Equalise the length of your in and out breathing before attempting kumbhaka. Read Ch. 13 on the bandhās thoroughly before starting kumbhaka.

(c) Learn to do antara kumbhaka by slow degrees. Start by holding the breath for only a few seconds without losing grip on the inner body. Watch the condition of the body, the nerves and the intellect. It takes some time before you can understand, experience and retain the precise inner grip over the intercostal muscles and diaphragm in the kumbhaka.

(d) When starting to learn internal retention (antara kumbhaka) allow some time to elapse after each kumbhaka. This enables the lungs to revert to the normal, natural and fresh condition before making another attempt. For instance, three or four cycles of normal or deep breathing should follow one cycle of kumbhaka until the session is over.

(e) If beginners perform internal retention after each inhalation, it will strain the lungs, harden the nerves and make the brain tense, and progress will be exceedingly slow.

(f) As you improve, shorten the interval between the cycles of normal breathing and antara kumbhaka.

(g) Increase the time you hold your breath in internal retention without exceeding your capacity.

(h) If the rhythm of inhalation and exhalation is disturbed by holding the breath, it shows that you have exceeded your capacity; therefore, reduce the length of internal retention. If the rhythm is undisturbed, then your practice is correct.

(i) Knowledge of the bandhās is essential for the proper practice of kumbhaka. They act as safety valves for distributing, regulating and absorbing energy, and prevent its dissipation. An electric motor burns out if its voltage is allowed to rise too high. Similarly, when the lungs are full and the energy in them is not checked by the bandhās, they will be damaged, nerves will be frayed and the brain made unduly tense. This will not happen if one practises jālandhara bandha.

(j) Never do antara kumbhaka while standing, as you may lose your balance and fall.

(k) When in a reclining position, place pillows under the head to keep it higher than the torso, so that no strain is felt in the head (Pl. 77).

(l) Do not raise the bridge of the nose in internal retention. If it moves up, the brain is caught up in the movement; it cannot then watch the trunk (Pl. 78).

(m) Throughout the practice of Prāṇāyāma, pivot the head and the cervical spine forwards and downwards and the erect dorsal spine and sternum upwards (Pl. 76). This helps the brain and cervical spinal-cord to move towards the sternum and relax the forehead. This makes the energy of the brain descend to the seat of the Self.

(n) Throughout each internal retention, keep a firm grip on the diaphragm and abdominal organs. There is a tendency, whether unconscious or deliberate, to tighten and loosen them in order to hold the breath longer. Avoid this as it dissipates energy.

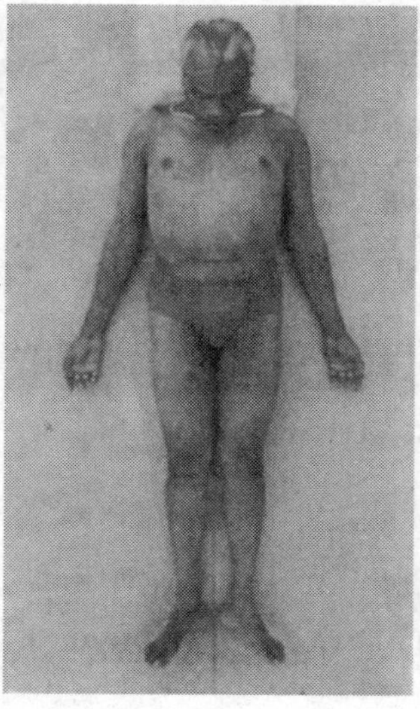

Pl.77

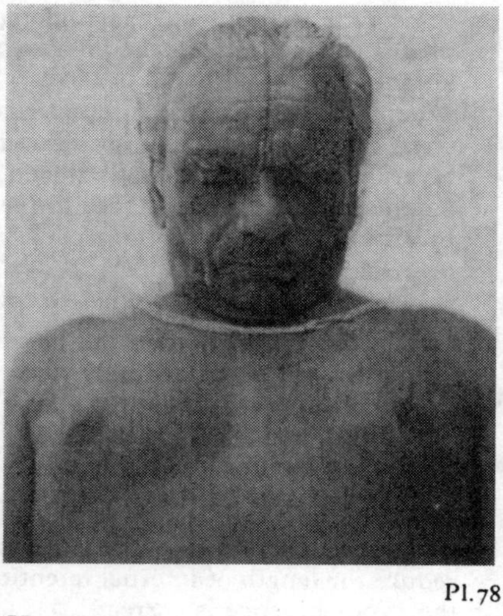

Pl.78

(o) If strain is felt in the lungs or heart, exhale, and take a few normal or deep breaths. This refreshes the lungs to restart antara kumbhaka. If you continue after having felt the strain, you disturb the harmonious functioning of both the body and the intellect. This leads to mental imbalance.

(p) When you are able to hold the breath in internal retention for a minimum of ten to fifteen seconds you may introduce mūla bandha. In the initial stages do mūla bandha at the end of inhalation and retain it throughout retention.

(q) In internal retention, pull the abdominal organs in and up, and simultaneously bring the lower spine forward (Pl. 69). Keep the trunk firm and the head, arms and legs relaxed throughout.

(r) Maintain the lift of the spine from the sacroiliac region and base of the liver and stomach throughout.

(s) Move the outer and inner spinal column forwards and upwards, rhythmically and evenly. As the spine moves anteriorly, roll the skin with it into the torso.

(t) If the skin of your chest slackens over the ribs, it is a sign that the breath has leaked from the lungs unawares.

(u) Do not overstretch or hollow the chest. Raise it in front, at the back and on both sides evenly. Hold the inner frame of the ribs firm and keep the outer body light. This will balance the body evenly and increase the duration of kumbhaka.

(v) See that the back and front intercostal muscles and the inner and outer layers on the sides move independently and uniformly.

(w) Adjust the skin of the armpits from back to front. Do not press the skin around the armpits of the chest but lift it up. If the skin of the armpits or the shoulders move up, this is a sign of tension. Release the skin and bring it down.

(x) At the end of inhalation (pūraka) and the start of retention (kumbhaka) the sādhaka experiences a spark of divinity. He feels the oneness of body, breath and self. In this state there is no awareness that time is passing. The sādhaka experiences freedom from cause and effect. He should retain this state throughout kumbhaka.

(y) The volatile contents of a well-sealed bottle do not leak, though the bottle be shaken. The vital energy of the sādhaka does not escape when kumbhaka is done with the bandhās. The trunk is sealed at the base by contracting the anus and the perineum and lifting them up from Mūlādhāra. The sādhaka then becomes full of vigour (tejas) and lustre (ojas).

(z) Beginners need pay no attention to uḍḍīyāna bandha and mūla bandha until they have mastered the rhythm of breathing. Advanced pupils should do all the bandhās after mastering them individually while holding their breath.

The Technique of Bāhya Kumbhaka

(a) Bāhya kumbhaka (retention of breath after complete exhalation) is of two kinds, pensive or dynamic. When pensive, it is practised without uḍḍīyāna. It is performed to keep oneself quiet and be done at any time, even after meals. When dynamic, it is done with uḍḍīyāna bandha, which massages the abdominal organs and heart and prevents dissipation of energy.

(b) Start by practising pensive external retention cycles. Then concentrate on external retention with uḍḍīyāna bandha.

(c) At the beginning, after each dynamic external retention, allow some time to elapse for the lungs and the abdominal organs to become normal.

(d) External retention with uḍḍīyāna should never be forced. If forced, one gasps, loses one's grip on the abdominal organs and feels a dryness in the lungs.

(e) Start external retention with uḍḍīyāna very gradually and maintain the grip of uḍḍīyāna for the same length of time in each cycle. Do six to eight cycles a day.

(f) Do a few cycles of normal or deep breething and one external retention with uḍḍīyāna. For instance, three or four cycles of normal breathing may be followed by one external retention with uḍḍīyāna. Repeat the sequence, reducing the number of cycles of normal breathing as stability is gained by practice.

(g) While practising, follow the techniques given in paragraphs b, d, e, f, h, l, m, p, s, t, u and w of the techniques of antara kumbhaka, substituting 'bāhya kumbhaka' for the words 'antara kumbhaka' wherever they occur.

(h) As one uses tweezers to remove a thorn and feels freedom from pain at once, use the intelligence as the tweezers to remove faulty grips and movements which act as thorns in practice.

(i) As the eyelids act instinctively to prevent foreign matter entering the eyes, the sādhaka should be always alert to prevent false grips, movements and habits entering into his practice of prāṇāyāma.

(j) Kumbhaka that reddens the face, burns the eyes and causes irritability is faulty. Never do kumbhaka with open eyes. Do not practice it if you have heart or chest problems, or when you are unwell.

(k) The body is the kingdom. The skin is its frontier. Its ruler is the Ātman, whose all-seeing eye (jñāna chaksu) watches every detail during prāṇāyāma.

(l) Mountain torrents dislodge rocks and gouge out canyons, yet when the energy of the flowing water is stilled and balanced against that of the rocks, each loses its separate identity. The result is a lake, reflecting the serene beauty of the mountains around. Emotions are the torrents, while the steady intellect forms the rock. In kumbhaka both are evenly balanced and the soul is reflected in its pristine state.

(m) Consciousness (chitta) wavers with the breath while kumbhaka stills and frees it from desires. The clouds disperse and the self shines like the sun.

(n) After practice of prāṇāyāma and kumbhaka relax in śavāsana (see Ch. 30).

Chapter 16

Grades of Sādhakas

1. Sādhakas are divided into three main groups in accordance with the progress they achieve in the practice of prāṇāyāma: These categories are: low (adhama), in which the breathing is coarse and rough; average (madhyama), in which it is half-soft, and high (uttama), in which it is soft and fine.

2. These groups are again sub-divided to show their subtle differences. Beginners are split into the lowest of the 'low' (adhamādhama), average among the 'low' (adhamamadhyama), and the best among the 'low' (adhamōttama). The 'average' (madhyama) and the 'high' (uttama) groups are similarly divided. But the final goal of every sādhaka is to join the highest of the 'high' (uttamōttama).

3. A beginner in prāṇāyāma (adhama) uses physical strength and lacks rhythm and poise. His body and brain are rigid, while his breath is forceful, jerky and superficial. An average (madhyama) sādhaka has some control in the art of sitting and a greater lung capacity than the beginner. He lacks the skill to maintain a steady posture or to breathe rhythmically. His practice is moderate, whereas that of the more perfect (uttama) sādhaka is disciplined; he sits erect and aware. His lungs are capable of sustaining prāṇāyāma for a longer time. His breath is rhythmic, soft and subtle, while his body, mind and intellect are poised. He is always ready to adjust his posture and to correct his own mistakes.

4. Very often, understanding and practice do not go together. One sādhaka may be better able to understand, while another may have better skill in practice. In each case, he has to develop uniformity in skill and intelligence and use them harmoniously for the better practice of prāṇāyāma.

5. Patanjali mentions the important part played in prāṇāyāma by place (deśa), time (kāla) and condition (saṁkhyā), whether internal or external, for the sādhaka. They may be regulated, lengthened or made subtle (*Yoga Sūtras* II, 50). His torso is the place, his age is the time, and his condition is the slow steady balance and even flow of his breathing.

6. The beginner may use the top of his lungs only, while the average performer will be concerned with his diaphragm or navel, and the adept

with his pelvic region. One has to learn to involve the whole torso when practising prāṇāyāma.

7. Time represents the length of each inhalation and exhalation, and circumstances, the controlled flow and subtlety of the breath.

8. Condition represents the number and length of the in-breaths, retentions, out-breaths and second retentions. The sādhaka has to determine their number and length for a given day and must keep to a regular schedule. The soft and delicate flow of breath in each cycle is the ideal condition (saṁkhyā).

9. The sādhaka may complete a cycle lasting ten seconds, another of twenty and a third of thirty. He may practise on three levels, the purely physical one, using his body as an instrument, the emotional one, using only his mental faculties, or the intellectual one, controlling his breath with intelligence. A beginner may reach perfection if his cycle is very short but soft and fine; on the other hand, an adept who takes pride in the length of his cycle, which is coarse and rough, is reduced to the level of a beginner.

10. The sādhaka should develop steadiness in the body, keep his mind and emotions in balance and his intellect sober. Then he is able to observe the subtle flow of his breath and feel its absorption within his system. His body, breath, mind, intellect and self become one and lose their individual identity. The knowable, the knower and the knowledge become one. (*Yoga Sūtra*, I, 41.)

11. A musician is lost in his ecstasy while displaying all the subtleties of the rāga (musical note, melody and harmony) in which he has specialised and experiences supreme consciousness. He may or may not be aware that his experience is shared by his audience. This is the quest of the sound (nādānusandhāna). The sādhaka likewise is lost in his ecstasy, but, his experience of prāṇāyāma is purely subjective. He alone listens to the subtle and soft sound of his own breathing and enjoys the absolute soundless state of kumbhaka. This is the quest of the Self (Ātmānusandhāna).

12. The intake of breath (pūraka) is the absorption of cosmic energy; inhalation-retention (antara kumbhaka) is the union of the Universal Self with the individual self; the outflow (rechaka) is the surrender of the individual energy, followed by exhalation-retention (bāhya kumbhaka), in which the individual and the Universal Self are merged. This is the state of nirvikalpa samādhi.

Chapter 17

Bīja Prāṇāyāma

What is Japa?

1. Though the soul is free from cause and effect, joy and sorrow, it is caught up with the turbulent activity of the mind. The purpose of mantra japa is to check and focus the disturbed mind upon a single point and is linked to a single thought. Mantra is a vedic hymn or musical verse, the repetition of which is japa or a prayer. This has to be done with sincerity, love and devotion, which develops the relationship between man and his Maker. When restricted to between one and twenty-four syllables it becomes a seed (bīja) mantra, the key word which unlocks his soul. The illumined guru, who has earned the grace of God, initiates and gives the key word to his deserving śiṣya, which unlocks the latter's soul. This is the seed for the śiṣya to study himself and to get himself initiated into all aspects of Yoga.

2. The mind takes the form of its thoughts and is shaped so that good thoughts make a good mind and evil thoughts a bad one. Japa (the repetition of a mantra) is used to disengage the mind from idle talk, jealous ideas and tale-bearing, so that the mind turns towards thoughts about the soul and God. It is the focusing of a wandering agitated mind upon a single thought, act or feeling.

3. Mantras are given for repeated continuous utterance, with reason, purpose and object. Constant repetition (japa) of a mantra with reflection upon its meaning (artha-bhāvana; artha = meaning, bhāvana = reflection) brings illumination. By such constant repetition and reflection, the thoughts of the sādhaka are churned, cleansed and clarified. He sees his soul reflected in the pool of his mind.

4. This japa transforms the sādhaka and transmutes his ego, thereby making him humble. He attains inner quietness and becomes one who has conquered his senses (jitēndriyan).

5. During the practice of prāṇāyāma, repeat the mantra, mentally synchronising its silent flow without moving the mouth or the tongue. This keeps the mind attentive and helps to increase the length of the three processes in breathing – inhalation, exhalation and retention. The flow of breath and the growth of the mind become smooth and steady.

6. The practice of prāṇāyāma is of two kinds: sabīja (with seed) and nirbīja (without seed). Sabīja prāṇayama includes the repetition of a mantra and is taught to four types of sādhakas, with varying stages of mental development, mūḍha, kṣipta, vikṣipta, and ekāgra (see Ch. 2).

7. The mantra should not be repeated quickly in order to complete a cycle of prāṇāyāma. It should be rhythmic, pacing the flow of breath equally in inhalation, exhalation and retention. Then the senses are silent. When perfection is achieved, the sādhaka becomes free and pure without the support of the mantra.

8. Nirbīja prāṇāyāma is taught to the fifth type of sādhaka, the one with the highest mental development, known as niruddha. It is done without the support of a mantra, wherein the sādhaka breathes, lives and experiences the state known as 'that thou art' (tattvam asi).

9. Sabīja, like a seed, sprouts thoughts, ideas and visions, while nirbīja, which is like a roasted seed, does not. Sabīja has a beginning and an end; it has shape, form and connotations, like lamp and light and light and flame. Nirbīja has no conditions, no beginning and no end.

10. Sabīja prāṇāyāma turns the mind and intellect of the sādhaka to the Lord, the seed of omniscience and the source of all being. The word that expresses Him is the mystic syllable ĀUṀ (praṇava). The Lord has been described by Patanjali as one who is untouched by the cycles of action and reaction, cause and effect, affliction and pleasure.

11. It is said in the *Chāndogya-Upaniṣad* that Prajāpati (the Creator) brooded on the worlds created by him. From them issued the three Vedas – Ṛg, Yajur and Sāma. From these, when brooded upon, came the three syllables: bhuḥ (earth), bhuvaḥ (atmosphere) and svaḥ (sky). From them, when they had been brooded upon, issued the syllable ĀUṀ. As leaves are held together by a branch, so is all speech held together by ĀUṀ.

12. ĀUṀ conveys concepts of omnipotence and universality. It contains everything that is auspicious as well as awe-inspiring. It is a symbol of serenity and majestic power. ĀUṀ is the everlasting spirit, the highest aim. When its connotations are fully known, all longings are fulfilled. It is the surest means of salvation and the supreme help. It connotes the fullness of human life, thought, experience and worship. It is the immortal sound. Those who enter and take refuge in it become immortal.

13. The Upanisads mention various triads of the soul, worshipped by the use of threefold ĀUM. In the realm of sex it symbolises the feminine,

masculine and neuter sexes, as well as their creator, who is beyond the sexes. With power and light, ĀUṀ symbolises fire, wind and sun, as well as the generator of these sources of power and light. In the form of the Lord, the symbol is worshipped as Brahmā, the creator, Viṣṇu, the protector, and Rudrā, the destroyer, synthesising the forces of all life and matter. As time, ĀUṀ stands for the past, the present and the future, together with the Almighty, who is beyond the reach of time. As thought, it represents the mind (manas), intellect or understanding (buddhi), and the self or ego (ahaṁkāra). The word ĀUṀ also represents the three states (guṇās) of illumination (sattva), activity (rajas), and inertia (tamas), and also anyone who has become free of them, a guṇātīta.

14. The three letters A, U and M, together with the dot over the M, are symbols of man's search for truth along the three paths of knowledge, action and devotion, and the evolution of a great soul into one who has achieved poise of the soul and whose intellect has attained a state of stability – a sthita prajñā. If he follows the path of wisdom (jñāna-mārga), his desires (ichhā), actions (kriyā) and learning (vidyā) are all under his control. If he follows the path of action (karma-mārga), he will undergo austere penance (tapas) to attain his goal in life, self study (svādhyāya), and then dedicate the fruits of his actions to the Lord (Īśvara-pranidhāna). If he follows the path of devotion (bhakti-mārga), he will be immersed in hearing the Lord's name (Śravaṇa), meditating upon His attributes (Manana), and thinking of His glory (Nididhyāsana). His state is one beyond that of sleep (nidrā), dream (svapna) or awakening (jāgṛti), for though his body is at rest as if in sleep, his mind is seemingly in a dream and his intellect is fully alert; he is in the fourth transcendental state, the turīyāvasthā.

15. One who has realised the manifold meanings of ĀUṀ becomes free from the shackles of life. His body, breath, senses, mind, intellect and the syllable ĀUṀ are fused together.

16. ĀUṀ is the word that all the Vedas glorify, and all self-sacrifice expresses. It is the goal of all sacred studies and the symbol of holy life. Fire is latent in dried wood and it can be generated by friction again and again. Even so, the latent divinity in the sādhaka is stirred into manifestation by the word ĀUṀ. By rubbing his intelligent awareness against the sacred word ĀUṀ, he sees the hidden divinity within himself.

17. By meditating upon AUṀ, the sādhaka remains steady, pure and faithful, and becomes great. As a cobra sheds its old skin, so he sheds all evil. He finds the peace of the Supreme Spirit, where there is no fear, dissolution or death.

18. Since the word ĀUṀ is one of supreme and majestic power, its force has to be diffused by adding it to the name of a deity, and making the combination into a mantra as a bīja for the practice of Prāṇāyāma, as for instance, eight syllables 'ĀUṀ NAMŌ NĀRĀYAṆĀYA' or five syllables 'ĀUṀ NAMAḤ ŚIVĀYA' or twelve syllables 'ĀUṀ NAMŌ BHAGAVATE VĀSUDEVĀYA' or GĀYATRI MANTRA with twenty-four syllables.

Chapter 18

Vṛtti Prāṇāyāma

1. Vṛtti means action, movement, a course of conduct or method.

2. There are two types of vṛtti prāṇāyāmas: Samavṛtti and Viṣamavṛtti. It is the former if the length of time in each inhalation, exhalation and retention of breath is the same, and it is the latter if the length is altered and varied.

SAMAVṚTTI PRĀṆĀYĀMA

3. Sama means equal, identical or in the same manner. In samavṛtti prāṇāyāma an attempt is made to achieve uniformity in the duration of all the four processes of breathing, namely, inhalation (pūraka), retention (antara kumbhaka), exhalation (rechaka) and retention (bāhya kumbhaka). If the duration of pūraka is say five seconds or ten seconds, it should be the same in rechaka and kumbhakas.

4. Start samavṛtti prāṇāyāma, conforming only to even duration of inhalation (pūraka) and exhalation (rechaka).

5. Achieve uniformity in length of time, maintaining the perfect soft rhythm in pūraka and rechaka.

6. Only then, attempt retention of breath after inhalation (antara kumbhaka). At first you will not be able to maintain the same length of time for internal retention as for pūraka and rechaka.

7. Start the internal retention gradually. At first the ratio of time between the three processes should be kept at 1 : $\frac{1}{4}$: 1. Slowly increase the proportions to 1 : $\frac{1}{2}$: 1. When this is firmly established, increase to 1 : $\frac{3}{4}$: 1. When this becomes easy, then increase the proportion of antara kumbhaka to the ratio of 1 : 1 : 1.

8. Do not attempt to restrain the breath after full exhalation (bāhya kumbhaka) until you have achieved this ratio.

9. Then start external retention (bāhya kumbhaka) gradually. At the beginning, keep the ratio of time for in-breath, internal retention, out-

breath and external retention at 1 : 1 : 1 : $\frac{1}{4}$. Slowly increase the proportions to 1 : 1 : 1 : $\frac{1}{2}$. After this is firmly established, attempt 1 : 1 : 1 : $\frac{3}{4}$ and lastly increase the proportions to achieve the ratio of 1 : 1 : 1 : 1.

10. First practice internal retention (antara kumbhaka) separately, interspacing one antara between three or four cycles of normal breathing. Repeat the antara cycle five or six times. When this becomes easy and comfortable, decrease the interspacing. When this comes with ease, do pūraka, antara kumbhaka and rechaka without interspersion.

11. When the uniform ratio of pūraka, antara kumbhaka and rechaka is maintained with ease, introduce bāhya kumbhaka once in three or four cycles.

12. Gradually decrease the number of cycles in between. Then perform pūraka, antara kumbhaka, rechaka and bāhya kumbhaka without interspersion.

VISAMAVṚTTI PRĀṆĀYĀMA

13. Visama means irregular. Viṣamavṛtti Prāṇāyāma is so-called because the duration of pūraka, antara kumbhaka, rechaka and bāhya kumbhaka are varied. This leads to interrupted rhythm, and the difference in ratio creates difficulty and danger for the pupil unless he is gifted with strong nerves and good lungs.

14. First start with inhalation, antara kumbhaka and exhalation only in the ratio of 1 : 2 : 1. Increase the ratios gradually to 1 : 3 : 1, and then to 1 : 4 : 1. Then adjust and adopt the ratio to 1 : 4 : 1$\frac{1}{4}$; 1 : 4 : 1$\frac{1}{2}$; 1 : 4 : 1$\frac{3}{4}$ and 1 : 4 : 2. When this is mastered, and only then, add bāhya kumbhaka gradually in the ratio of 1 : 4 : 2 : $\frac{1}{4}$; 1 : 4 : 2 : $\frac{1}{2}$; 1 : 4 : 2 : $\frac{3}{4}$; and 1 : 4 : 2 : 1. These four ratios constitute one cycle of viṣamavṛtti prāṇāyāma.

15. At first the pupil will find it hard to maintain rhythm during rechaka, bāhya kumbhaka and pūraka, as gasping will ensue. But it all eases with long and uninterrupted practice.

16. In viṣamavṛtti prāṇāyāma the ideal ratio is as follows: if full inhalation takes five seconds the breath is held (antara kumbhaka) for twenty seconds, exhalation takes ten seconds, and bāhya kumbhaka five seconds, the ratio being 1 : 4 : 2 : 1.

17. When this has been achieved, reverse the process. Inhale for ten seconds, hold for twenty seconds and exhale for five seconds, the ratio being

2 : 4 : 1. Then add bāhya kumbhaka 2 : 4 : 1 : $\frac{1}{4}$, and gradually increase the duration of bāhya kumbhaka ratio to 2 : 4 : 1 : $\frac{1}{2}$, 2 : 4 : 1 : $\frac{3}{4}$ and 2 : 4 : 1 : 1.

18. The length of time can be varied. For instance, if inhalation is twenty seconds, retention ten seconds and exhalation five seconds, minimise bāhya kumbhaka to 2$\frac{1}{2}$ seconds, so as to make the ratio 4 : 2 : 1 : $\frac{1}{2}$.

19. The length of time can be varied in viṣamavṛtti prāṇāyāma in different ratios, as for instance, 1 : 2 : 4 : $\frac{1}{2}$; 2 : 4 : $\frac{1}{2}$: 1; 4 : $\frac{1}{2}$: 2 : 1; $\frac{1}{2}$: 1 : 4 : 2. The permutations and combinations in viṣamavṛtti prāṇāyāma are numerous and no mortal can perform all possible combinations in his or her lifetime. An example of such permutations and combinations is given in the note on sūrya and chandra bhedana prāṇāyāmas in Ch. 27.

Note
20. The path of viṣamavṛtti prāṇāyāma is fraught with danger. So do not practise it on your own without the personal supervision of an experienced guru.

21. Due to different ratios for inhalation, inhalation-retention, exhalation and exhalation-retention, all the systems of the body, especially the respiratory organs, the heart and nerves are overtaxed and strained. This may cause tension in the brain and in the blood vessels, which in turn may create hypertension, restlessness and irritation.

22. This caution regarding viṣamavṛtti prānāyāma and the practice of kumbhakas applies with greater force than to samavṛtti prāṇāyāma. Remember Svātmārama's words in his *Haṭha Yoga Pradīpikā*, that prāṇa should be tamed more gradually than lions, elephants and tigers; otherwise it will kill the practitioner.

Section III

The Techniques of Prāṇāyāma

Chapter 19

Ujjāyī Prāṇāyāma

The prefix 'uḍ' means upwards or expanding. It also conveys the sense of pre-eminence and power. 'Jaya' means conquest or success, and, from another point of view, restraint. In ujjāyī the lungs are fully expanded, with the chest thrust out like that of a mighty conqueror.

All stages of this prāṇāyāma except those with retentions (kumbhaka) may be done at any time. However, if the heart feels heavy, full or painful, or the diaphragm is hard, and if you are agitated or the heart-beat is abnormal, lie down after laying two wooden planks on the floor, (each about one foot square and 1½ inches thick) on top of each other. Rest the back on the planks, with your buttocks below them and arms stretched downwards. (Pls 79 to 81). You can also lie with a bolster as in Pl. 82. Keep the weight on the legs for comfort and relaxation, as shown in Pl. 83. Two cushions may be used instead of planks (Pl. 84). If the legs cannot be stretched out, because of infirmity or disease, bend the knees and rest the lower legs on a bolster or a stool (Pls 85 and 86).

When the back is thus rested, the pelvic muscles initiate inhalation. This relieves any tension and softens the diaphragm. The lungs and the respiratory muscles function smoothly and breathing becomes deep. The practice of this prāṇāyāma brings amazing relief to patients with enlarged ventricles and congenital heart defects. Moreover, it stills the fears that beset heart patients who are afraid to make the least movement lest they aggravate their condition.

Pl. 79

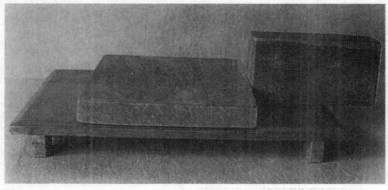

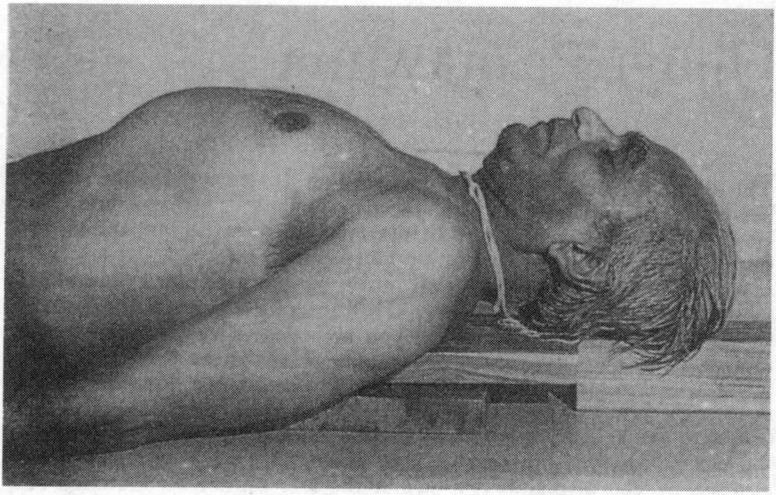

Pl.80

Pl.81

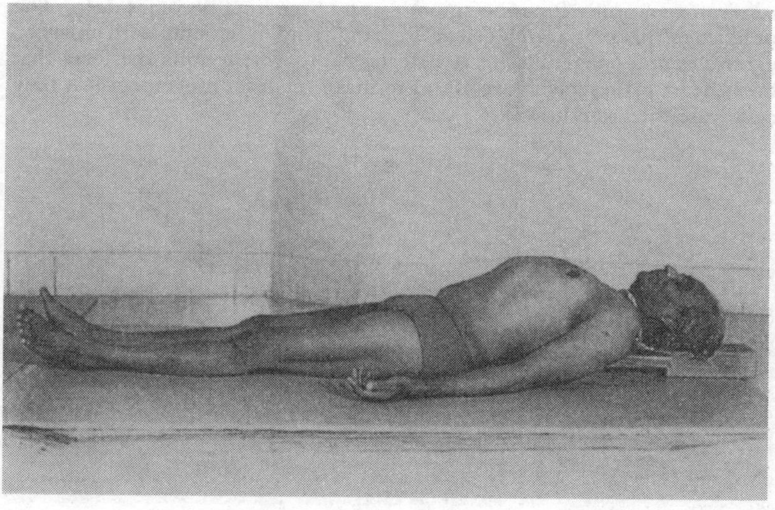

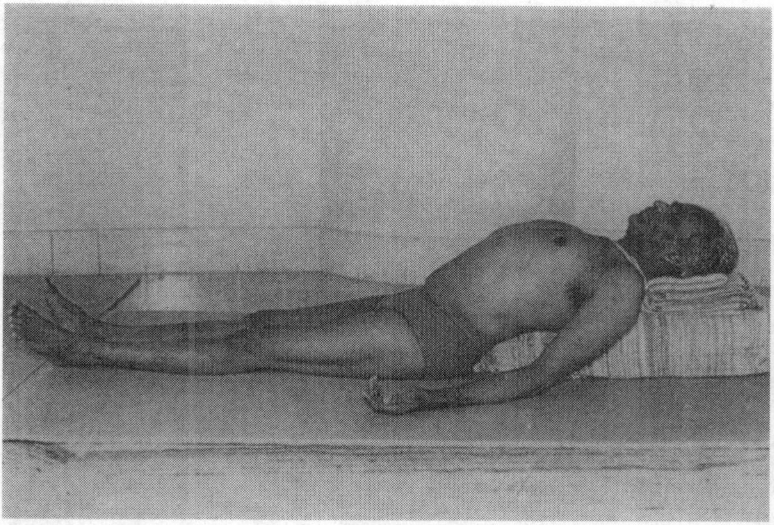

Pl.82

Pl.83

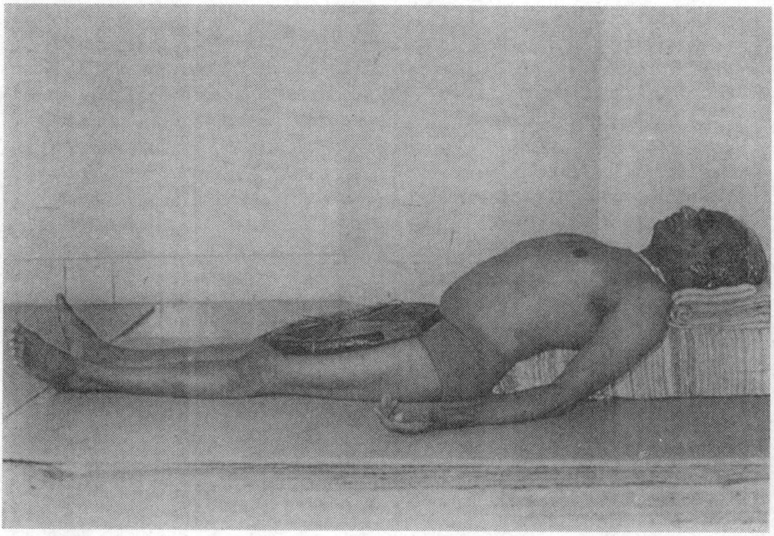

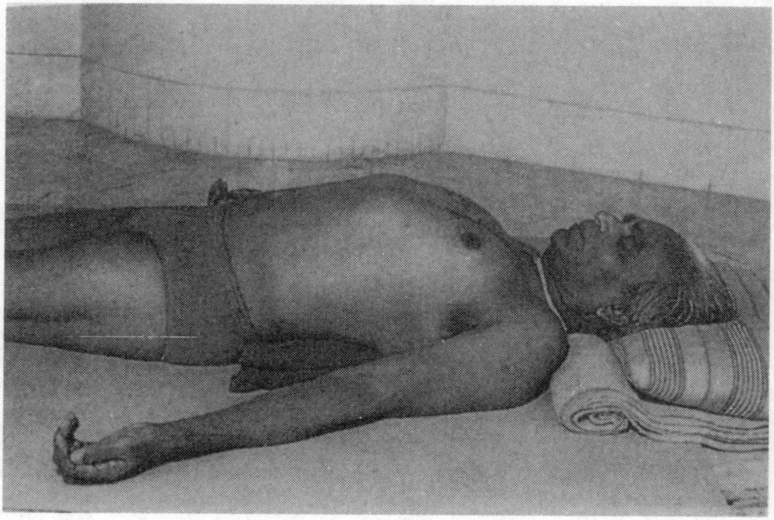

Pl.84

Pl.85

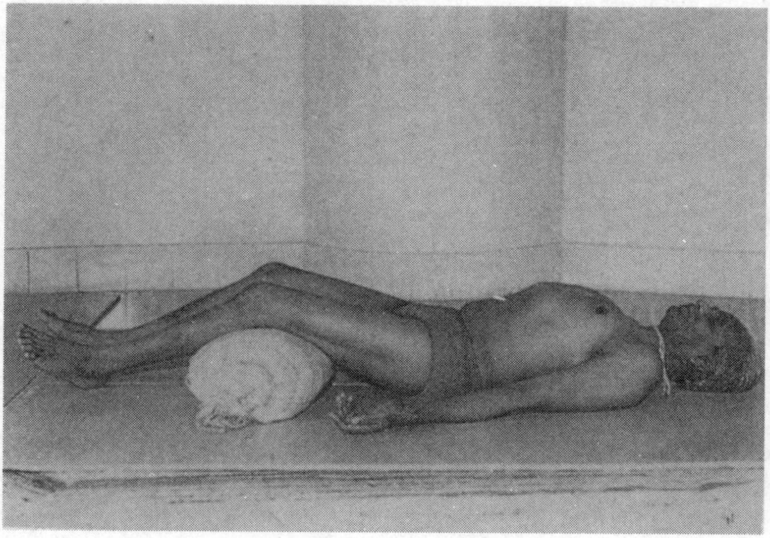

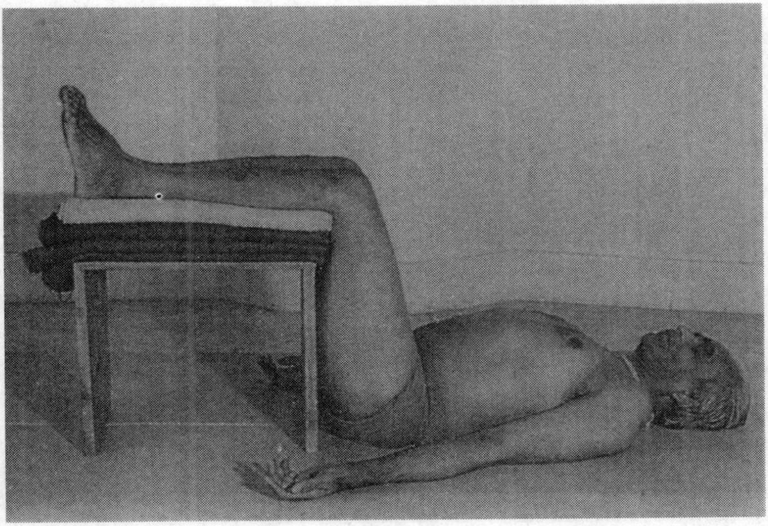

Pl.86

Note

1. All stages of all prāṇāyāmas begin with exhalation (rechaka) and end with inhalation (pūraka). First, you must breathe out whatever tidal air remains in the lungs, then start prāṇāyāma. Do not end it with exhalation, as this strains the heart, but take a normal inhalation at the end of each stage of prāṇāyāma. Do not use force.

2. The passages for in and out breaths differ in the sinus areas. In inhalation the breath touches the inner surface of the sinus passages at the bottom (Pl. 87). In exhalation it touches the outer surface at the top (Pl. 88).

3. All inhalations are made with a sibilant sound 'ssss' and all exhalations with aspirate 'hhhh'.

4. When sitting for prāṇāyāma in the initial stages, use a support as explained in Ch. 11, Para. 30 (Pls 42 and 43).

5. Though śavāsana is suggested at the end of each prāṇāyāma, if you want to do more than one stage or different prāṇāyāmas in succession, it should be done only at the end of the practice.

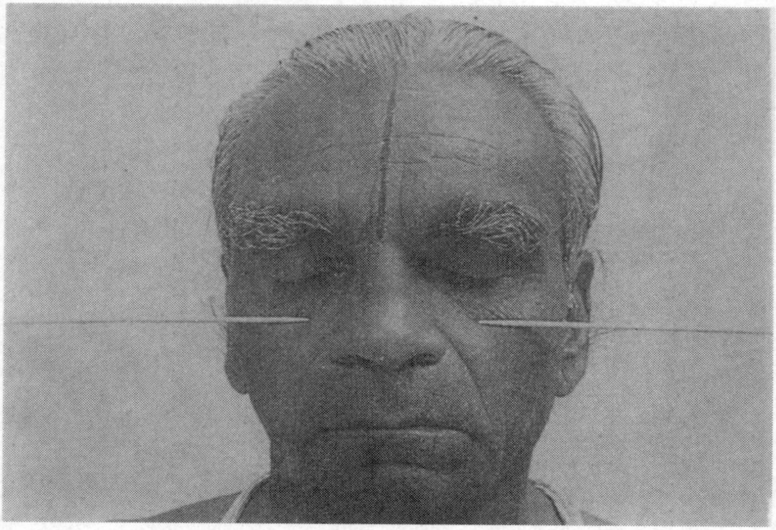

Pl.87

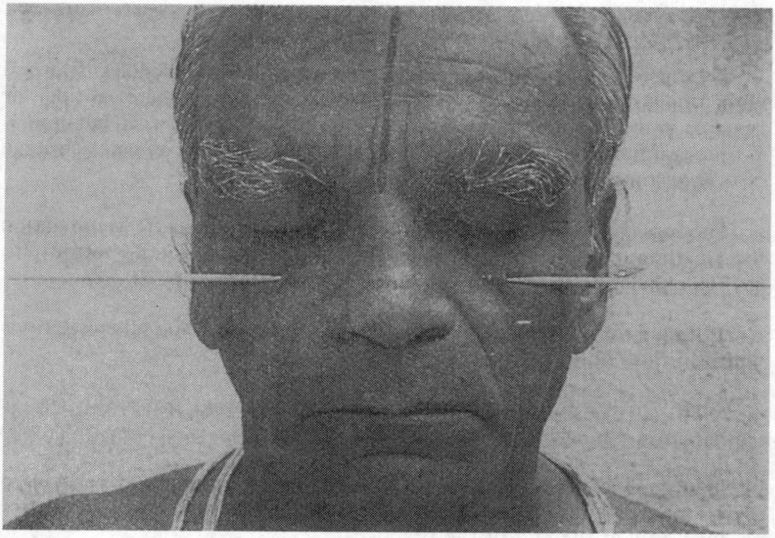

Pl.88

STAGE I

This preparatory stage trains one in the art of being aware of sensations in the lungs; it leads to even breathing.

Technique

1. Spread a blanket, folded lengthwise, on the floor. Over it, at the head and exactly in line with the edge, lay another blanket folded three or four times so that it fits the back of the head and trunk (Pl. 89).

2. Lie flat on the back on the folded blanket, keeping the body in a straight line. Do not cave in the rib-cage. Close the eyes and lie quietly for a minute or two (Pl. 50). Cover the eyes with a soft cloth for quick relaxation of the facial muscles (Pl. 90).

3. Breathe normally. Consciously observe and feel the flow of breath throughout.

4. As you breathe in, make sure that both lungs fill evenly. Feel the chest expand upwards and outwards. Synchronise the two movements.

5. Breathe out quietly, emptying the lungs evenly on both sides. Correct it if the lungs move unevenly.

6. Continue in this way for ten minutes, keeping the eyes closed throughout.

Effects

The above practice makes one attentive, invigorates the nerves, loosens any hardness in the lungs and prepares them for deep breathing.

STAGE II

This preparatory stage trains one to lengthen the duration of each out-breath and to learn the art of exhalation.

Technique

1. Lie down, following the instructions given in Paras 1 and 2 of Stage I (Pl. 89).

2. Close the eyes without tensing the eye-balls, keep them passive and receptive, and direct the gaze inwards (Pl. 54).

3. Keep the inner ears alert and receptive.

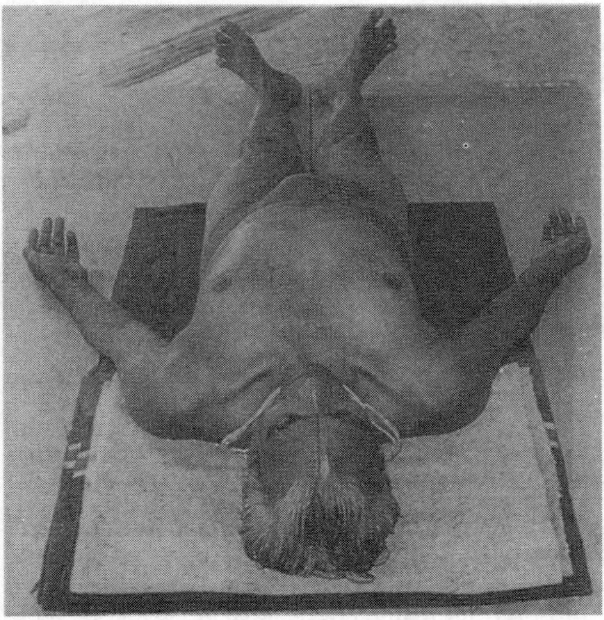

Pl.89

Pl.90

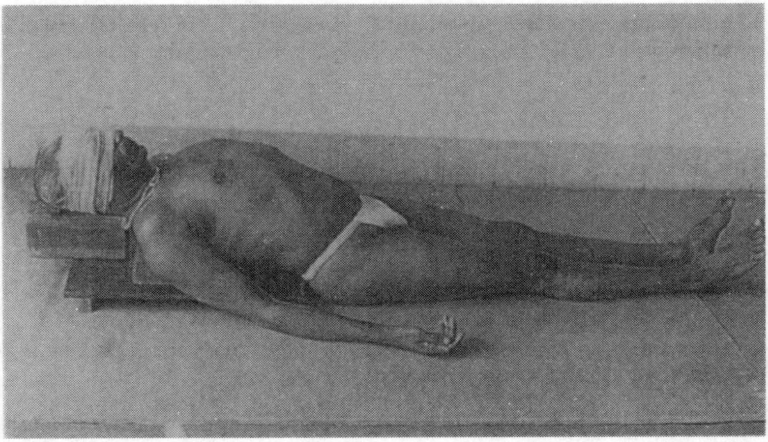

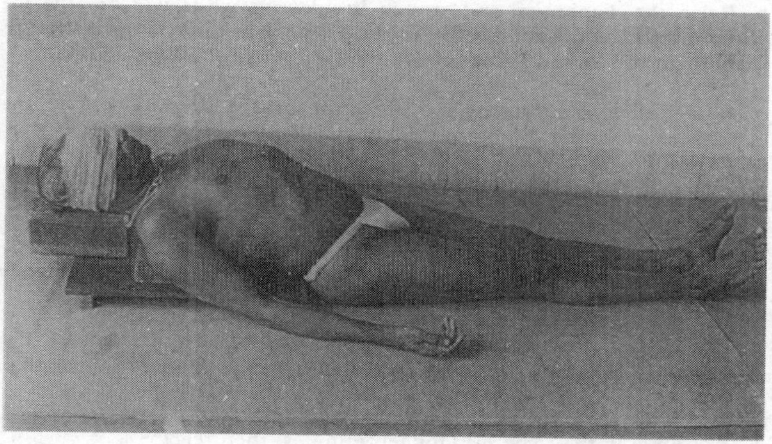

Pl.91

4. First exhale quietly until lungs feel empty, but without pressing down upon the abdominal organs (Pl. 91).

5. Inhale normally through the nose. This is inhalation (pūraka).

6. Exhale slowly, deeply and steadily until the lungs feel empty. This is exhalation (rechaka).

7. Continue for ten minutes and then relax.

The emphasis here is on slow, deep and steady exhalation.

Effects
This stage soothes the nerves and calms the brain. Its slow, steady and deep exhalations are ideal for sufferers from cardiac disorders and hypertension.

STAGE III

This preparatory stage trains one to lengthen the duration of each in-breath and to learn the art of inhalation.

Technique
1. Lie, as described in Stage I, Paras 1 and 2. Then follow the instructions given in Stage II, Paras 2 to 4.

2. Relax the diaphragm and stretch it sideways while you breathe in, without inflating the abdomen (Pl. 92). To prevent this, do not allow the diaphragm to roll or to move above the floating ribs (Pls 93 and 94).

3. Take a slow, deep, steady and sibilant in-breath carefully through the nose. Make sure that both lungs fill evenly.

4. Listen to the sound attentively, and maintain its rhythm throughout.

5. Fill the lungs completely till the sound of inhalation becomes inaudible.

6. Deep inhalation tends to move the eye-balls up (Pl. 95). Consciously draw them down and gaze into the lungs (see Pl. 54).

7. At the start of exhalation immobilise the diaphragm, then breathe out slowly but not deeply. Here the out-breath will be slightly longer than normal.

8. Continue in the same way for ten minutes, then relax.

The emphasis here is on slow, deep and steady inhalations. Once more, listen to the sound and maintain its rhythm throughout. In order to get better rhythmic deep breathing, it is advisable to use two planks for the back, as described at the beginning of this chapter (see Pls 80 to 86).

Effects
This preliminary practice is good for those suffering from low blood pressure, asthma and depression. It invigorates the nervous system and instils confidence.

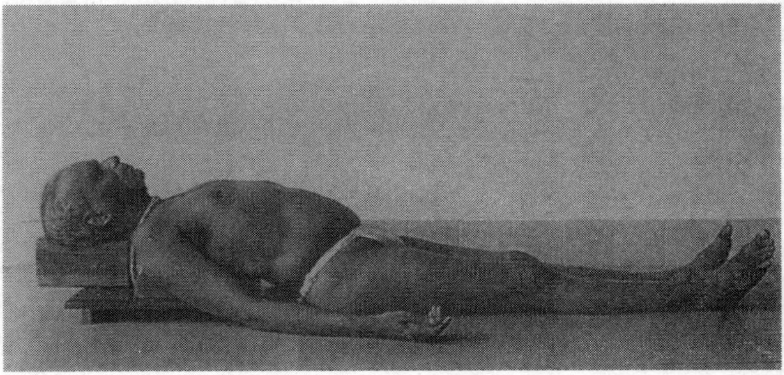

Pl.92

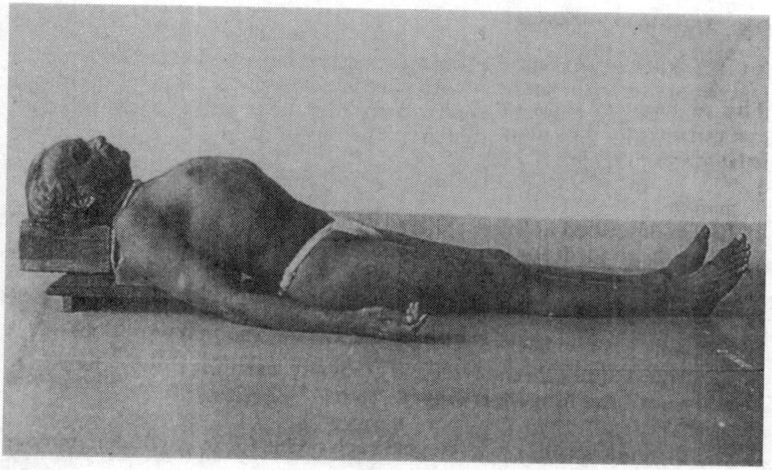
Pl.93

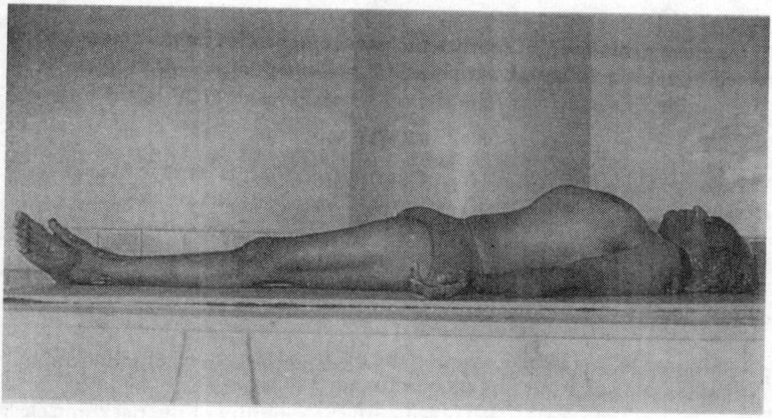
Pl.94

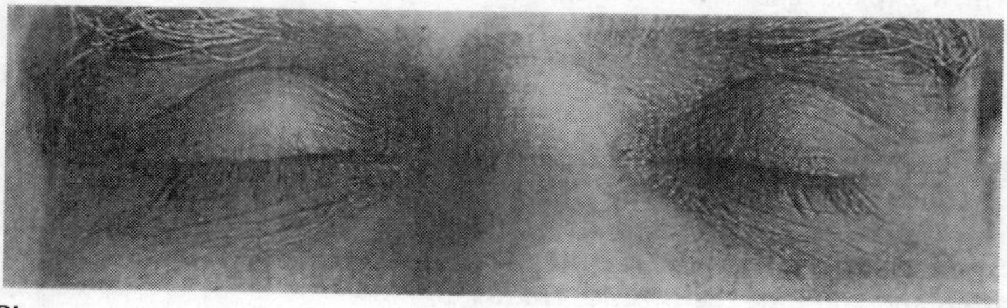
Pl.95

STAGE IV

This preparatory stage trains one to prolong the length of each in-breath and out-breath. This helps to master the arts of deep inhalation and deep exhalation.

Technique

1. Lie, as described in Stage 1, Paras 1 and 2. Then follow the instructions given in Stage II, Paras 2 to 4.

2. Now breathe in, following the techniques given in Paras 2 to 5 of Stage III.

3. Grip the diaphragm and release it gradually, exhaling slowly, deeply and steadily until the lungs feel empty.

4. This completes one cycle. Repeat such cycles for ten to fifteen minutes, then relax.

Effects.

This stage gives energy, soothes the nerves and tones them. Stages I to IV are preparatory to ujjāyī prāṇāyāma, performed while lying down.

STAGE V

The breathing here is similar to that in Stage I but is done while sitting. It trains one in the art of observation and leads to even breathing.

Technique

1. Sit in padmāsana, siddhāsana, swastikāsana or vīrāsana, or in any convenient and comfortable position.

2. Sit quietly for a while, keeping the back and the spinal column firm, but the spinal muscles soft and mobile for adjusting the torso. The firmness of the spine has to be evenly balanced with the mobility of the back muscles, which expand and contract with the flow of in and out breaths. The absorption of the breath should synchronise with the mobility of the back muscles. The slower their movement, the better the absorption of the breath.

3. Lower the head towards the trunk and lift up the inner frame of the chest towards the descending chin. Rest the chin in the notch just above the breastbone. This is the chin-lock (jālandhara bandha) (Pl. 57). If you cannot do it completely, keep the head down as low as you can without strain and continue the practice (Pl. 63).

4. Keep the arms down and rest the back of the wrists on the knees (Pl. 32) or join the tip of the index finger of each hand with the tip of the thumb and keep the other fingers extended (jñāna mudra) (Pl. 13).

5. Do not tense the eye-balls as in Pl. 95, but keep them passive as well as receptive. Close the eyes and direct the gaze inwards (Pl. 54).

6. Keep the inner ears alert and receptive.

7. First exhale quietly as far as possible, without pressing down upon the abdominal organs (Pls 96 and 97). Note the dots on the torso, which show skin movements for out-breath, in-breath and retention.

8. Follow the techniques given in Paras 3 to 6 of Stage I, observing the flow of breath. Do this for ten minutes and then rest in śavāsana (Pl. 182) for a few minutes.

STAGE VI

Here, the breathing is similar to that in Stage II, but done while sitting. It trains one to lengthen the duration of each out-breath and to learn the art of exhalation.

Technique

1. Sit in any comfortable position, following the techniques given in Paras 1 to 7 of Stage V. Exhale whatever breath is in the lungs (Pl. 96).

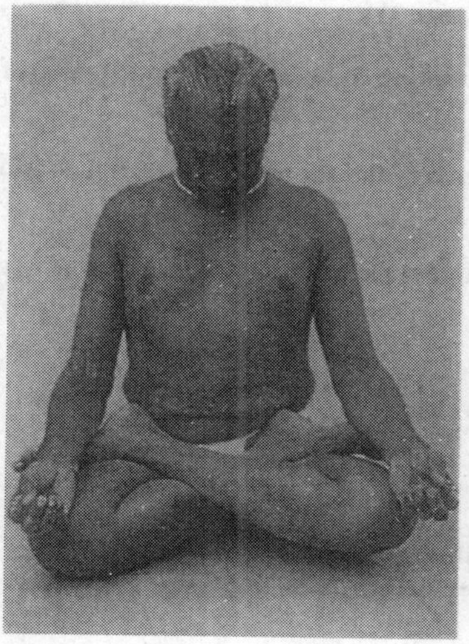

Pl.96

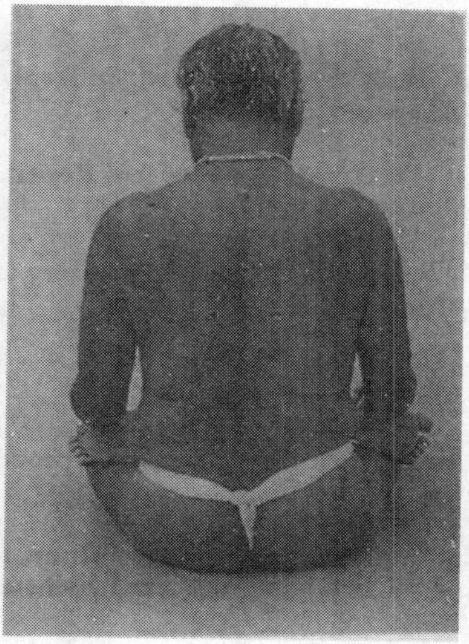

Pl.97

2. Inhale normally through the nose.

3. Exhale slowly, deeply and steadily until the lungs feel empty.

4. Attend to the posture while exhaling and listen carefully to aspirate sound of the breath. Maintain its rhythm and smoothness throughout.

5. This completes one cycle. Repeat such cycles for ten minutes, inhale, then rest in śavāsana (Pl. 182).

The emphasis here is on slow, deep and steady exhalations.

STAGE VII

The breathing here is similar to that in Stage II, but performed while sitting. It trains one to lengthen the duration of each in-breath and to learn the art of inhalation.

Technique

1. Sit in any comfortable position, following the techniques given in Paras 1 to 7 of Stage V and exhale (Pl. 96).

2. Take a slow, deep in-breath carefully through the nose, following the techniques given in Paras 3 to 7 of Stage III.

3. Breathe out slowly but not deeply, making the exhalation slightly longer than normal.

4. This completes one cycle. Repeat such cycles for ten minutes, inhale and then rest in śavāsana (Pl. 182).

Stages V to VII are preparatory to ujjāyī prāṇāyāma practices, done in a sitting position.

STAGE VIII

Now begin ujjāyī prāṇāyāma proper, with deep in and out breaths.

Technique

1. Sit in any comfortable position, following the techniques given in Paras 1 to 7 of Stage V and exhale whatever breath is in the lungs (Pl. 96).

2. Take a slow, deep, steady in-breath through the nose.

3. Listen to the sibilant sound of the breath. Control, adjust and synchronise its flow, tone and rhythm. The flow is controlled by the resonance of the sound, and the tone by the flow. This is the key to success in prāṇāyāma.

4. Fill the lungs from the bottom to the top, right up to the collar-bones. Consciously try to channel the breath to the remotest parts of the lungs (Pls: front view, 98; back view, 99; side view, 100).

5. Be continuously aware of the inflow of breath.

6. As you breathe in, your body, lungs, brain and consciousness should be receptive rather than active. Breath is received as a divine gift and should not be drawn in forcefully.

7. Do not inflate the abdomen as you inhale. Keep the diaphragm below the ribs throughout. Observe this in all types of prāṇāyāma. If the diaphragm is lifted above the floating ribs, the abdomen gets inflated instead of the chest.

8. The movements described in Paras 4, 6, and 7 above are made by drawing the entire abdominal area from the pubis to the breastbone

Pl.98

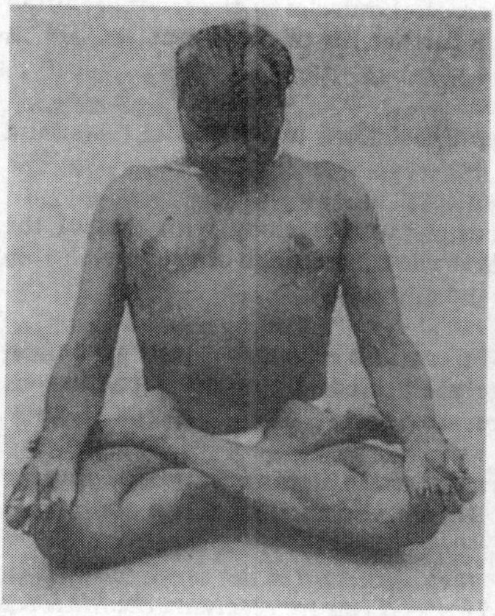

Pl.99

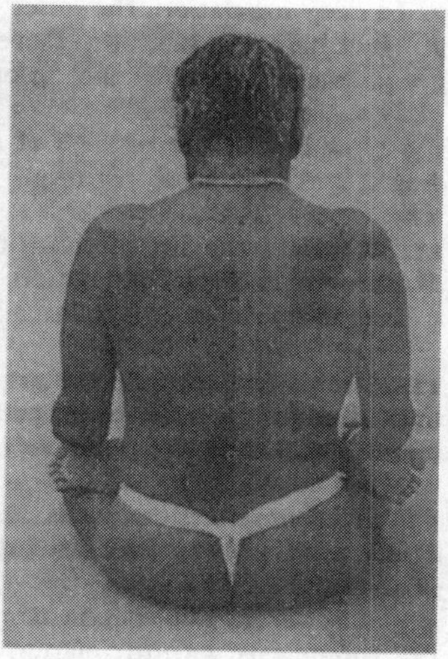

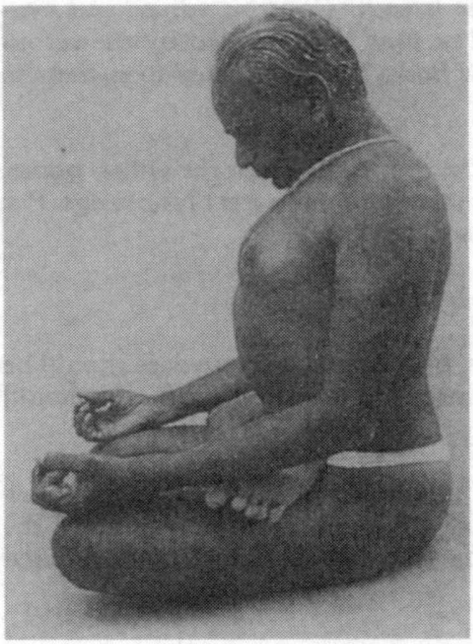

Pl. 100

towards the spine, and then up towards the head. This automatically massages the internal organs.

9. In deep inhalation, the inner intercostal muscles at the front are lifted up. Just before exhalation, there is a further lift of these muscles, which prepares one before breathing out.

10. Now begins the process of deep exhalation, in which the trunk and diaphragm play an active role.

11. Maintain the lift of the intercostal muscles along with that of the diaphragm, and start exhalation. Allow the breath to go out slowly, deeply and steadily.

12. After a few seconds the grip of the trunk relaxes by itself gradually, until the lungs have been passively emptied. Maintain a continuous awareness during the out-flow of breath.

13. This completes one cycle. Repeat for ten to fifteen minutes keeping the eyes closed and the limbs relaxed. Inhale and then lie down and rest in śavāsana (Pl. 182).

14. Inhale with warmth, elation and joy as if you are receiving the life force

as a gift from God. Exhale with a sense of gratitude, silently expressing your humbleness as a surrender to the Lord.

15. At each inhalation and exhalation there is a fractional pause when the muscles of the torso adjust themselves. Learn to be aware of this.

Effects

This prāṇāyāma aerates the lungs, soothes and tones the nervous system. As a result of the deep respiratory action, the blood carries the supply of life-giving energy to the minutest parts of the tissues. It reduces phlegm, relieves pain in the chest, and the voice becomes melodious.

STAGE IX

This is a stage for beginners, introducing retention of the breath when the lungs are full. It is a deliberate internal retention (sahita antara kumbhaka).

Technique

1. Sit in any comfortable position following the techniques given in Paras 1 to 7 of Stage V, and exhale (Pl. 96).

2. Breathe in and hold the breath. Keep the trunk firm and alert. (Pls: front view, 101; back view, 102; side view, 103).

3. Do not raise the bridge of the nose or the eyes or the head throughout retention (Pl. 78).

4. Feel the breath percolating to the remotest pores of the skin of the torso and become aware of the process.

5. After a few seconds, this awareness begins to lose its grip. The moment this happens, exhale normally. This is one cycle, so practise ten to fifteen of them.

6. If any fatigue is felt during this practice, these cycles may be alternated with normal breathing.

7. When this practice becomes easy, intensify it until you can comfortably hold the breath for ten to fifteen seconds at a time. To increase the length of retention, lift the diaphragm towards the lungs, hold it firmly, and draw the abdomen in and up towards the spine. Then hold the breath without raising the bridge of the nose (Pl. 78).

8. If hardness is felt in the lungs, or tension in and around the temples or in the head, it is a sign that you are exceeding your capacity; if so, reduce the

length of the internal retention. The transition from internal retention to exhalation should be smooth.

9. Breathe out slowly, without losing control of the trunk, diaphragm, and lungs. After completing the practice take a few deep breaths and then rest in śavāsana (Pl. 182).

Note
Internal retention may also be done while lying down, keeping pillows below the head to simulate jālandhara bandha (Pl. 77).

Effects
The practice of sahita antara kumbhaka develops harmony between the breath and the lungs, and between the nerves and the mind. If correctly performed, it induces a dynamic state in which the body feels filled to the brim with energy. It increases one's capacity for work, removes despair and creates hope. Through the creation of energy, it invigorates the nervous system and develops endurance. It is ideal for those who suffer from low blood pressure, languor, laziness and doubt.

However, antara kumbhaka is not advisable for those suffering from high blood pressure, hyper-tension and cardiac disorders.

STAGE X

This is a stage for beginners, introducing retention of the breath when the lungs are empty. It is called deliberate external retention (sahita bāhya kumbhaka).

Technique
1. Sit in any comfortable position, following the techniques described in Paras 1 to 7 of Stage V, and exhale whatever breath is in the lungs (Pl. 96).

2. Breathe in normally and out steadily and slowly, emptying the lungs as far as possible without straining.

3. Remain passive and hold the breath as long as possible (Pl. 96), then inhale normally. This is one cycle. Repeat ten to twelve of them or continue for ten minutes.

4. Constriction in the abdomen, pressure at the temples or gasping for air indicate that you have reached your capacity in external retention (bāhya kumbhaka); in which case reduce the length of the retention. The transition to inhalation should be smooth. If any fatigue is felt during this practice, cycles of this stage may be alternated with normal breathing.

5. Take a few deep breaths and lie down in śavāsana (Pl. 182).

Note
External retention may also be done while lying down, keeping pillows under the head (Pl. 77).

Effects
Bāhya kumbhaka is especially good for people who are overtense or suffering from high blood pressure, as it relieves nervous tension. It brings about a passive state, a feeling of quietness, as if one were an empty vessel floating on water. However, it is not advisable for those suffering from depression, malancholia and low blood pressure.

STAGE XI

This is internal retention (antara kumbhaka) for advanced students.

Technique
1. Sit in any comfortable position, following the techniques described in Paras 1 to 7 of Stage V, and exhale (Pl. 96).

2. Take a strong, deep breath without any force, jerk or harshness, keeping the trunk alert.

Pl. 101

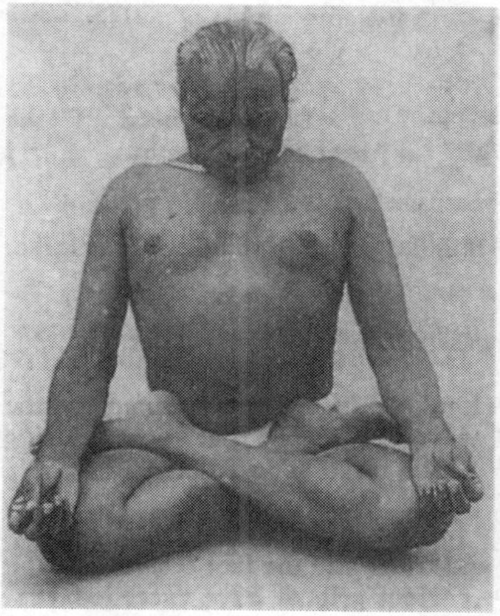

Pl. 102

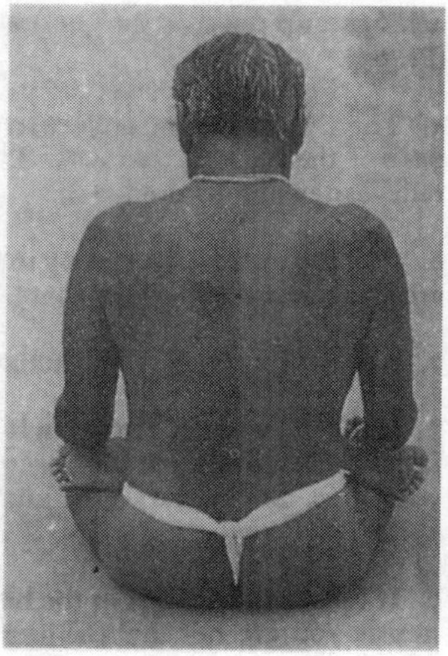

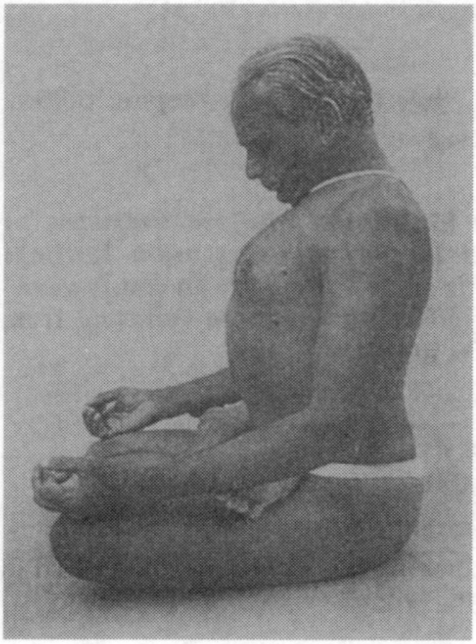

Pl. 103

3. Hold the breath for ten to fifteen seconds (Pls 101 and 103)

4. In a few moments the body loses its grip. To maintain this grip, raise the side ribs. Now contract the lower trunk from the pubis, perineum and anus and lift it up towards the chest along with the spine. This is mūla bandha (Pl. 69).

5. This lift of the torso creates tension in the head. Lower the head from the base of the back of the neck. This gives a better jālandhara bandha and relieves tension in the head.

6. Feel the breath percolating to the remotest pores of the skin of the torso, arousing awareness everywhere.

7. Keep the eyes, ears and tongue passive, and the brain quiet.

8. If the duration of retention is too long, the throat feels strained and the facial muscles and temples become taut. This means that you are losing your grip. So, recharge the energy of the torso as instructed in Para. 4 above.

9. If tension is still felt in the head and trunk and the face feels flushed, it means you are not maintaining the correct grip or have exceeded your

capacity. This may lead to injury to the nervous system. In which case, do not continue the retention.

10. Breathe out normally or deeply without losing grip on the trunk, diaphragm and the lungs.

11. This is one cycle of retention. Practise ten to twelve such cycles, maintaining the same awareness throughout as in the first cycle. Since the capacity for retention varies with individuals, it is not possible to mention the duration of breath retention. It is advisable to do internal retention after an interval of three or four breaths.

12. After completing the practice, inhale and lie in śavāsana (Pl. 182).

In this stage the emphasis is on retention of breath rather than on in and out breath.

Effects
This stage is good for persons suffering from dullness, nausea, and physical fatigue. It keeps the body warm, removes phlegm, and creates exhilaration and confidence. It leads to better concentration. Faulty practice causes irritation, throbbing, short temper and exhaustion.

STAGE XII

This is external retention (bāhya kumbhaka) for advanced students.

Technique
1. Sit in any comfortable position, following the techniques given in Paras 1 to 7 of Stage V, and exhale (Pl. 96).

2. Breathe in normally, and out steadily and strongly. Empty the lungs as far as you can without force, jerk or harshness.

3. When exhalation is complete do not inhale, but pause and draw in the entire abdominal area back towards the spine and up towards the chest. This is uḍḍīyāna bandha (Pl. 104).

4. Retain this grip as long as you can. When tension is felt, relax the abdomen, bring it to normal and then breathe in.

5. This is one cycle. Repeat eight to ten such cycles, then inhale and lie in śavāsana (Pl. 182).

6. As the practice improves, increase the duration of retention after

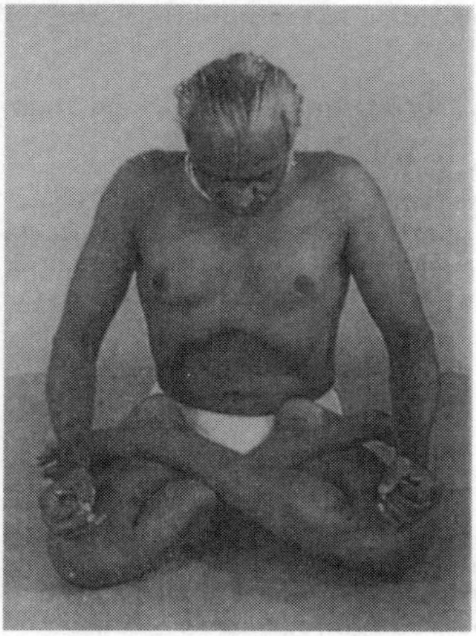

Pl. 104

exhalation. The duration varies with each individual. Watch your own capacity to increase it.

7. Never breathe in during uḍḍīyāna bandha, as this may make you gasp and strain the heart.

8. At the beginning it is advisable to do external retention after an interval of three or four deep breaths.

Effects
This stage cleanses the abdominal organs and prevents their prolapse.

STAGE XIII

This advanced stage combines both internal (antara) and external (bāhya) retentions (kumbhakas) with two or three in and out breaths.

Technique
1. Here, first exhale (Pl. 96).

2. Breathe in deeply. After full inhalation, retain the breath (antara kumbhaka) for ten seconds (Pl. 101).

3. Breathe out deeply. After full exhalation, hold the breath (bāhya kumbhaka) with uḍḍīyāna bandha for five seconds (Pl. 104) and inhale deeply. This completes one cycle.

4. Exhale, and take two or three deep in and out breaths. Then repeat the cycles of kumbhakas, followed again by two or three deep in and out breaths.

5. Do five to six cycles, ending with inhalation. Then lie down in śavāsana (Pl. 182).

Table of Ujjāyī Prāṇāyāma

Stage	*Pūraka*		*Antara Kumbhaka*		*Rechaka*		*Bāhya Kumbhaka*	
	N	*D*	*No MB*	*MB*	*N*	*D*	*No UB*	*UB*
Lying:								
I	✓				✓			
II	✓					✓		
III		✓			✓			
IV		✓				✓		
Sitting:								
V	✓				✓			
VI	✓					✓		
VII		✓			✓			
VIII		✓				✓		
IX	✓		AFS		✓			
X	✓					✓	ALAP	
XI		SD		10–15 sec	N or D			
XII	✓					SD		ALAP
XIII		SD		10–15 sec	N or D			ALAP

AFS = A few seconds
ALAP = As long as possible
D = Deep
MB = Mula bandha
N = Normal
UB = Uḍḍiyāna bandha
SD = Strong deep

Chapter 20

Viloma Prāṇāyāma

Loma means hair, the 'vi' denotes disjunction or negation. Viloma means anti-hair or against the natural order of things.

In viloma prāṇāyāma inhalation or exhalation is not a continuous process, but one that is interrupted by several pauses. For instance, if one complete inhalation were to take fifteen seconds, then in viloma it would be interrupted every two or three seconds, thus bringing the length of the in-breath to twenty-five or thirty seconds. Similarly, with interrupted exhalation the out-breath is lengthened from twenty-five to thirty seconds. This prāṇāyāma may be compared to climbing up or down a tall ladder, with a pause at each step. See that there is no unconscious out or in breath during the pauses of interrupted inhalation or exhalation. The techniques given below are in nine stages.

STAGE I

This stage is an introduction to interrupted in-breathing (pūraka) in a lying position. It is suitable for beginners and invalids, or when suffering from fatigue, weakness, strain or low blood pressure.

Technique

1. Lie quietly for a few minutes as in ujjāyī Stage I, preferably using planks or cushions as explained at the beginning of Ch. 19.

2. Follow the techniques given in Paras 2, 3 and 4 of ujjāyī, Stage II, and exhale whatever breath is in the lungs (Pl. 91).

3. Now start with interrupted inhalation, as follows. Inhale for two or three seconds, pause, and hold the breath for two or three seconds and do this again. To pause, the diaphragm is lightly immobilised. When you breathe in again, do not let the diaphragm loose after each pause. Continue in this way until the lungs are completely full, which may involve four or five pauses. No strain should be felt throughout the practice.

4. Now exhale slowly and deeply, as in ujjāyī, Stage II, gradually releasing the grip of the diaphragm.

5. This completes one cycle of viloma, Stage I. Repeat them for seven to ten minutes, or for as long as you do not feel fatigue; breathe normally two or three times, then rest in śavāsana (Pl. 182).

STAGE II

This is an introduction to interrupted out-breath (rechaka) when lying down. It is suitable for beginners, weak persons and invalids, or when suffering from fatigue, strain, high blood pressure or a heart complaint.

Technique

1. Lie quietly for a few minutes as in ujjāyī Stage I, then follow the techniques given in Paras 2, 3 and 4 of ujjāyī Stage II. Exhale whatever breath is in the lungs (Pl. 91).

2. Take a long deep breath without any pause, as in ujjāyī, filling the lungs completely, but do not over-strain.

3. Exhale for two or three seconds, pause, hold the breath for two or three seconds and repeat. Continue in this way until the lungs feel completely emptied, which may involve four or five pauses. Gradually release the grip on the abdomen.

4. This completes one cycle of viloma Stage II. Repeat them for seven to ten minutes or for as long as fatigue is not felt. Inhale, then do śavāsana (Pl. 182).

Effects

This practice brings a feeling of ease and lightness to the body.

STAGE III

This stage is a combination of Stages I and II, in a lying down position.

Technique

1. Lie quietly for a few minutes as in ujjāyī Stage I, then follow the techniques given in Paras 2, 3 and 4 of ujjāyī Stage II, and exhale (Pl. 91).

2. Now start interrupted inhalation as described in Para. 3 of Stage I above.

3. Hold the breath for a second or two.

4. Now start interrupted exhalation, following the techniques given in Para. 3 of Stage II above, gradually releasing the grip on the diaphragm.

5. This completes one cycle of viloma, Stage III. Repeat them for eight to twelve minutes or for as long as no strain is felt. Inhale, then rest in śavāsana (Pl. 182).

STAGE IV

This stage is an introduction to interrupted in-breathing (pūraka) in a sitting position. It is suitable for beginners.

Technique

1. Sit in any comfortable position, following the techniques given in Paras 1 to 7 of ujjāyī, Stage V. Exhale without strain. (Pl. 96).

2. Now start interrupted inhalation, as follows: Inhale for two or three seconds, pause and hold the breath for two or three seconds; again inhale for two or three seconds, pause and hold the breath for two or three seconds. To pause, the diaphragm is lightly gripped. Do not let the diaphragm loose when you breathe in again after each pause. Continue in this way until the lungs are completely full, which may involve four or five pauses. No strain should be felt throughout.

3. Gently draw the abdominal organs towards the spine and up. Then exhale slowly and deeply, as in ujjāyī, Stage VI, gradually releasing the grip on the abdomen.

4. This completes one cycle of viloma, Stage IV. Repeat such cycles for seven to ten minutes, or for as long as you do not feel fatigue. Breathe normally two or three times, then rest in śavāsana (Pl. 182).

Effects

The effects are similar to those of Stage I.

STAGE V

This stage is an introduction to interrupted out-breaths (rechaka) in a sitting position. It is suitable for beginners of normal health.

Technique

1. Sit in any comfortable position, following the techniques given in Paras 1 to 7 of ujjāyī, Stage V. Exhale without strain (Pl. 96).

2. Take a long, deep breath at one stretch, without any pauses. Fill the lungs to the brim.

3. Now start interrupted exhalation as in Stage II but immobilising the diaphragm, as follows: Exhale for two seconds, pause, grip the diaphragm and hold the breath for two or three seconds and repeat. Continue in this way until the lungs feel completely emptied, which may take four or five pauses. Allow the grip on the diaphragm to release gradually.

4. This completes one cycle of viloma Stage V. Repeat them for eight to ten minutes or for as long as no strain is felt. Take two or three normal breaths, then lie in śavāsana (Pl. 182).

Effects
This practice brings a feeling of exhilaration and calmness.

STAGE VI

This stage is a combination of Stages IV and V, done when sitting.

Technique
1. Sit in any comfortable position, following the techniques given in Paras 1 to 7 of ujjāyī, Stage V. Exhale without straining (Pl. 96).

2. Now start interrupted inhalation, following the technique of Para. 2 of Stage IV above.

3. Hold the breath for two or three seconds. Grip the abdomen, then start interrupted exhalation, following the technique of Para. 3 of Stage V above.

4. This completes one cycle of viloma, Stage VI. Repeat for ten to fifteen minutes or for as long as no strain is felt. Take two or three breaths, then lie in śavāsana (Pl. 182).

Effects
This develops endurance and a sense of exhilaration.

STAGE VII

Here internal retention (antara kumbhaka) is introduced, following an interrupted in-breath. It is for intermediate and more intensive students who have acquired some strength and stability in their practice.

Technique
1. Sit in any comfortable position, following the techniques given in Paras 1 to 7 of ujjāyī, Stage V. Exhale deeply, without straining (Pl. 96).

2. Start interrupted inhalation, as described in Para. 2 of Stage IV above.

3. Now hold the breath for ten to fifteen seconds. This is internal retention (antara kumbhaka) (Pl. 101). Grip the diaphragm, then exhale slowly and deeply, gradually relaxing the hold of the diaphragm.

4. This completes one cycle of viloma, Stage VII. Repeat them for fifteen to twenty minutes or longer, as long as no fatigue or strain is felt. Take two or three breaths, then lie in śavāsana (Pl. 182).

Effects
This stage helps those suffering from low blood pressure. The lungs cells are aerated, elasticity is created in the lungs, and the art of deep breathing is learnt with precision, ease and comfort.

STAGE VIII

Here external retention (bāhya kumbhaka) is introduced, followed by an interrupted out-breath. It is for students who have acquired strength and stability in their practice.

Technique
1. Sit for some time, following the techniques given in Paras 1 to 7 of ujjāyī, Stage V. Slowly exhale until the lungs feel empty, without straining (Pl. 96).

2. Take a long deep breath without any pause. Fill the lungs completely, but do not over strain.

3. Hold the breath for two to three seconds.

4. Now do interrupted exhalation, as described in Para. 3 of Stage V above.

5. Hold the breath for five or six seconds before inhaling.

6. This completes one cycle of viloma, Stage VIII. Repeat for fifteen to twenty minutes, or for as long as you do not feel fatigue. Take two or three normal breaths, then lie in śavāsana (Pl. 182).

Effects
This rests the nerves and soothes the brain.

STAGE IX

This stage combines Stages VII and VIII, including (a) interrupted in and out breaths, (b) internal and external retentions, and (c) the bandhās. It is only for advanced students who have practiced Yoga for many years.

Technique
1. Sit in any comfortable position, following the techniques given in Paras

1 to 7 of ujjāyī, Stage V. Exhale until the lungs feel empty, without straining (Pl. 96).

2. Start interrupted inhalation as described in Para. 2 of Stage IV.

3. Then hold the breath with mūla bandha for ten to fifteen seconds or for as long as you can (Pl. 101).

4. Now start interrupted exhalation as described in Para. 3 of Stage V.

5. When the lungs feel empty, hold the breath for five or six seconds. Perform uḍḍīyāna bandha as described in Para. 3 of Stage XII of ujjāyī, but take care not to overstrain (Pl. 104).

6. This completes one cycle of viloma, Stage IX. Repeat them for fifteen to twenty minutes or for as long as you do not feel fatigue. Take two or three normal breaths, then lie in śavāsana (Pl. 182).

Effects
This stage combines the effects of Stages VII and VIII.

Table of Viloma Prāṇāyāma

Stage	*Pūraka*		*Antara Kumbhaka*		*Rechaka*		*Bāhya Kumbhaka*	
	No P	*P*	*No MB*	*MB*	*No P*	*P*	*No UB*	*UB*
Lying:								
I		√			√			
II	√					√		
III		√				√		
Sitting:								
IV		√			√			
V	√					√		
VI		√				√		
VII		√	10–15 sec		√			
VIII	√					√	5–6 sec	
IX		√		10 sec		√		5–6 sec

MB = Mūla bandha
P = Pauses
UB = Uḍḍīyāna bandha

Chapter 21

Bhrāmarī, Mūrchhā and Plāvinī Prāṇāyāma

BHRĀMARĪ PRĀṆĀYĀMA

Bhramara means a large black bumble-bee and this prāṇāyāma is so called because during exhalation a soft humming sound like that of a bumble-bee is made. The best time to perform it is in the silence and quiet of the night. Bhrāmarī prāṇāyāma may be done in two stages, one lying, one sitting.

Technique

Here deep inhalations are done as in Ujjāyī Prāṇāyāma and deep exhalations with a humming or murmuring sound. However, it is not advisable to hold the breath (kumbhakas) in this prāṇāyāma. Bhrāmarī may also be done while performing ṣaṇmukhī mudrā without jālandhara bandha, as there is no retention of breath here.

ṢAṆMUKHĪ MUDRĀ (Pls 105 and 106)

Raise the hands to the face and the elbows to the level of the shoulders. Place the thumb-tips in the ear-holes to keep out external sounds. If the thumb-tips cause pain, reduce the pressure or push the tragi (the small protuberances at the entrance of the ears) over the ear-holes and press them in.

Pl. 105

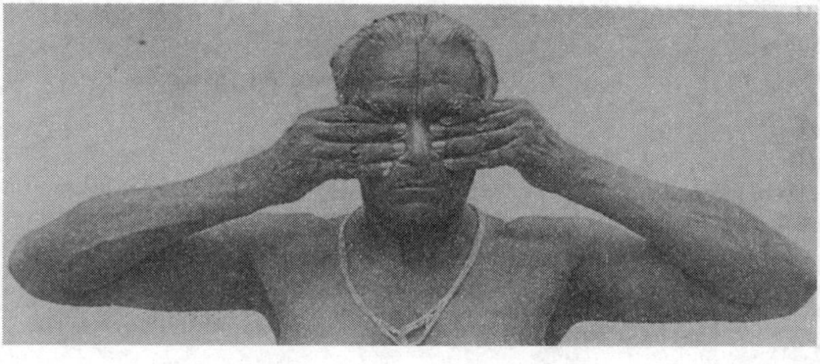

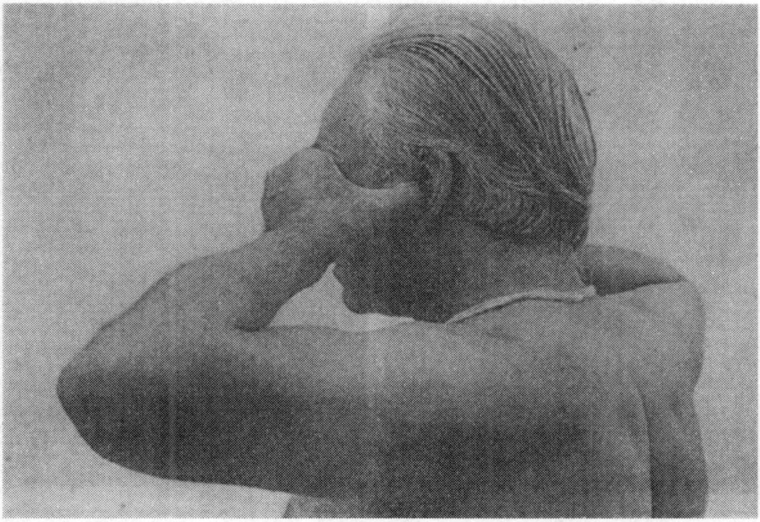

Pl. 106

Close the eyes. Bring the fore and middle fingers over the eyelids. Draw the upper lids down with the pads of the middle finger-tips and cover the remaining space above it with the pads of the forefinger tips to keep out the light. Keep the eye-balls passive and receptive and press them gently with the fingers.

Now press the nostrils with the ring finger-tips to narrow the nasal passages for slow, steady, rhythmic and subtle breathing. Keep the little fingers on the upper lips to feel the flow of breath.

The sādhaka can hear the inner sound as the ears are closed by the thumbs. Through pressure on the eye-balls, he also sees various colours of dazzling light, sometimes steady like that of the sun. If it is difficult to hold ṣaṇmukhī mudrā, then wrap a cloth round the head and over the ears and temples (Pl. 107).

After completing practice of bhrāmarī prāṇāyāma, inhale, then do śavāsana (Pl. 182).

Note

Kumbhakas can be attempted, wrapping a cloth round the head with jālandhara bandha in all the other Prāṇāyāmas (Pl. 108).

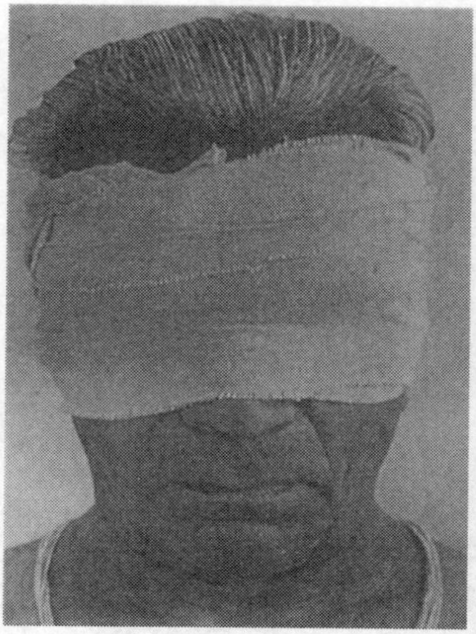

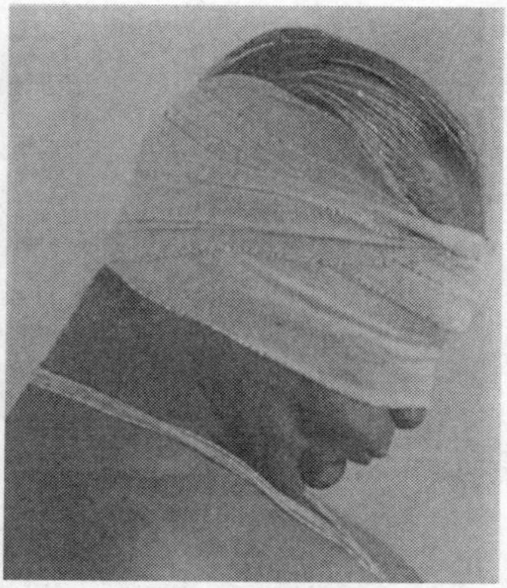

Pl. 108

Pl. 107

Effects

The humming sound induces sleep and is good for persons suffering from insomnia.

MŪRCHHĀ PRĀṆĀYĀMA

Mūrchhā means a state of swoon. This prāṇāyāma is done as in ujjāyī and the internal retention is held till faintness is felt. It makes the mind inactive and brings sensual tranquillity.

PLĀVINĪ PRĀṆĀYĀMA

Plāva means swimming or floating. Very little is known of this prāṇāyāma. It is said to help the sādhaka to float on water with ease.

Mūrchhā and plāvinī prāṇāyāma are no longer in vogue.

Table of Bhrāmarī Prāṇāyāma

Stage		*Pūraka* N	*Pūraka* D	*Rechaka* DHS	*Ṣaṇmukhī mudrā*
Lying:					
I	A	√		√	
	B	√		√	√
II	A		√	√	
	B		√	√	√
Sitting:					
III	A	√		√	
	B	√		√	√
IV	A		√	√	
	B		√	√	√

D = Deep
HS = Humming sound
N = Normal

Chapter 22

Digital Prāṇāyāma and the Art of Placing the Fingers on the Nose

THE NOSE

1. The nose is a cone-shaped chamber, supported by bone and cartilage, lined on the outside by skin and on the inside by mucous membranes, while the nostrils are supported and partitioned by the septum. The inner sides of the nostrils are irregular and connected by small holes to the sinuses in the skull.

2. Air entering the nostrils is filtered and passed down the wind-pipe to the lungs. The flow is slowed down slightly when air enters the wider passages halfway up the nose. The sides of the nasal chamber in the skull are lined by three whorled and porous bones called conchae. Shaped like the wings of a bird, they cause the air currents to spiral so that they brush the mucous membrane lining in complex and variable patterns. Pressure from the thumb and two fingers on the nose widens or narrows the nasal passages. This helps to control the shape, direction and flow of these currents. The close attention required to monitor this flow develops inner awareness. This awareness is also enhanced by learning to hear the subtle vibrations set up by the air flow. Hence the important part played by the ears in prāṇāyāma.

3. The air currents also influence the organs of smell through the ethmoid bone at the base of the skull. This bone is perforated for the filaments of the olfactory nerve which stimulates the limbic system of the brain concerned with transforming perception into feeling.

4. Inhaled air circulates over the areas of the mucous membranes (the mucosa). Unless these function efficiently, breathing is strained and irregular. They may be congested by changes of atmosphere, or their secretion affected by various factors such as tobacco, smoke, infections, emotional states and so on. The flow of air is diverted periodically from one nostril to the other due to changes in the blood circulation, as well as

through injury, disease or a cold. Such changes alter the shape and size of the nose, the nostrils and the nasal passages.

5. Muscles attached to the cartilages are accessories which dilate or compress the nostrils. Being part of the muscle system of the face connected with the lips and eye-brows they can express emotional states like anger, disgust or danger and reveal inner personality.

6. According to *Śiva Svarodaya*, a Yoga text, the five basic elements of earth (pṛthvi), water (ap), light (tejas), air (vāyu) and ether (ākaśa) are located in the nose (Pl. 109). In prāṇāyāma, the flow of vital energy (prāṇa) in the breath contacts these elements, when it passes over or through their sites and influences the behaviour of the practitioner. These sites or areas shift every few minutes or so. For instance when the current of air brushes the earth site in the right nostril, it brushes the water site in the left nostril. The pattern is:

Right nostril	Left nostril
Earth	Water
Water	Fire
Fire	Air
Air	Ether
Ether	Earth

The shift from one site to the other is gradual. Many years of practice are needed to locate and distinguish the sites or areas of the five elements or energies and when and where the air is in touch with each nostril. It may

Pl. 109

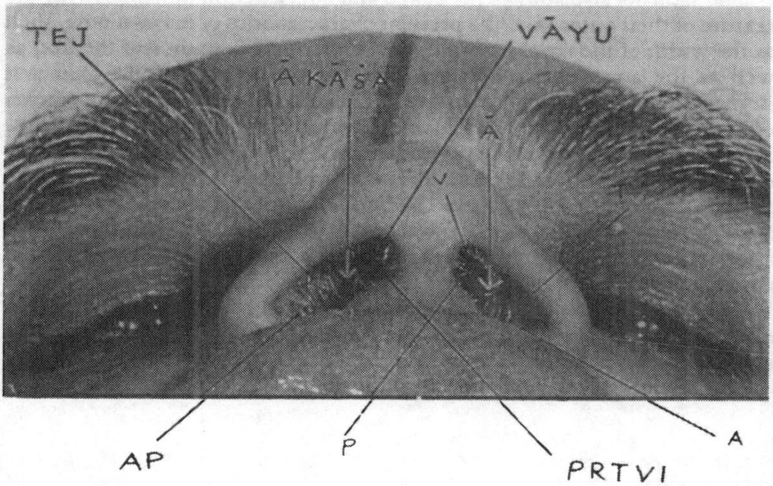

take less time to locate the above areas under an experienced teacher. Precise and sensitive adjustments with the thumb and the ring and little fingers of the right hand on the nose will make the breath flow simultaneously over the same location in both nostrils creating clarity in the brain and stability in mind. The text further explains that the best and ideal time for meditation (dhyāna) is when the breath flows in the central part of both the nostrils – the ether element.

THE ART OF FINGERING

7. The training required of a sādhaka for prāṇāyāma may be compared to that for becoming a master musician. Krṣna the divine cowherd, charmed the gopis and conquered their hearts by playing his flute, manipulating it and creating a world of mystic sounds. In his practice of prāṇāyāma, the sādhaka subdues and conquers his senses by 'playing' on his nostrils, delicately fingering them to manipulate breath patterns as if playing the flute.

There are several openings in wind instruments, but only two in the nose, so that the sādhaka requires greater dexterity than the flautist to control the infinitely fine and subtle tones and shades of his breath.

A good musician studies the construction, shape, stops, and other characteristics of his instrument, as well as the atmospheric changes that affects it. By constantly practising with his fingers, he trains their virtuosity for delicate adjustments, and his ears to listen for the minutest variation in sound and learns to co-ordinate the skill of his fingers with his ears. Only then can he begin to capture the strains – the tone, the pitch, the resonance and the cadence – of the music.

The sādhaka also studies the shape and construction of his nostrils, the texture of their outer skin, the peculiar characteristics of his own nose, such as the width of the nasal passages, deviation of the septum and the like, as well as the atmospheric changes affecting the texture of the skin and dryness or otherwise in the passages. He regularly practises the movements of his wrist and fingers till he becomes dexterous and is able to refine them. He adjusts the finger-tips over the outer nasal skin surface covering the sites of the five elements (earth, water, fire, wind and ether) in the nostrils. These five sites act as stops. He adjusts the flow, rhythm and resonance of breath by narrowing or widening the nasal passages at these locations by delicate fingering and by attentively listening to the sound of the breath which he modulates and corrects.

The door-keepers of a temple sanctum (dvārapālas) regulate the stream of devotees, the fingers regulate the volume and flow of breath, and by narrowing the passages filter out impurities during respiration.

Due to controlled inhalation through the narrowed nasal passages, the lungs have more time to absorb oxygen, whilst in controlled exhalation unused oxygen is re-absorbed and waste matter is ejected.

By narrowing the nasal passages through digital control the sādhaka develops greater sensitivity and awareness. By practising ujjāyī and viloma Prāṇāyāmas, the sādhaka's knowledge of prāṇāyāma deepens while his body derives practical knowledge through what it has experienced.

In the practice of prāṇāyāma by digital control the sādhaka unites his theoretical with practical knowledge. This co-ordination kindles his knowledge until it bursts into the flame of intelligence, which is full of resolution and energy (vyavasāyātmika buddhi).

8. Prāṇāyāma may be broadly divided into two categories:

(a) When there is no digital control over the nostrils.
(b) When the thumb and two fingers of the right hand are used to regulate and control the flow of breath through the nose. This is called digitally controlled prāṇāyāma. Moreover, this prāṇāyāma is of two types:
   (i) Inhalation and exhalation are practised on both sides of the nostrils, partially closing them to learn to use pressure and balance on the thumb and fingers for an even flow of breath from both nostrils (Pl. 110).
   (ii) Wherein one nostril is kept blocked with the finger tips, while the breath is made to flow from the thumb side and vice versa. For example, if the breath is drawn from the right side, the ring and little fingers should be made to close the left nostril without

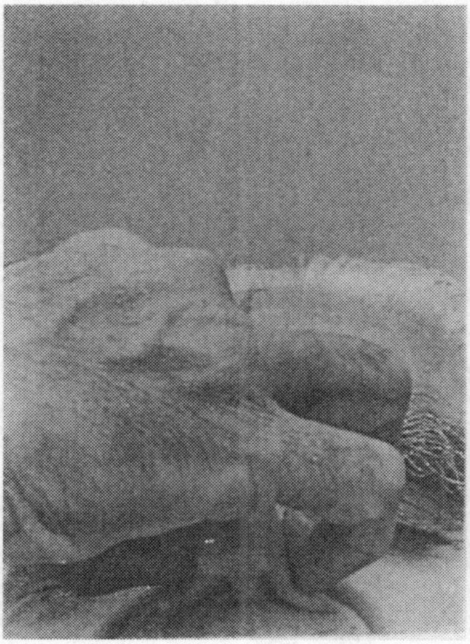

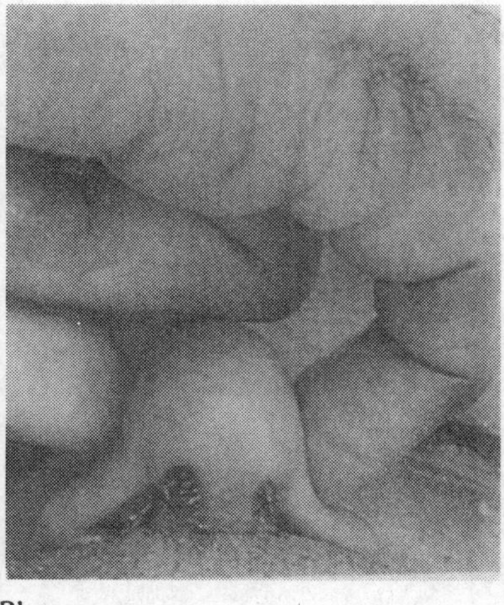

Pl. 111

Pl. 110

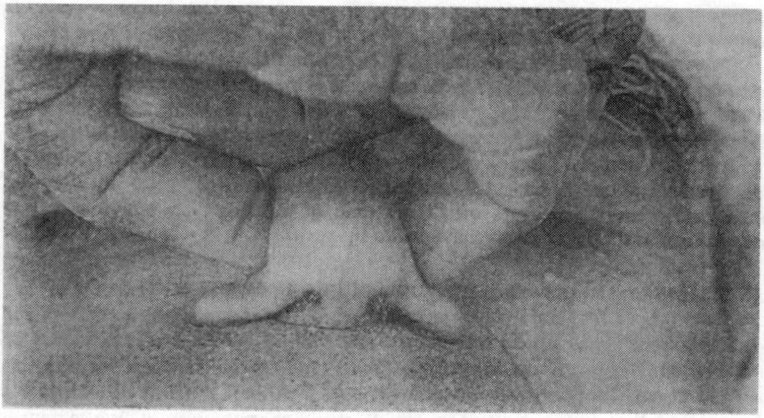

Pl. 112

disturbing the position of the septum (Pl. 111) and vice versa (Pl. 112). Care is taken that the breath should not flow in the blocked nostril.

In the first category (a) only the physical body is involved. The second (b) is a more advanced Prāṇāyāma in which the passage of air is regulated manually with skill and subtlety and delicate control of the fingers.

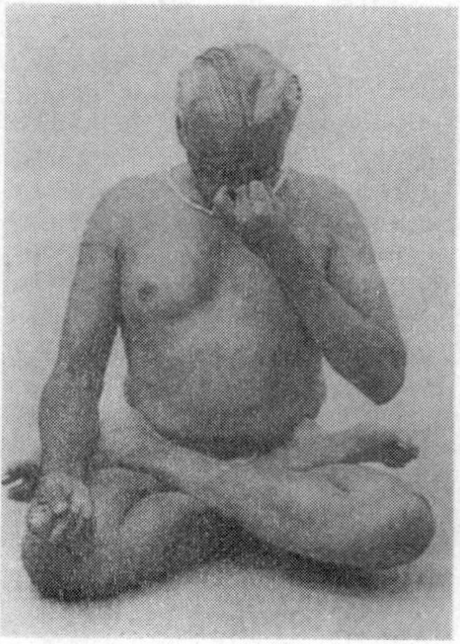

Pl. 113

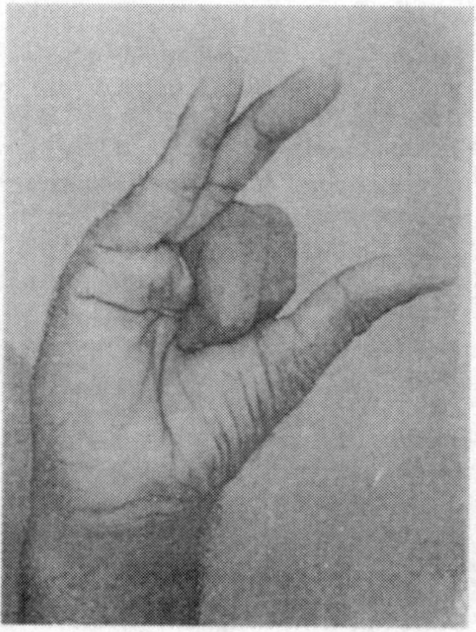

Pl. 114

Pl. 115

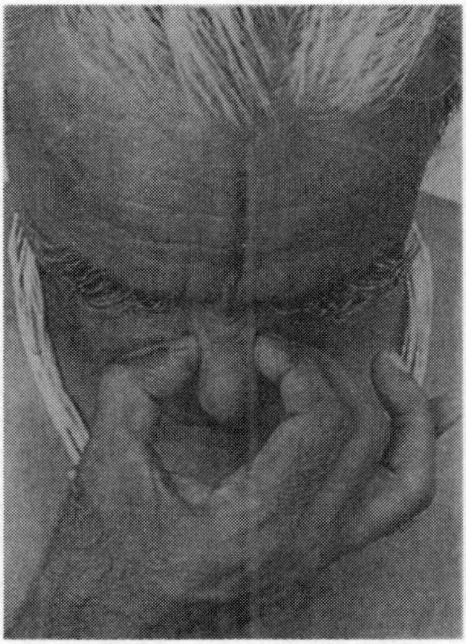

Pl. 116

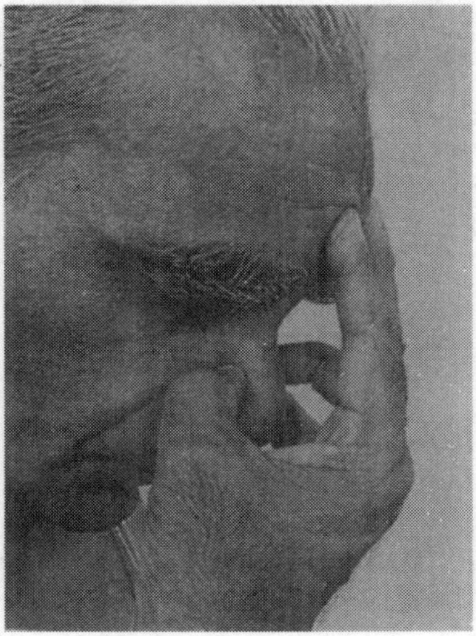

9. In ancient India, as in most of the older civilisations, the auspicious and ritual ceremonials were performed with the right hand. All left-handed actions and ceremonials were regarded as being sinister. Hence the left hand may only be used in prāṇāyāma if the right hand or arm is out of action (Pl. 113).

10. Yoga texts like *Gheraṇḍa saṁhitā* recommend the use of the thumb, ring and little fingers of the right hand on the nose without defining their correct placement (Pl. 114). They stress that the fore and middle fingers are not to be used. If the fore and middle fingers were used, the forearm and wrist would tilt and become heavy (Pl. 115). Moreover, correct and accurate pressure could not be applied to the nostrils since the nose would pull the fingers down and accuracy in the performance of prāṇāyāma would be lost. Similarly keeping the fore and middle fingers on the centre of the forehead (Pl. 116) or extended outwards (Pl. 117) would create varying pressures on the thumb, ring and little fingers, which in turn would create uneven curvature of the digits and irregular flow of breath.

11. If the fore and middle fingers are folded into the hollow of the palm, the thumb rests on the right side of the nose (Pl. 118) and the ring and little fingers on the left (Pl. 119), while the wrist is placed centrally (Pl. 120). This enables the thumb, ring and little fingers to move on either side smoothly and freely, while the palm is balanced evenly there as well. The

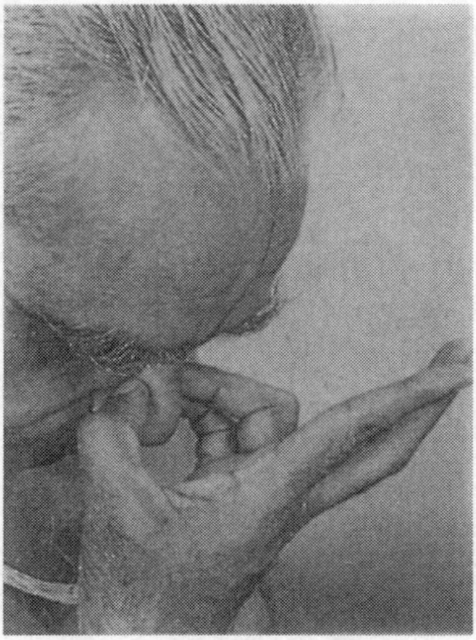

Pl. 117

Pl. 118

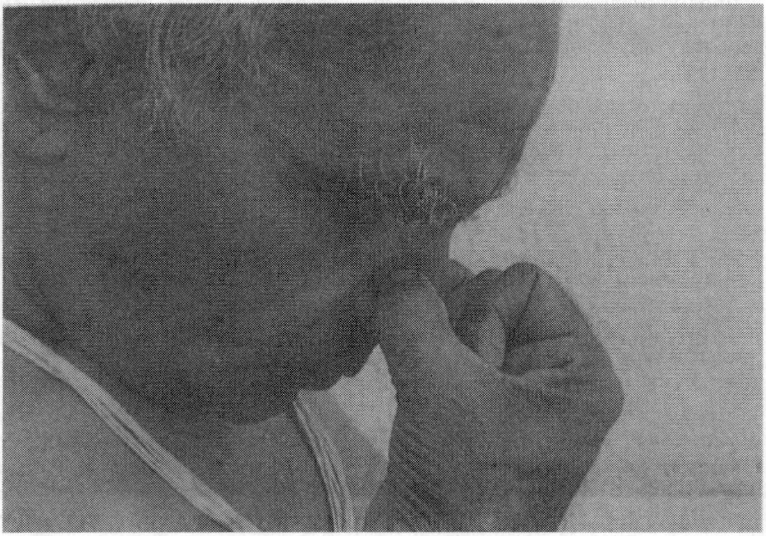

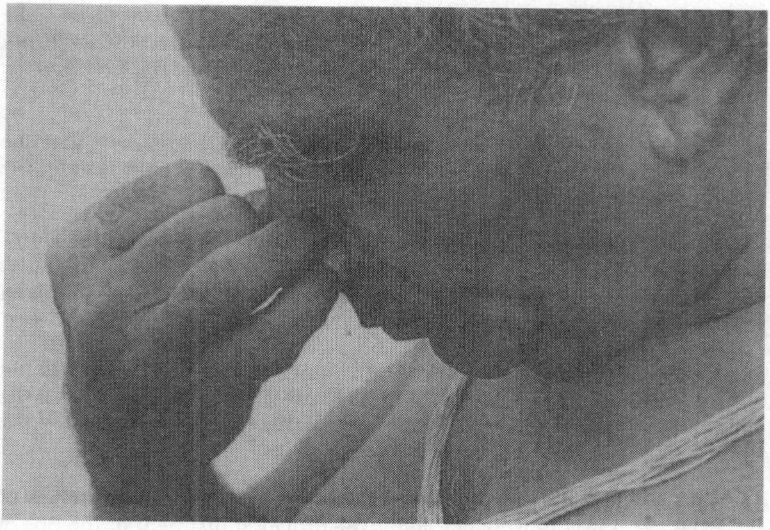

Pl. 119

Pl. 120

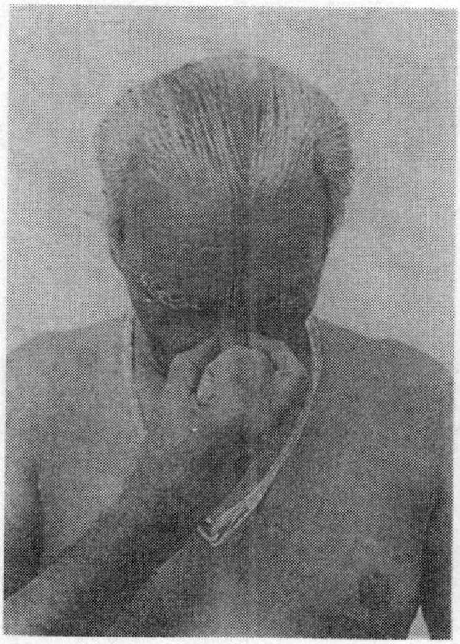

Pl. 121

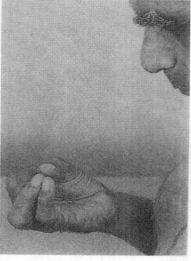

nerves and muscles of the middle portion of the right forearm make it the crucial place for the digital control of the breath through the nostrils. From here the middle portion of the right forearm, movements of the wrist and the fingers are regulated.

12. When seated to practise digital or manual prāṇāyāma, see that the shoulders are level and parallel to the floor and that the chin rests in the notch between the collar-bones (Pl. 57).

13. Resting the left hand on the left knee, bend the right arm at the elbow without tightening the biceps, forearm or wrist (Pls 121 and 122). Stability, skill and sensitivity are required for controlling the width of the nasal passages, but not strength or tension.

14. Do not allow the flexed right hand to touch the chest (Pl. 123). Do not close the armpits. Do not allow the arms to press upon the chest. Keep the shoulders down and the arms passive and light, except for the tips of the thumb, ring and little fingers (Pl. 120).

15. Flex and fold the tips of the fore and middle fingers into the hollow of the palm (Pl. 124). This brings about the proper adjustment of the tips of the ring and little fingers against the tip of the thumb, creating space between the fingers and the thumb. This makes the palm soft.

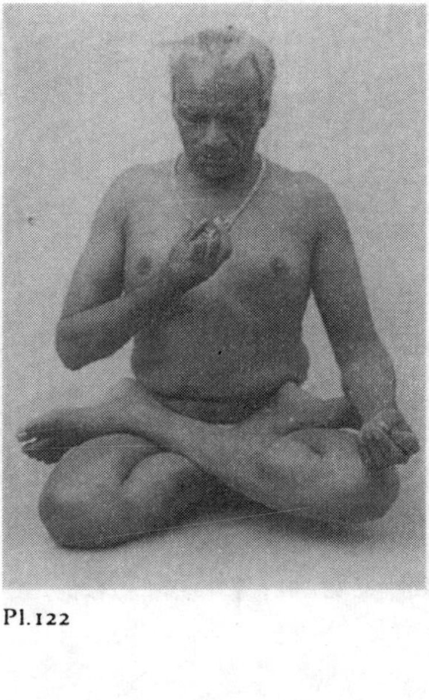

Pl. 122

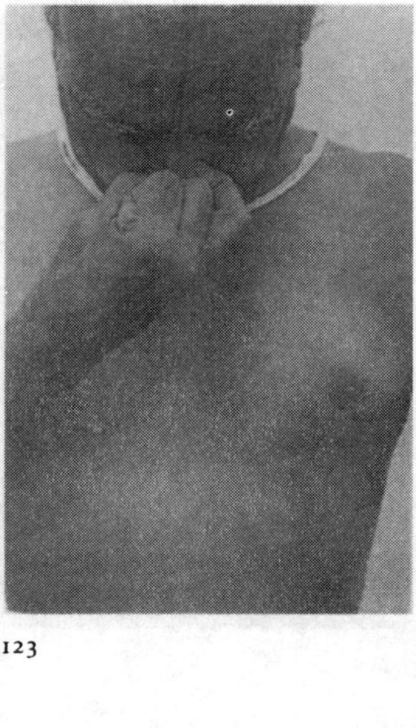

Pl. 123

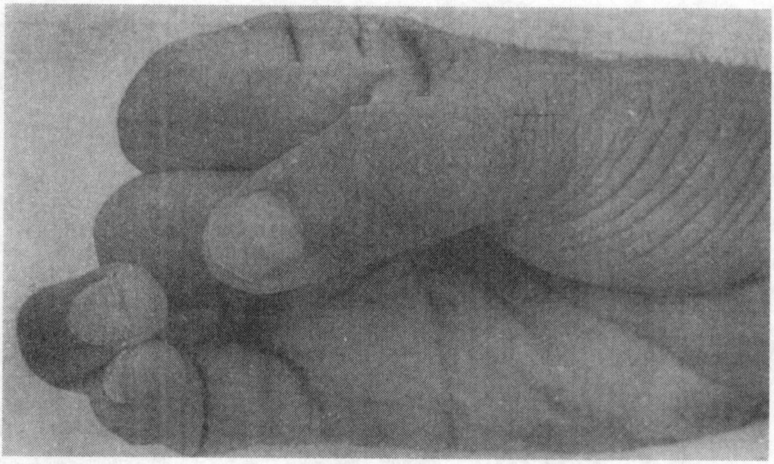

Pl. 124

Pl. 125

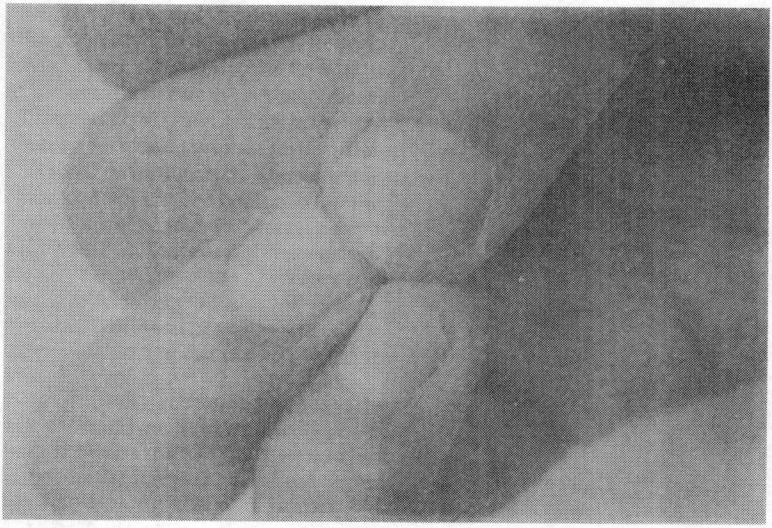

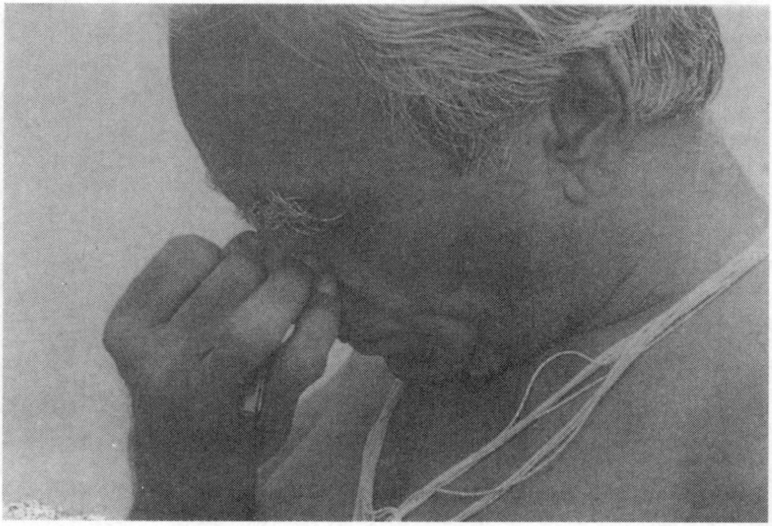

Pl. 126

Pl. 127

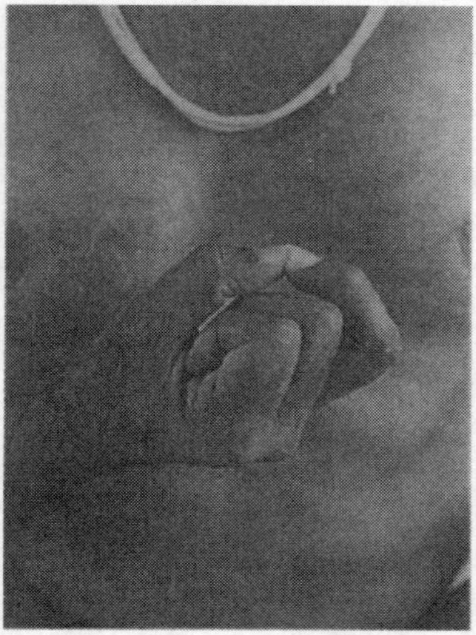

16. The individual widths of the tips of the ring and little fingers are much less than that of the thumb. To equalise them curve the fingers to meet the thumb, join their tips, keeping space between the knuckles (Pl. 125). If this is difficult, place a round object, such as a cork, about half an inch wide, between the knuckles (Pl. 126). The fingers will then become accustomed to their new position. The centre of the thumb should lie opposite the joined tips of the two fingers (Pl. 127). Normally the skin of the thumb tip is harder and thicker than that of the two finger tips. Press the thumb tip lightly against the tips of the ring and little fingers to make it soft.

17. Raise the right wrist until the tips of the thumb and the ring and little fingers are opposite the nose. Keep the front of the wrist away from the chin, and bring the tips of the thumb and of the ring and little fingers horizontally against the nostrils (Pl. 128).

18. Between the nasal bone and the cartilage there are tiny inverted V-shaped notches. The skin below the V-shaped notches of the nose is concave. The tips of the thumb and digits are convex in shape. Therefore, place the thumb and digits to rest there evenly as shown in Pl. 129. Keep the walls of the nasal passages parallel with the septum, using pressure from the top and bottom corners of the thumb and of the finger-tips throughout the practice of prāṇāyāma. Never keep the fingers on the nostrils as shown in Pl. 130, but gently rotate the tips on the root of the nose towards the nostrils to feel the passage of the breath (Pls 131 and 132). Partially close the passage of both nostrils to measure in them the even flow of breath (see Pl. 110). If the digits are not steady, the flow of breath becomes uneven, creating strain on the nervous system and heaviness in the brain cells. Fine adjustment of the digital tips is necessary to widen or narrow the nasal passages from moment to moment according to the movement of breath and also to suit individual requirements. The widening or narrowing of the nasal passages by digital control may be compared to the fine adjustment of the aperture of the iris of a camera lens for correct exposure of a colour film. If the aperture adjustment is inaccurate, the result will not show correct rendering of colours. Similarly, if the apertures of the nasal passages are not manipulated with subtlety, the results of prāṇāyāma will be distorted. The correct adjustment of nasal passages will control the flow of breath from the external, measurable area of the nostrils to the immeasurable depth within.

19. In digitally controlled Prāṇāyāma the thumb and opposing fingers of the right hand are manipulated like a pair of calipers (Pl. 127). Control is by the tips of the thumb on the right nostril and those of the ring and little fingers on the left nostril. These three digits are those used for the practice of prāṇāyāma for the best results.

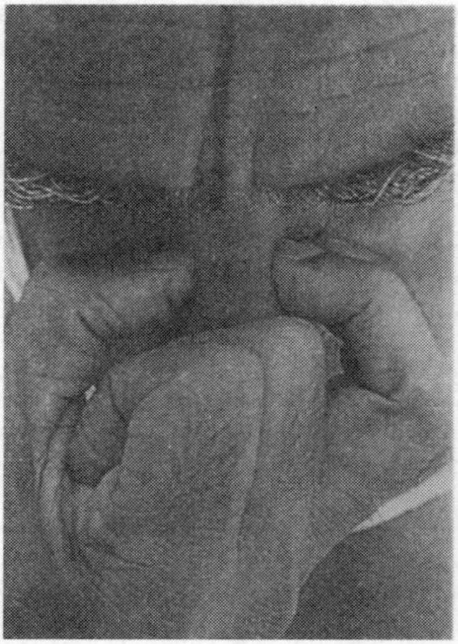

Pl. 128

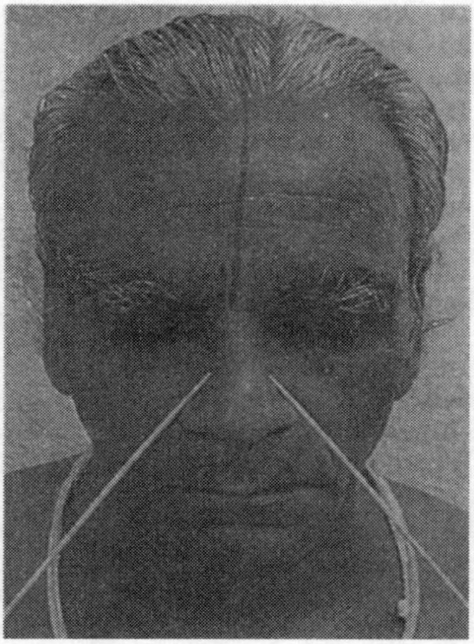

Pl. 129

Pl. 130

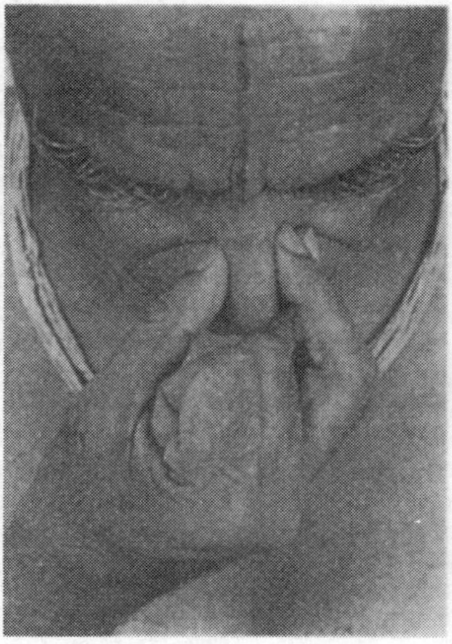

Pl. 131

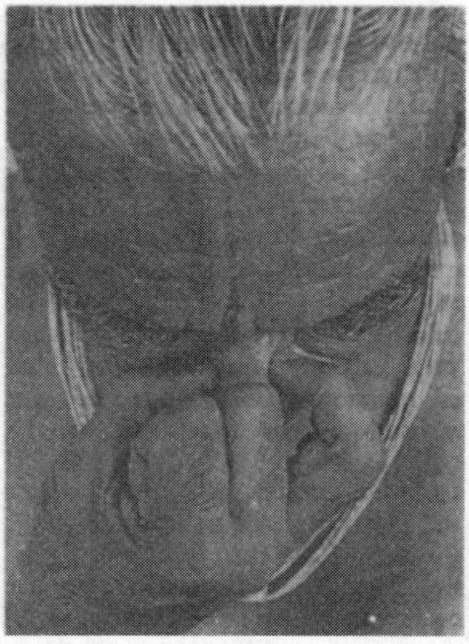

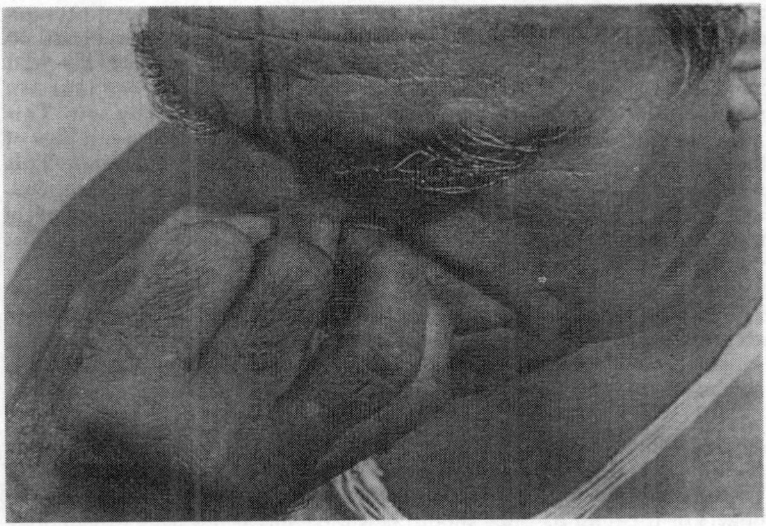

Pl. 132

Pl. 133

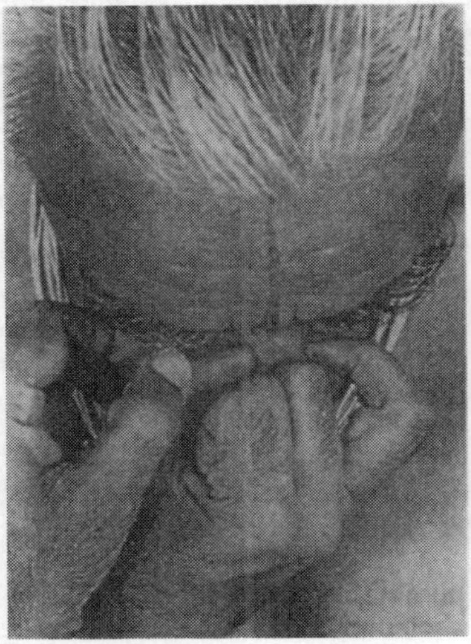

Pl. 134

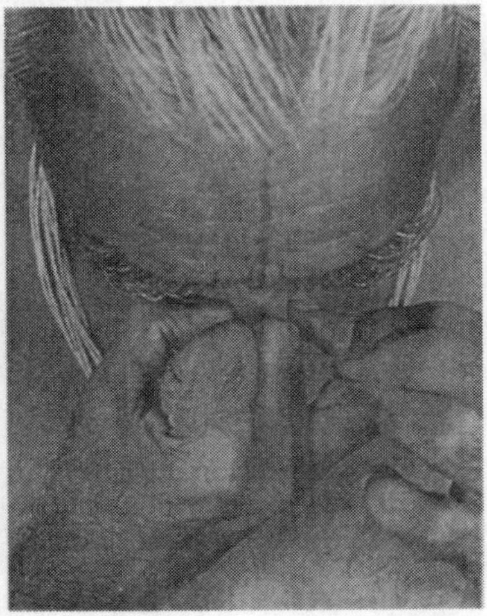

20. Normally the skin of the nose is softer than that of the tips of the thumb and the fingers. The tips get further tensed when the fingers are placed on the nose. To reduce this tension, pull back the skin of the fingers of the right hand, from the tips to the knuckles, with the left hand (Pls 133 and 134). See that the skin of the nostrils and of the finger-tips are equally soft. This makes the membranes passive and receptive. Then the in-and-out flow of breath moves smoothly, softly and in fine form over the membranes. This receptivity in the membranes helps the thumb and fingers to learn, feel, check, control and prolong the flow of breath as well as the duration of time. For the smooth and soft flow of the breath over the membranes, adjust the digits on the nasal skin delicately.

21. The softer and more sensitive the skin of the finger-tips, the more accurately can the breath be controlled. The passage in each nostril is widened or narrowed by very light sensitive pressure so as to regulate the flow of breath and the subtle forms of energy associated with it.

22. Do not pinch or irritate the nose (Pl. 135), nor move the position of the septum (Pl. 136). This not only disturbs the flow of breath on the sides of the nose, but also makes the chin lean to the stronger side. Do not jerk the fingers or the thumb. They should be subtle and at the same time mobile enough to make the fine adjustments needed to broaden or narrow the nasal passages.

23. Whenever dryness or irritation is felt on the membranes, lighten the finger pressure on them without losing the contact that makes the blood flow. This keeps the skin of the nose and of the finger-tips fresh, clean and sensitive. Sometimes, if it is sticky, one may have to pull the outer skin of the nose down with the left hand (Pls 137 and 138).

24. See that the chin does not move to the right as you bring your hand up to your nostrils.

25. Those using the right hand tend to lean the chin and head towards the right while changing the finger pressures from left to right. Those who use the left hand may lean them towards the left. Learn to keep the middle of the chin in line with the middle of the sternum.

26. During inhalation the flow of air through the nasal membranes moves upwards, and in exhalation downwards. Unconsciously the digits follow the breath. Adjust and move the fingers against the current of breath.

27. In prāṇāyāma the breath enters the nose at the centre by the sides of the septum, gliding effortlessly over it and then moving down to the lungs. It

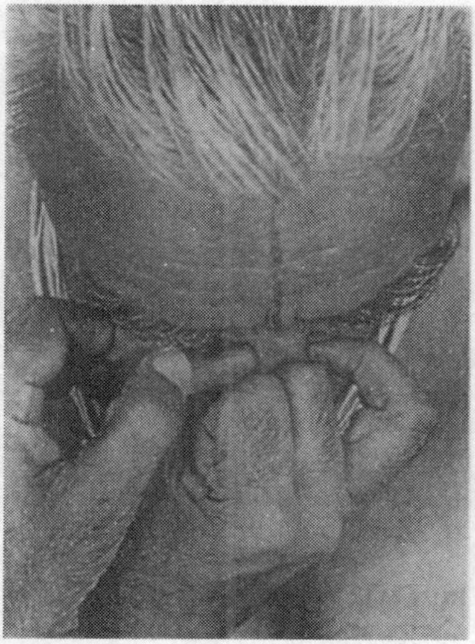

Pl. 135

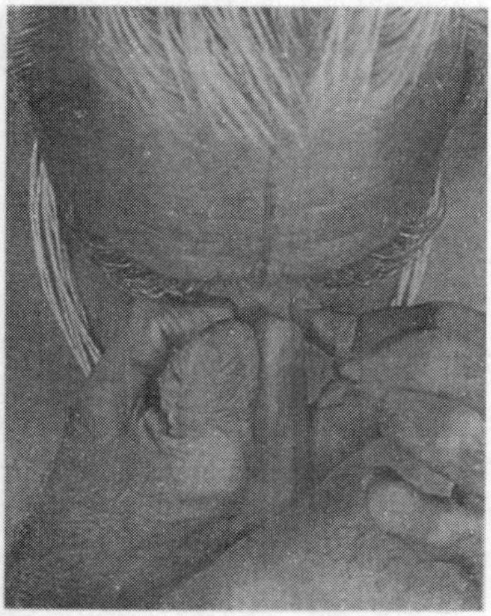

Pl. 136

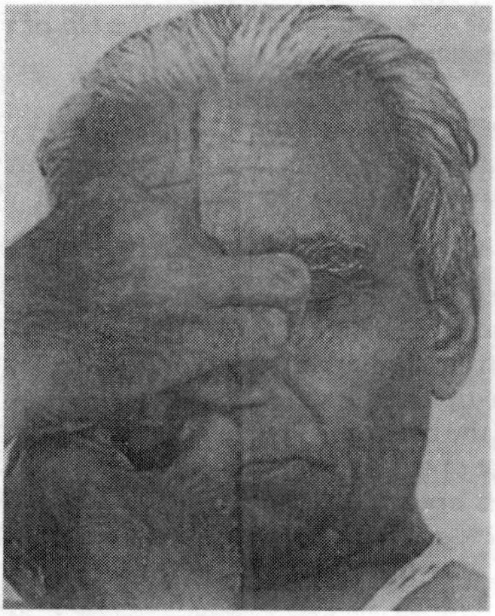

Pl. 137

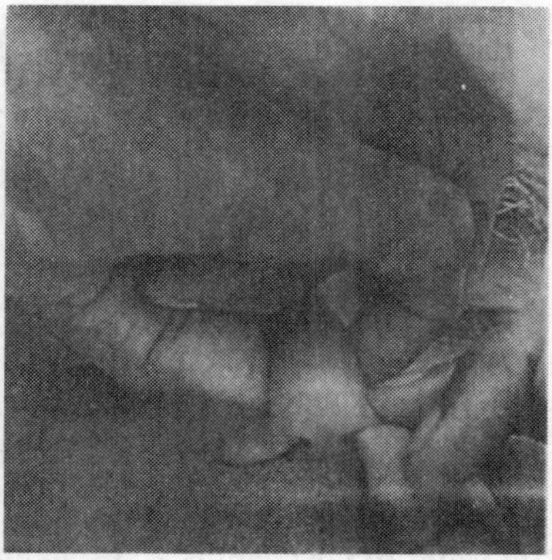

Pl. 138

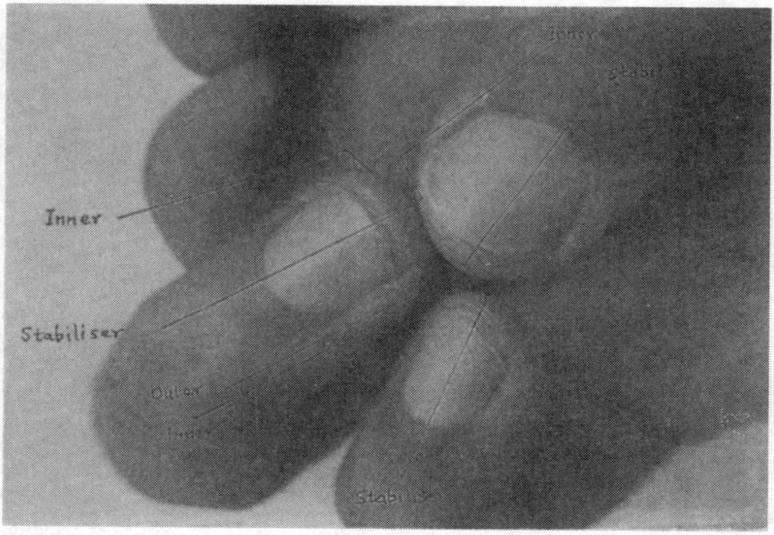

Pl. 139

leaves by the outerside of the nostrils near the cheeks. Use the tip of the thumb and digits differently for inhalation and exhalation.

28. Divide the tips into three portions, outer, middle and inner (Pl. 139). During inhalation the outer finger-tip is used to control the incoming breath, the middle to stabilise it and the inner to channel it into the bronchi.

29. In inhalation the top (inner) part of the digital tip is pressed lightly to narrow the passage at the root of the nose. The digital manipulation required may be compared to diverting water from a reservoir to surrounding fields. Air acts as the reservoir and the finger-tips as the sluice gates through which water passes into irrigation channels, the bronchi. The flow is controlled by the sluice gates, which break the force of the current and stabilise the level of water in the channel. The channels branch off into irrigation ditches to take the water into the fields for crops. The bronchi branch off into bronchioles to take the inhaled air into the furthermost corners of the alveoli.

30. In exhalation, the inner digital tips are used for control, the middle for stabilising and breaking the force, and the outer for channeling the breath. In exhalation, if the narrow (inner) tips of the digits are used as in inhalation,

there will be a choking sensation. Lighten the pressure of the inner tips of the digits and make the outer ones narrow and steady. This will smooth the outflow of beath. Exhalation may be likened to the flow of a river to the sea. The flow of breath from the alveoli is like the flow of water in the mountain streams that merge into rivulets, the bronchioles. The rivulets join the tributaries and finally a great river spreads into a delta to meet the sea. The air in the bronchioles flows into the bronchi and thence into the nasal cavity, the delta, to merge into the ocean of the atmosphere.

31. If the sound of the breath is rough, or if the breathing is quick, it is because the nasal passages are too wide. The flow will become smoother if the passage be narrowed. If the flow is correct and even, soft vibration will be felt by the finger-tips. Listen to the resonant sound of breath and refine it. If the sound is not resonant, but harsh, it is a sign that the finger-tips are vertical to the nostrils (see Pl. 130). Adjust them at once to face the nostrils horizontally.

32. Act with perfect understanding between the finger tips and the nasal membranes. Touch, balance and sustained pressure, by the finger tips tracing the flow of breath will alone lead to perfection in digital Prāṇāyāma.

33. As we gently take in the delicate fragrance of a flower, practise Prāṇāyāma as if drawing in the fragrance of the air.

34. If inhalation is longer than exhalation, it indicates that the nasal passages were more blocked during inhalation than exhalation. In order to increase the length of time for exhalation, gently lessen digital pressure during inhalation, but increase it for exhalation. If it is the other way, then vice-versa. After achieving equality in both over a period of time, narrow the nasal passages to make respiration deep and long as well as smooth and subtle. Too much or no digital pressure makes the finger-tips insensitive. Correct sensitivity can be achieved only by training and experience.

35. Measure the smoothness and length of time taken by the first inhalation and try to maintain it when you breathe out. The first breath is always the guide. The same applies when you increase the duration and also throughout your prāṇāyāma practices, for rhythm and balance is the secret of Yoga.

36. We unconsciously breathe the prayer 'So 'haṁ': 'He (Sah) the Immortal Spirit am I (Ahaṁ) in respiration.' Inhalation flows with the sound of 'Sah' and exhalation with 'Ahaṁ'. This unconscious prayer (japa) is said without realising its meaning (artha) and feeling (bhāvana). When Prāṇāyāma is practised, listen to this prayer with meaning and feeling when this realisation becomes nādānusandhāna (nāda = sound,

anusandhāna = quest) in which the sādhaka gets absorbed in the sound of his own breath. This enables him to receive the incoming breath as life's elixir and a blessing from the Lord, and the outgoing breath as his surrender to Him.

37. Keep the eyes, jaws, cheeks and the skin around the temples soft and relaxed. Do not raise the eye-brows when inhaling.

38. Forceful in and out breathing fosters the ego. If the flow is smooth and almost inaudible to the sādhaka, he will be filled with humility. This is the beginning of self-culture (Ātma-sādhana).

39. If the bone in your nose has been broken or the septum is not straight, adjust the digits somewhat differently. Find the opening of the nasal passage near the bone and keep the finger tips on the skin just above the opening. If the bend or deviation is to the right, the middle tip of the thumb should be moved up with the nasal skin (Pl. 140); if to the left, then move the tip of the ring finger with the nasal skin (Pl. 141).

40. The ala nasi are the fleshy curved parts at the tip of the nose which flare and dilate the nostrils. Sometimes the skin there is very soft, with the result that the nostrils get blocked at the slightest pressure. If you feel this has happened to the left nostril, insert the little finger to dilate it (Pl. 142); but if to the right nostril, move the inner tip of the thumb up towards the root of the nose (Pl. 140).

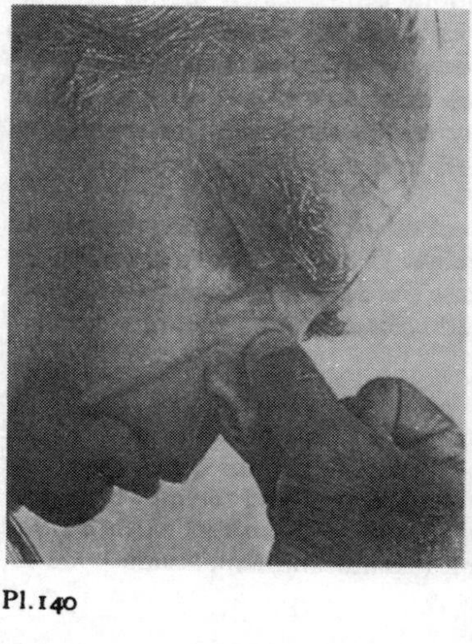

Pl. 140

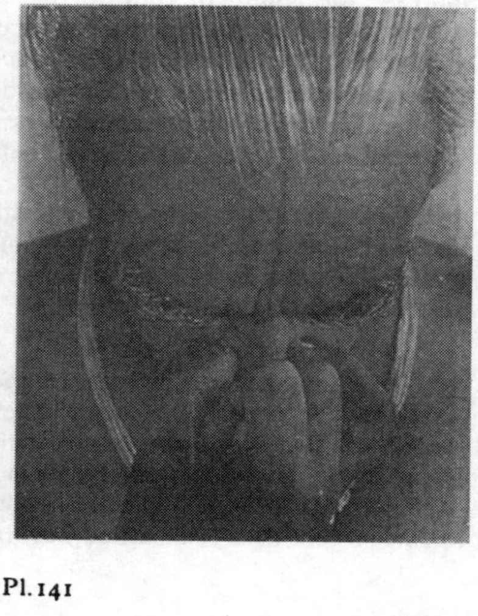

Pl. 141

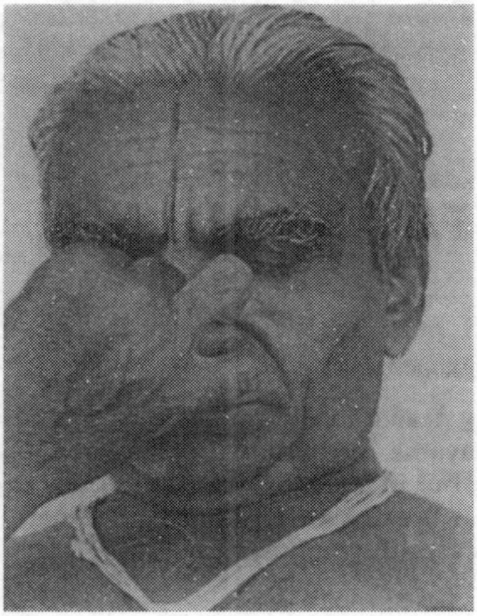

Pl. 142

41. If the nasal skin feels very dry, lift it with the finger tips and gently push it towards the septum as you breathe in. If the nostrils feel dry, ease the pressure on the nostrils. If the digital tips do not react to the flow of breath, stop practice for the day.

42. Measure the extent and fineness of the breath at the start. When the volume or the length of breath begins to vary or when the outer nostrils become hard and rough, stop practice for the day.

43. Never practise digital prāṇāyāma during headache, or when worried, anxious or restless, nor when the nose is blocked or ṛunning, when you have a fever or immediately afterwards. At such times practise śavāsana (Pl. 182), inhaling normally, exhaling slowly and deeply.

Chapter 23

Bhastrikā and Kapālabhāti Prāṇāyāma

BHASTRIKĀ PRĀṆĀYĀMA

Bhastrikā means bellows: air is forcibly drawn in and out as if using a pair of bellows. In all other types of prāṇāyāma inhalation sets the pace, the pattern and the rhythm for exhalation, but in bhastrikā exhalation sets the force and the pace. Here both out and in-breaths are vigorous and forceful. The sound is like that made by a blacksmith's bellows.

STAGE I

The nostrils are kept open throughout.

Technique

1. Sit in any comfortable position, following the techniques given in Paras 1 to 7 of ujjāyī, Stage V. Exhale whatever breath is in the lungs (Pl. 96).

2. Take a short, strong breath and expel it with a quick strong blast. Repeat this and you will find the second in-breath quicker and more forceful than the first one, due to the forceful character of the preceding out-breath.

3. One quick in and out breath, taken together, completes one blast of bhastrikā.

4. Do four to eight such blasts at a stretch to complete one cycle, ending with an out-breath.

5. Now take a few slow and deep breaths as in ujjāyī, or if you wish you may hold your breath within, with mūla bandha, for five to eight seconds (Pl. 101). Then exhale slowly and deeply as in ujjāyī. This rests the lungs and the diaphragm and prepares them for fresh blasts of bhastrikā.

6. Repeat cycles of bhastrikā blasts interspersed with ujjāyī, with or without retention, three or four times. Then take a deep breath and lie in śavāsana (Pl. 182).

7. As stamina improves, the number of blasts in each cycle, as well as the number of cycles, may be increased. However, immediately the tone of the breathing changes, stop at once.

STAGE II

Both nostrils are kept partially closed throughout.

Technique

1. Sit in any comfortable position, following the techniques of Paras 1 to 7 of ujjāyī, Stage V. Exhale whatever breath is in the lungs (Pl. 96).

2. Bring the right hand to the nostrils as explained in Paras 12 to 22 in Ch. 22 on digital prāṇāyāma.

3. Partially close both nostrils with the tips of the thumb, ring and little fingers. Make sure that both sides of each nostril are even (Pl. 110).

4. Now perform bhastrikā blasts following the techniques given in Paras 2 to 7 of Stage I above.

5. Repeat five or six times, take a few deep breaths, then lie in śavāsana (Pl. 182).

STAGE III

Here bhastrikā is done through alternate nostrils, with interspersion of ujjāyī breaths. Advanced students may do this without the interspersions.

Technique

1. Sit in any comfortable position, following the techniques given in Paras 1 to 7 of ujjāyī, Stage V. Exhale whatever breath is in the lungs (Pl. 96).

2. Bring the right hand to the nostrils as explained in Paras 12 to 22 of Ch. 22 on digital prāṇāyāma.

3. With the help of digital control, block the left nostril completely and the right one partially (Pl. 111).

4. Inhale and exhale through the right nostril vigorously, doing four to eight blasts at a stretch, making sure the pressure is the same with each blast. See that no breath escapes from the left nostril and end with a blast of out-breath.

5. Now block the right nostril, partially open the left (Pl. 112) and breathe vigorously through it with the same number of blasts as on the right and keeping the same pressure for each blast. See that no breath escapes from the right nostril. End the blast with an out-breath.

6. These two together complete one cycle of Stage III.

7. Repeat them on both sides three or four times, take a few deep breaths and then lie in śavāsana (Pl. 182).

8. If you cannot do several cycles at a stretch, then after each cycle take a few breaths as in ujjāyī to rest the lungs.

STAGE IV

In stage III one cycle of bhastrikā blasts is done through the right nostril, the other from the left. In this stage the in-and-out blasts are done through alternate nostrils; that is, if the in-breath is done from the right, then the out-breath is from the left and then the other way round. Four or five such blasts form one half-cycle. The other one starts with an in-breath from the left and is followed by an out-breath from the right, with an equal number of blasts. These two make one cycle of Stage IV.

Technique

1. Sit in any comfortable position, following the techniques given in Paras 1 to 7 of ujjāyī, Stage V. Exhale whatever breath is in the lungs (Pl. 96).

2. Bring the right hand to the nostrils as explained in Paras 12 to 22 in Ch. 22 on digital prāṇāyāma.

3. Block the left nostril, half-open the right (Pl. 111) and take a quick strong in-breath through it. Quickly close the right nostril, half-open the left and breathe out quickly and vigorously through it (Pl. 112). Do four or five blasts in quick succession. This forms the first half-cycle.

4. Now do the other half-cycle, repeating the same procedure as above, but breathing in from the left and out through the right. This completes the second half-cycle. Do an equal number of blasts as above, maintaining the same rhythm, tone and volume throughout.

5. Do three to four such full cycles, take a few breaths of ujjāyī to rest the lungs, and then rest in śavāsana (Pl. 182).

KAPĀLABHĀTI PRĀṆĀYĀMA

Some call kapālabhāti a prāṇāyāma, while others call it a kriyā (kapāla means skull and bhāti means light or lustre). This is similar to bhastrikā but milder. In it inhalation is slow and exhalation vigorous, but there is a split second of retention after each out-breath. Do kapālabhāti instead of bhastrikā if the latter proves too strenuous.

Kapālabhāti may be divided into stages similar to bhastrikā, and practised accordingly.

Effects of Bhastrikā and Kapālabhāti

Both these activate and invigorate the liver, spleen, pancreas and abdominal muscles, and improve digestion. They drain the sinuses and stop the nose running. They also create a feeling of exhilaration.

Notes and cautions

1. Bhastrikā generates prāṇa to activate the entire body. Just as too much stoking burns out the boiler of an engine, too long a practice of bhastrikā endangers the lungs and wears out the system, since the breathing process is so forceful.

2. As soon as the sound diminishes, stop and start afresh or reduce the number of blasts and cycles, or stop for the day.

3. Stop the practice the moment irritation or strain is felt.

4. Do not practise if the sound of the out-breath is incorrect or if the blasts fail to come. Any force will lead to injury or a nose-bleed.

5. Persons with weak constitutions and poor lung capacity should not attempt bhastrikā or kapālabhāti, since they may damage the blood vessels or brain.

6. They should not be performed by the following:

(a) Women, since the vigorous blasts may cause prolapse of the abdominal organs and of the uterus while the breasts may sag.

(b) Those suffering from ear or eye complaints (such as pus in the ear, a detached retina, or glaucoma).

(c) Persons with high or low blood pressure.

(d) Those suffering from bleeding of the nose, or throbbing or aching of the ears. If this happens, stop immediately for some days. Then try again and, if any of these signs recur, these practices are not for you.

7. Many people misconceive that bhastrikā prāṇāyāma awakens the kuṇḍalinī śakti. The authoritative books have said the same regarding

many Prāṇāyāmas and āsanas, but this is far from true. There is no doubt that bhastrikā and kapalabhāti refresh the brain and stir it to activity, but if people perform them because they believe that they awaken the kuṇḍalinī, disaster to body, nerves and brain may result.

Table of Bhastrikā Prāṇāyāma

Stage I	PR	PR	PR	PR	P	R	P	R	or	PR	PR	PR	PR	P	AK	R
(ON)	BH	BH	BH	BH	U	U	U	U		BH	BH	BH	BH	U	MB	U
Stage II	PR	PR	PR	PR	P	R	P	R	or	PR	PR	PR	PR	P	AK	R
(BNPC)	BH	BH	BH	BH	U	U	U	U		BH	BH	BH	BH	U	MB	U
Stage III	PR	PR	PR	PR	PR	PR	PR	PR	PR	PR	PR	PR	or	P	AK	R
(RNPC/	BH	BH	BH	BH	BH	BH	BH	BH	U	U	U	U		U	MB	U
LNPC)	RR	RR	RR	RR	LL	LL	LL	LL								
Stage IV	PR	PR	PR	PR	PR	PR	PR	PR	P	R	P	R	or	P	AK	R
(RNPC/	BH	BH	BH	BH	BH	BH	BH	BH	U	U	U	U		U	MB	U
LNPC)	RL	RL	RL	RL	LR	LR	LR	LR								

AK	=	Antara kumbhaka
BH	=	Bhastrikā (pūraka short strong, rechaka quick strong)
BNPC	=	Both nostrils partially closed
LNPC	=	Left nostril partially closed
MB	=	Mūla bandha
ON	=	Open nostrils
PR	=	Pūraka, rechaka
RNPC	=	Right nostril partially closed
R	=	Right
L	=	Left
U	=	Ujjāyī

Chapter 24

Śītalī and Śītakārī Prāṇāyāma

In these two prāṇāyāmas inhalation is done through the mouth and not the nostrils without jālandhara bandha.

ŚĪTALĪ PRĀṆĀYĀMA

This prāṇāyāma cools the system, hence the name.

STAGE I

In this stage, inhalation is through the curled tongue, while retention and exhalation are done as in ujjāyī.

Technique

1. Sit in any comfortable position, following the techniques given in Paras 1 to 7 of ujjāyī, Stage V. Exhale whatever breath is in the lungs (Pl. 96).

2. Keep the head level. Open the mouth and form the lips into an O.

3. Push out the tongue and curl it lengthwise so that its shape resembles a fresh curled leaf about to open (Pl. 143).

4. Stretch the curled tongue further out (Pl. 144) and draw in air through it as if drinking with a straw, and fill the lungs completely. The breath is moistened by passing through the curl of wet tongue.

5. After a full in-breath, withdraw the tongue and close the mouth.

6. Lower the head and perform jālandhara bandha (Pl. 57). Hold the breath for five to ten seconds, with or without mūla bandha (Pl. 101).

7. Exhale as in ujjāyī.

8. This completes one cycle of śītalī. Repeat them for five to ten minutes at a stretch. At the end of the last one, inhale normally through both nostrils and then lie in śavāsana (Pl. 182).

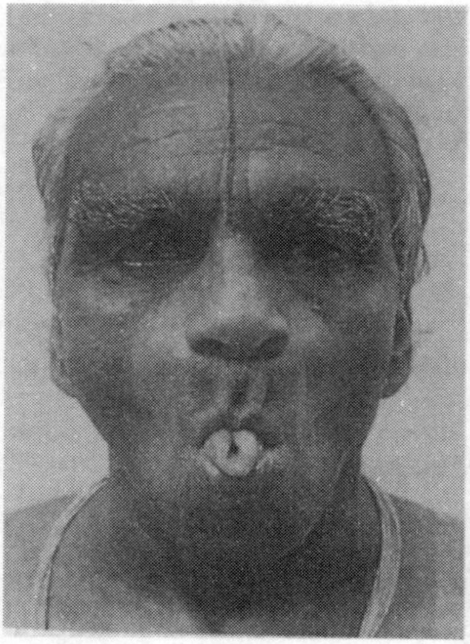

Pl. 143

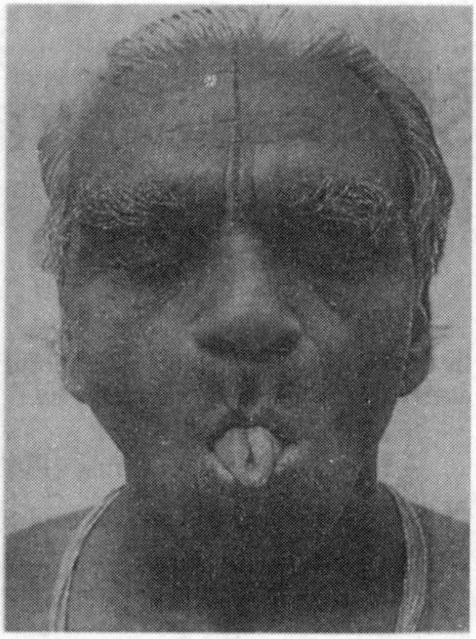

Pl. 144

STAGE II

In this stage inhalation is done as above, but exhalation is done with both nostrils partially closed.

Technique

1. Sit in any comfortable position, following the techniques given in Paras 1 to 7 of ujjāyī, Stage V. Exhale whatever breath is in the lungs (Pl. 96).

2. Now inhale, following all the techniques in Paras 2 to 6 of Stage I above (Pl. 144) and ending with mūla bandha (Pl. 69).

3. Bring the right hand to the nostrils, as explained in Paras 12 to 22 of Ch. 22 on digital prāṇāyāma.

4. Partially close both nostrils with the tips of the thumb, the ring and little fingers, keeping the pressure even on both nostrils so that the walls of the nasal passages remain parallel to the septum (Pl. 110).

5. Exhale slowly, steadily and completely, without strain. Adjust the fingers on the nostrils delicately to control the volume and to regulate the flow of the out-breath evenly on both sides.

6. When the lungs feel completely empty, lower the hand and rest it on the knee.

7. This completes one cycle. Repeat for five to ten minutes. At the end of the last cycle, inhale normally through both nostrils, then lie down in śavasana (Pl. 182).

STAGE III

Here inhalation is done as in Stages I and II, and exhalation through alternate nostrils, keeping one side blocked and the other partially closed.

Technique

1. Sit in any comfortable position, following the techniques given in Paras 1 to 7 of ujjāyī, Stage V. Exhale deeply (Pl. 96).

2. Now inhale, following the techniques in Paras 2 to 6 of Stage I above (Pl. 144) and ending with internal retention and mūla bandha (Pl. 101).

3. Bring the right hand to the nostrils as explained in paras 12 to 22 of Ch. 22 on digital prāṇāyāma.

4. Block the left nostril completely, partially close the right (Pl. 111) and exhale slowly, steadily and completely through it without straining.

5. When the lungs feel completely empty, lower the hand and rest it on the knee. Inhale again, as in paras 2 to 6 of Stage I.

6. Bring the right hand to the nose and block the right nostril completely, partially close the left one (Pl. 112) and exhale slowly, steadily and completely without straining. Then lower the hand.

7. This completes one cycle. Repeat for five to ten minutes. At the end of the last cycle, inhale normally with open nostrils, then lie down in śavāsana (Pl. 182).

ŚITAKARI PRANAYAMA

Śītakārī is that which causes cold. It is a variation of śītalī prāṇāyāma. It is also called śītakārī prāṇāyāma as the breath is drawn with a hissing sound between the two lips.

Technique

Follow the same techniques and stages of śītalī as described above, but without curling the tongue. The lips are kept slightly apart and the tip of the tongue protrudes only slightly, but is kept flat.

Śītakārī, like śītalī, is performed in three stages, following the same techniques as in all stages of śītalī.

Effects

These two prāṇāyāmas are exhilarating. They cool the system and soothe the eyes and ears. They are beneficial in cases of low fever and biliousness. They activate the liver and spleen, improve digestion and relieve thirst. They are beneficial to halitosis. These prāṇāyāmas may be done by the sādhaka, even when the nostrils are blocked.

Table of Śītalī and Sītakārī Prāṇāyāma

Śītalī

Stage	*Pūraka*		*Antara kumbhaka*		*Rechaka*
	Head	*Straight*	*JB*		
	D	*CT*	*No MB*	*MB*	*D*
I	√	√	Either (MB 5–10 sec)		ON
II	√	√		√	BNPC
III	√	√		√	ANPC

Sītakārī

Stage	*Pūraka*		*Antara Kumbhaka*		*Rechaka*
	Head	*Straight*	*JB*		
	D	*FT*	*No MB*	*MB*	*D*
I	√	√	Either (MB 5–10 sec)		ON
II	√	√		√	BNPC
III	√	√		√	ANPC

ANPC = Alternate nostrils partially closed
BNPC = Both nostrils partially closed
D = Deep
CT = Curled tongue
FT = Flat tongue
JB = Jālandhara bandha
MB = Mūla bandha
ON = Open nostrils

Chapter 25

Anuloma Prāṇāyāma

'Anu' means 'along with', or in orderly succession, and 'loma' is hair or in natural order. Here the fingers control the nostrils to discharge delicately the flow of the out-going breath.

Master the techniques of ujjāyī and viloma Prāṇāyāma before attempting anuloma.

In anuloma, inhalation is done through open nostrils, with or without pauses, and with mūla bandha in the advanced stages. Exhalation is done either with both nostrils partially open or alternatively with one nostril completely blocked and the other partially closed; uḍḍīyāna is used in the advanced stages.

In all stages, the in-breath is shorter than the out-breath, the emphasis being on delicate prolongation of the latter.

This prāṇāyāma, as well as those that follow, are done only when sitting, especially in an āsana, as explained in Ch. 11.

STAGE Ia

In this stage a deep inhalation is made with open nostrils, followed by a deep exhalation with both nostrils partially closed. This is to prolong the length of exhalation, to train the finger-tips to control both nostrils evenly, and to refine the flow of the out-breath.

Technique

1. Sit in any āsana, following the techniques given in Paras 1 to 7 of ujjāyī, Stage V. Exhale whatever breath is in the lungs (Pl. 96).

2. Inhale deeply through both nostrils until the lungs are full (Pl. 98).

3. Hold the breath for a second or two in order to bring the right hand to the nostrils, as explained in Paras 12 to 22 of Ch. 22 on digital prāṇāyāma.

4. Now begins the process of digitally controlled exhalation.

5. Partially open both nostrils with the tips of the thumb and fingers, making the inner walls of the nasal passages parallel to and equidistant from the septum (Pl. 110).

6. Keep the pressure evenly on both sides so that the nostrils are ready to discharge the subtle flow of the out-breath evenly.

7. Exhale slowly, carefully and deeply, without using any force.

8. Keep the fingers firm and sensitive to adjust the nostrils and to monitor and equalise the volume of out-flow on each side.

9. When the lungs are completely empty, lower the right hand and rest it on the knee.

10. This completes one cycle. Repeat them for fifteen to twenty minutes. Inhale with open nostrils, then lie in śavāsana (Pl. 182).

Effects
This prāṇāyāma cleanses the nasal passages.

STAGE Ib

In this stage deep inhalation is done with open nostrils; exhalation is through alternate nostrils, keeping one completely blocked and the other partially open. Here each nostril is trained to develop awareness and sensitivity independently during exhalation.

Remember to keep the walls of the nasal passages parallel to the septum, even if they are both partially closed or blocked on one side and partially open on the other side.

Technique
1. Sit in any āsana, following the technique given in Paras 1 to 7 of ujjāyī, Stage V. Exhale (Pl. 96).

2. Inhale, following the techniques given in Paras 2 and 3 of Stage Ia (Pl. 98).

3. Now the process of exhalation through the right nostril starts. Block the left nostril completely with the tips of the ring and little fingers, without altering the position of the septum.

4. Partially open the right nostril with the tip of the thumb, keeping its inner wall parallel to the septum (Pl. 111).

5. Breathe out slowly and carefully through the partially open right nostril. Control the smooth out-flow of breath with the help of the thumb-tip, and see that no breath escapes through the left nostril.

6. When the lungs feel completely empty, lower the right hand and rest it on the right knee.

7. Now inhale deeply through open nostrils until the lungs are completely full, and hold the breath for a second or two (Pl. 98).

8. Now starts the process of exhalation through the left nostril. Bring the right hand to the nostrils. With the tip of the thumb block the right nostril completely, without altering the position of the septum.

9. With the tips of the ring and little fingers, open the left nostril partially, keeping its inner wall parallel to the septum (Pl. 112).

10. Breathe out slowly and completely through the partially open left nostril. Control the smooth out-flow of breath with the help of the two finger-tips. See that no breath escapes through the right nostril.

11. When the lungs feel empty, lower the right hand and rest it on the knee.

12. This completes one cycle. Repeat them for fifteen to twenty minutes. Inhale, then lie in śavāsana (Pl. 182).

Effects

This prāṇāyāma is exhilarating and good for controlling hyper-tension and high blood pressure.

STAGE IIa

This stage is similar to that of Ia; with the introduction of internal retention (antara kumbhaka), and is for intermediate students.

Technique

1. Sit in any āsana, following the techniques given in Paras 1 to 7 of ujjāyī, Stage V. Exhale whatever breath is in the lungs (Pl. 96).

2. Inhale, following the techniques given in Para. 2 of Stage Ia. (Pl. 98).

3. When the lungs are full, hold the breath for ten to fifteen seconds or for as long as you can (Pl. 101).

4. Now exhale, following the techniques of Paras 5 to 8 of Stage Ia (Pl. 110), then lower the right hand.

5. This completes one cycle. Repeat them for ten to fifteen minutes. Inhale, then lie in śavāsana (Pl. 182).

Effects
This sharpens inner awareness and concentration.

STAGE IIb

This stage is similar to Ib, but with the introduction of internal retention (antara kumbhaka).

Technique
1. Sit in any āsana, following the techniques given in Paras 1 to 7 of ujjāyī, Stage V. Exhale deeply (Pl. 96).

2. Inhale, following the technique given in Para. 2 of Stage Ia (Pl. 98).

3. When the lungs are full, hold the breath for fifteen to twenty seconds, or for as long as you can (Pl. 101).

4. Now exhale through the right nostril, as in Paras 3 to 5 of Stage Ib (Pl. 111).

5. When the lungs are completely empty, lower the right hand and rest it on the knee.

6. Now inhale deeply with open nostrils as in Para. 2 above, till the lungs are full (Pl. 98).

7. Hold the breath for the same length of time as in Para. 3 above (Pl. 101).

8. Exhale through the left nostril, following the techniques given in Paras 8 to 10 of Stage Ib (Pl. 112). Then lower the right hand.

9. This completes one cycle. Repeat them for ten to fifteen minutes. Inhale, then lie in śavāsana (Pl. 182).

Effects
This leads to fine control and lengthening of exhalation.

STAGE IIIa

This is similar to Stage Ia, with the introduction of pensive external retention (bāhya kumbhaka without uḍḍīyāna).

Technique
1. Sit in any āsana, following the same techniques as in Paras 1 to 7 of ujjāyī, Stage V. Exhale (Pl. 96).

2. Inhale, following the technique given in Para. 2 of Stage Ia (Pl. 98).

3. Now start exhalation through partially opened nostrils, as described in Paras 4 to 8 of Stage Ia (Pl. 110).

4. When the lungs feel completely empty, lower the right hand and rest it on the knee. Remain passive without inhalation for five seconds. This is pensive external retention (Pl. 96).

5. This completes one cycle. Repeat them for ten to fifteen minutes. Inhale through open nostrils, then lie in śavāsana (Pl. 182).

Effects
This cleanses the nasal passages and creates quietness and calmness in the sādhaka.

STAGE IIIb

This is similar to Stage Ib, with the introduction of pensive external retention (bāhya kumbhaka without uḍḍīyāna).

Technique
1. Sit in any āsana, following the techniques given in Paras 1 to 7 of ujjāyī, Stage V, and exhale (Pl. 96).

2. Inhale, following the technique given in Para. 2 of Stage Ia (Pl. 98).

3. Now exhale through the right nostril, as explained in Paras 3 to 5 of Stage Ib (Pl. 111).

4. When the lungs feel completely empty, lower the right hand and rest it on the knee. Remain passive (without inhalation) for five seconds (Pl. 96).

5. Then inhale deeply through open nostrils, as described in Para. 2 above (Pl. 98).

6. Now starts the process of exhalation through the left nostril, as explained in Paras 8 to 10 of Stage Ib (Pl. 112).

7. When the lungs feel empty, lower the right hand and remain passive (Pl. 96) for five seconds.

8. This completes one cycle. Repeat them for ten to fifteen minutes, ending with an in-breath. Then lie in śavāsana (Pl. 182).

Effects
This takes the sādhaka towards inner awareness, leading to finer control of exhalation.

STAGE IVa

Bandhās are introduced in these two stages: internal retention with mūla bandha and external retention with uḍḍīyāna bandha.

Technique
1. Sit in any āsana, following the techniques given in Paras 1 to 7 of ujjāyī, Stage V. Exhale (Pl. 96).

2. Inhale, following the technique given in Para. 2 of Stage Ia (Pl. 98).

3. When the lungs are full, hold the breath with mūla bandha for ten to twelve seconds, or for as long as you can (Pl. 101).

4. Exhale slowly, following the techniques given in Paras 5 to 8 of Stage Ia (Pl. 110), releasing the abdominal grip gradually.

5. When the lungs feel empty, lower the right hand and rest it on the knee. Then do external retention with uḍḍīyāna bandha for five to six seconds (Pl. 104).

6. Release the uḍḍīyāna grip.

7. This completes one cycle. Repeat such cycles for fifteen to twenty minutes. Inhale, then lie in śavāsana (Pl. 182).

Effects
This creates endurance, makes the mind reflective and prepares the sādhaka for dhyāna.

STAGE IVb

This is similar to Stage Ib, with the introduction of bandhās as in Stage IVa.

Technique
1. Sit in any āsana, following the techniques given in Paras 1 to 7 of ujjāyī, Stage V. Exhale (Pl. 96).

2. Inhale, following the technique given in Para. 2 of Stage Ia (Pl. 98).

3. When the lungs are full, hold the breath with mūla bandha (Pl. 101) as described in Para. 3 Stage IVa.

4. Exhale through the right nostril, keeping the left one blocked (Pl. 111); follow the techniques given in Paras 3 to 5 of Stage Ib, relaxing the abdominal grip gradually.

5. When the lungs feel completely empty, lower the right hand and rest it on the knee. Then do external retention with uḍḍīyāna for five to six seconds (Pl. 104).

6. Release the uḍḍīyāna grip, then inhale deeply with open nostrils, as in Para. 2 above (Pl. 98).

7. Hold the breath with mūla bandha for ten to fifteen seconds (Pl. 101) or for the same length of time as in Para. 3 above.

8. Now exhale through the left nostril (Pl. 112), keeping the right completely blocked, following the techniques given in Paras 8 to 10 of Stage Ib.

9. When the lungs feel completely empty, lower the right hand and do external retention with uḍḍīyāna for five to six seconds (Pl. 104).

10. Release the uḍḍīyāna grip.

11. Two inhalations with open nostrils, two internal retentions with mūla bandha, two exhalations through alternate nostrils and two external retentions with uḍḍīyāna constitute one cycle. Repeat them for ten to fifteen minutes, ending with inhalation. Then lie in śavāsana (Pl. 182).

Effects

As this stage is intense, so are the effects.

STAGES Va to VIIIb

In all the following stages from V to VIII, use viloma techniques for inhalations and anuloma ones for exhalations.

STAGE Va

This stage is similar to Stage Ia above, of which the techniques of exhalation should be followed, but an interrupted inhalation with pauses as in viloma, Stage I should be substituted for in-breath.

STAGE Vb

This stage is similar to Ib, but with interrupted in-breaths with pauses.

STAGES VIa and VIb

These stages are similar to IIa and IIb respectively, except that the inhalations are interrupted by pauses.

STAGES VIIa and VIIb

These stages are similar to IIIa and IIIb respectively, except that the inhalations are interrupted by pauses.

STAGES VIIIa and VIIIb

These stages are similar to IVa and IVb respectively, except that the inhalations are interrupted by pauses.

Effects of Stages V to VIII

These stages are more intense than the preceding Prāṇāyāmas and their effects are correspondingly intense and efficacious. Stage VIII is the most intensive of all. It requires great strength, application, persistence, endurance and determination.

Table of Anuloma Prāṇāyāma

Stage		*Pūraka*		*Antara Kumbhaka*		*Rechaka*		*Bāhya Kumbhaka*	
		U	*V*	*No MB*	*MB*	*BNPC*	*ANPC*	*No UB*	*UB*
I	A	✓				✓			
	B	✓					✓		
II	A	✓		10–15 sec		✓			
	B	✓		10–15 sec			✓		
III	A	✓				✓		5 sec	
	B	✓					✓	5 sec	
IV	A	✓			10 sec	✓			5–8 sec
	B	✓			10 sec		✓		5–8 sec
V	A		✓			✓			
	B		✓				✓		
VI	A		✓	10 sec		✓			
	B		✓	10 sec			✓		
VII	A		✓			✓		5 sec	
	B		✓				✓	5 sec	
VIII	A		✓		10 sec	✓			5–8 sec
	B		✓		10 sec		✓		5–8 sec

ANPC = Alternate nostrils partially closed
BNPC = Both nostrils partially closed
MB = Mūla bandha
UB = Uḍḍīyāna bandha
U = Ujjāyī
V = Viloma

Chapter 26

Pratiloma Prāṇāyāma

Prati means opposite or against and loma means hair. Pratiloma therefore implies going against the natural order. It is the converse of anuloma. Here, the nostrils are controlled for inhalation and narrowed by the finger-tips to enable the in-breath to flow with delicacy.

In all 'a' stages inhalation is drawn through both partially open but controlled nostrils and in 'b' stages it takes place through alternate nostrils. All exhalations are done with open nostrils as in ujjāyī.

In this prāṇāyāma the in-breath lasts longer than the out-breath, the emphasis being on the slow, delicate prolongation of each in-breath. Anuloma and pratiloma prāṇāyāma are the foundations for viṣama vṛtti prāṇāyāma and a stepping stone to advance in this art.

STAGE Ia

In this stage inhalation is done through narrowly open but controlled nostrils and is followed by exhalation through open nostrils. This is to train the finger-tips in even control of both nostrils for the fine and delicate flow of inhalation.

Technique

1. Sit in any āsana, following the techniques given in Paras 1 to 7 to ujjāyī, Stage V. Exhale (Pl. 96).

2. Bring the right hand to the nostrils as explained in Paras 12 to 22 of Ch. 22 on digital prāṇāyāma.

3. Control both nostrils with the tips of the thumb and fingers, making the nasal passages as narrow as possible and parallel to the septum (Pl. 110).

4. Keep an even pressure on both sides of the nostrils so as to make the two passages even in width. Do not disturb the septum. Now the nostrils are ready to receive the flow of the in-breath.

5. Inhale slowly, carefully and deeply, without using any force. Feel the air as it enters the nasal passages. Keep the fingers firm and sensitive, adjusting their tips evenly on both sides of the nostrils to observe, guide and equalise the volume and the smooth in-flow of air.

6. When the lungs are completely full, hold the breath for a second or two, then lower the right hand and rest it on the right knee.

7. Exhale with open nostrils slowly, steadily and smoothly till the lungs feel completely empty.

8. This completes one cycle. Repeat the cycle for ten to fifteen minutes or for as long as you feel no strain. After completing the last cycle, inhale with open nostrils, then lie in śavāsana (Pl. 182).

Effects
This is effective for removing sluggishness and moodiness.

STAGE Ib

In this stage inhalation is done through digitally controlled alternate nostrils, followed by deep exhalation with open nostrils. The aim is to create intelligence and develop awareness in order to refine and lengthen the flow of the in-breath in each nostril. This prepares the sādhaka for nādī śodhana prāṇāyāma.

Technique
1. Sit in any āsana, following the techniques given in Paras 1 to 7 of ujjāyī, Stage V. Exhale (Pl. 96).

2. Bring the right hand to the nostrils as explained in Paras 12 to 22 of Ch. 22 on digital prāṇāyāma.

3. Block the left nostril completely with the tips of the ring and little fingers, without altering the position of the septum.

4. Control the right nostril with the tip of the thumb and make the passage as narrow as possible as in Pl. 111. This decreases the velocity and volume of the in-breath, and refines its tone.

5. Keep the inner wall of the right passage parallel to the septum.

6. Now inhale slowly, deeply and as delicately as possible through the partially open but controlled right nostril, till the lungs are completely full. Hold the breath for a second or two.

7. Lower the hand and rest it on the knee. Exhale slowly, softly, steadily and delicately with open nostrils until the lungs feel empty.

8. Again raise the hand to the nose and inhale through the left nostril, following the techniques given in Paras 2 to 6 above, but block the right nostril and breathe through the left (Pl. 112).

9. Lower the hand and rest it on the knee. Exhale as in Para. 7.

10. This completes one cycle. Repeat them for ten to fifteen minutes. After completing the last cycle, inhale through open nostrils, then lie in śavāsana (Pl. 182).

Effects
This develops tremendous sensitivity in the nasal membranes and dexterity in the finger-tips.

STAGE IIa

In this stage inhalation is done through controlled and narrowly open nostrils. This is followed by internal retention with blocked nostrils and mūla bandha, then exhalation is through open nostrils.

Technique
1. Sit in any āsana, following the techniques of Paras 1 to 7 of ujjāyī, Stage V. Exhale (Pl. 96).

2. Bring the right hand to the nostrils and inhale, following the techniques given in Paras 3 to 5 of Stage Ia above (Pl. 110).

3. When the lungs are completely full, block both nostrils with the centres of the tips of the thumb and of the fingers (Pl. 145), not allowing any air to escape. Hold the breath with mūla bandha (Pl. 69) for fifteen to twenty seconds or for as long as you can.

4. Lower the right hand and rest it on the right knee.

5. Exhale with open nostrils softly, slowly, steadily and smoothly till the lungs feel completely empty.

6. This completes one cycle. Repeat them for fifteen to twenty minutes, or for as long as you feel no strain. After completing the last cycle, inhale through open nostrils, then lie in śavāsana (Pl. 182).

STAGE IIb

This is similar to Stage Ib, with the addition of internal retention with mūla bandha, as in Stage IIa.

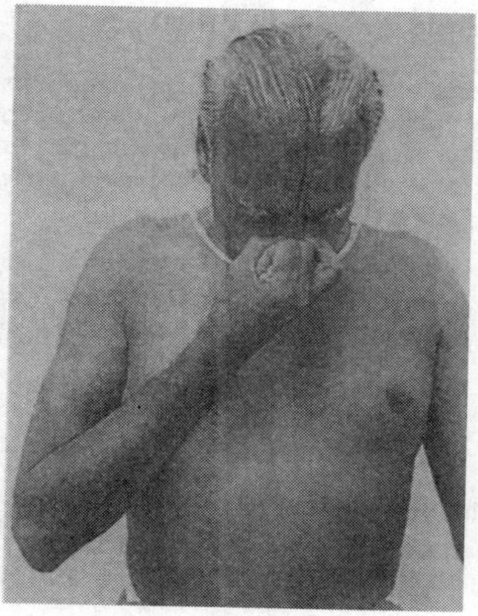

Pl. 145

Technique

1. Sit in any āsana, following the techniques given in Paras 1 to 7 of ujjāyī, Stage V. Exhale (Pl. 96).

2. Bring the right hand to the nostrils. Now inhale, following the techniques given in Paras 3 to 6 of Stage Ib above (Pl. 111).

3. After full inhalation, block both the nostrils (Pl. 145) and hold the breath with mūla bandha (Pl. 69) for fifteen to twenty seconds or as long as you can.

4. Lower the right hand to the knee. Exhale with open nostrils softly, slowly, steadily and smoothly till the lungs feel completely empty.

5. Again raise the right hand to the nose and block the right nostril completely, but control the left one and open it partially (Pl. 112).

6. Inhale through the left nostril, following the techniques in Paras 4 to 6 of Stage Ib, reading left for right and vice versa.

7. At the end of inhalation, hold the breath as in Para. 3 above.

8. Then lower the right hand and exhale slowly as in Para. 4 above.

9. Two inhalations done through alternate nostrils, two internal retentions with blocked nostrils and with mūla bandha, and two exhalations with open nostrils complete one cycle. Repeat them for fifteen to twenty minutes, or for as long as you feel no strain. After completing the last cycle, inhale through open nostrils, then lie in śavāsana (Pl. 182).

Effects of Stages IIa and IIb

These stages teach the sādhaka accurate finger placement for retentions. As the nostrils are completely blocked, no tension is felt in the head and facial muscles.

STAGE IIIa

This is similar to Stage IIa, with the introduction of external retention performed with uḍḍīyāna bandha.

Technique

1. Sit in any āsana following the techniques given in Paras 1 to 7 of ujjāyī, Stage V. Exhale (Pl. 96).

2. Bring the hands to the nostrils as explained in Paras 12 to 22 of Ch. 22 on digital prāṇāyāma.

3. Inhale, following the techniques given in Paras 3 to 5 of Stage Ia above (Pl. 110).

4. Exhale with open nostrils slowly, steadily and smoothly until the lungs feel completely empty.

5 Then do external retention with uḍḍīyāna for ten to fifteen seconds, or for as long as you can (Pl. 104). Finally, release the uḍḍīyāna grip.

6. One inhalation, one exhalation and one external retention with uḍḍīyāna bandha completes one cycle. Repeat them for ten to fifteen minutes, or for as long as you feel no strain. After the last cycle, inhale through open nostrils, then lie in śavāsana (Pl. 182).

STAGE IIIb

This is similar to Stage IIb, with the addition of external retention and uḍḍīyāna bandha as in Stage IIIa.

Technique

1. Sit in any āsana, following the techniques given in Paras 1 to 7 of ujjāyī, Stage V. Exhale whatever breath is in the lungs (Pl. 96).

2. Bring the right hand to the nostrils as explained in Paras 12 to 22 of Ch. 22 on digital prāṇāyāma.

3. Block the left nostril completely and inhale through the controlled and partially open right nostril (Pl. 111), following the techniques given in Paras 4 to 6 of Stage Ib above.

4. Lower the hand, rest it on the knee, and exhale with open nostrils, slowly, steadily and smoothly, until the lungs feel completely empty.

5. Now do external retention with uḍḍīyāna for ten to fifteen seconds, or for as long as you can (Pl. 104), then release the grip.

6. Raise the right hand to the nostrils, blocking the right completely and the left partially (Pl. 112). Inhale slowly, delicately and deeply through the left nostril, following the techniques given in Paras 4 to 6 of Stage Ib, but reading right for left and vice versa.

7. Lower the hand, rest it on the knee and exhale as in Para. 4 above.

8. When the lungs feel completely empty, do external retention with uḍḍīyāna bandha for ten to fifteen seconds, or for the same length of time as before (Pl. 104). Then release the grip.

9. Two inhalations (once through each nostril), two exhalations with open nostrils, and two external retentions with uḍḍīyāna bandha complete one cycle of this Stage. Repeat them for ten to fifteen minutes according to your capacity. At the end of the last cycle inhale with open nostrils, then lie in śavāsana (Pl. 182).

Effects of Stages IIIa and IIIb

With the addition of strengthening the abdominal muscles and organs, the effects are similar to those of Stages IIa and IIb.

STAGE IVa

This is a stage for highly advanced students. It is a combination of Stages IIa and IIIa, in which both internal retention with mūla bandha and external retention with uḍḍīyāna bandha are practised alternately.

Technique

1. Sit in any āsana, following the techniques given in Paras 1 to 7 of ujjāyī, Stage V. Exhale (Pl. 96).

2. Bring the right hand to the nostrils as described in Paras 12 to 22 of Ch. 22 on digital prāṇāyāma.

3. Inhale through partially open nostrils, as described in Paras 3 to 5 of Stage Ia above (Pl. 110).

4. When the lungs are full, block the nostrils and do internal retention with mūla bandha for fifteen to twenty seconds (Pl. 69), or for as long as you can, as explained in Para. 3 of Stage IIa (Pl. 145).

5. Lower the right hand and rest it on the knee.

6. Exhale with open nostrils softly, steadily, slowly and smoothly until the lungs feel completely empty.

7. Then do external retention with uḍḍīyāna for ten to fifteen seconds, or for as long as you can (Pl. 104). Finally release the grip.

8. Again repeat the process of inhalation, internal retention with mūla bandha, exhalation and external retention with uḍḍīyāna bandha as stated above.

9. One inhalation, one internal retention with mūla bandha, one exhalation and one external retention with uḍḍīyāna bandha completes one cycle. Repeat them according to your ability. After completing the last cycle, inhale through open nostrils and lie in śavāsana (Pl. 182). If any strain is felt, stop practice for the day.

STAGE IVb

This stage is more strenuous and complicated than the previous one. It combines Stages IIb and IIIb, but with internal retention with mūla bandha and external retention with uḍḍīyāna performed with each in and out breath respectively

Technique

1. Sit in any āsana, following the techniques given in Paras 1 to 7 of ujjāyī, Stage V. Exhale (Pl. 96).

2. Bring the right hand to the nostrils as explained in Paras 12 to 22 of Ch. 22 on digital prāṇāyāma.

3. Inhale, following the techniques given in Paras 3 to 6 of Stage Ib above (Pl. 111).

4. After full inhalation, do internal retention with mūla bandha as in Para. 3 of Stage IIb (Pl. 145).

5. Lower the right hand and exhale as in Para. 4 of Stage IIb.

6. When the lungs feel completely empty, do external retention with uḍḍīyāna for ten to fifteen seconds, or for as long as you can (Pl. 104).

7. Again bring the right hand to the nostrils and inhale through the left as in Para. 6 of Stage IIIb (Pl. 112).

8. When the lungs are full, hold the breath with mūla bandha for the same length of time as in Para. 4 above (Pl. 145).

9. Lower the hand and exhale as in Para. 5 above.

10. When the lungs feel completely empty, do external retention with uḍḍīyāna as in Para. 6 above (Pl. 104). Then release the grip and repeat.

11. Two inhalations (one through the right and another through the left nostril), two internal retentions with mūla bandha, two exhalations with open nostrils, and external retentions with uḍḍīyāna bandha, complete one cycle. Repeat them according to your capacity. After completing the last cycle, inhale normally through open nostrils and lie down in śavāsana (Pl. 182). If any strain is felt, stop prāṇāyāma practice for the day.

Effects of Stages IVa and IVb
These intense stages combine the effects of Stages IIa and IIb, and IIIa and IIIb.

Note
It is possible to combine viloma Prāṇāyāma techniques with those of pratiloma, that is, to introduce pauses during inhalations, exhalations or both. However, such combinations are not recommended since they cause undue strain and reduce the sensitivity of the nasal membranes and the dexterity of the finger-tips.

Table of Pratiloma Prāṇāyāma

Stage		*Pūraka* BNPC	*Pūraka* ANPC	*Antara Kumbhaka* MB	*Rechaka* ON	*Bāhya Kumbhaka* UB
I	A	√			√	
	B		√		√	
II	A	√		15–20 sec	√	
	B		√	15–20 sec	√	
III	A	√			√	10–15 sec
	B		√		√	10–15 sec
IV	A	√		15–20 sec	√	10–15 sec
	B		√	15–20 sec	√	10–15 sec

ANPC = Alternate nostrils partially closed
BNPC = Both nostrils partially closed
MB = Mūla bandha
ON = Open nostrils
UB = Uḍḍīyāna bandha

Chapter 27

Sūrya Bhedana and Chandra Bhedana Prāṇāyāma

SŪRYA BHEDANA PRĀṆĀYĀMA

Sūrya is the sun, and bhid, the root of bhedana, means to pierce or pass through.

In sūrya bhedana prāṇāyāma all inhalations are done through the right nostril and all exhalations through the left. Prāṇic energy in all inhalations is channelled through the pingalā or sūrya nāḍī and in all exhalations through the īḍā or chandra nāḍī.

In sūrya bhedana the flow of breath is digitally controlled and the lungs absorb more energy from the in-breath.

STAGE I

This stage consists of deep inhalation through the right nostril and deep exhalation through the left.

Technique

1. Sit in any āsana following the techniques given in Paras 1 to 7 of ujjāyī, Stage V. Exhale deeply (Pl. 96).

2. Bring the right hand to the nostrils as explained in Paras 12 to 22 of Ch. 22 on digital prāṇāyāma.

3. Block the left nostril completely with the tips of the ring and little fingers, without disturbing the septum. Partially close the right nostril with the right thumb, keeping the inner wall of the outer right nostril parallel to the septum (Pl. 111).

4. Inhale slowly, carefully and deeply through the partially closed right nostril, without using force, until the lungs are completely full.

5. Completely block the right nostril, without disturbing the septum Release the pressure on the left nostril and open it partially (Pl. 112).

6. Exhale slowly, steadily and deeply through the partially open left nostril, till the lungs feel empty.

7. This completes one cycle. Repeat for ten to fifteen minutes, inhale with open nostrils, then lie in śavāsana (Pl. 182).

8. As the practice improves, make the nasal apertures narrower by carefully manipulating the finger-tips to prolong the flow of breath.

STAGE II

This stage is similar to Stage I, with the addition of internal retention with mūla bandha, blocking both nostrils.

Technique

1. Sit in any āsana, following the techniques of Paras 1 to 7 of ujjāyī, Stage V. Exhale deeply (Pl. 96).

2. Inhale through the right nostril, slowly, deeply and fully, following the techniques of Paras 2, 3 and 4 of Stage I (Pl. 111).

3. Then block both nostrils and do internal retention with mūla bandha for fifteen to twenty seconds (Pl. 145), not allowing any air to escape. Gradually increase the length by five seconds. When this becomes stabilised without disturbing the flow and the smoothness of the in and out breaths, lengthen the duration of retention. In this way the sādhaka trains himself to attain his maximum capacity.

4. Now exhale slowly, steadily and deeply through the partially opened left nostril, till the lungs feel completely empty (Pl. 112).

5. This completes one cycle. Repeat for ten to fifteen minutes, inhale with open nostrils, then lie in śavāsana (Pl. 182).

STAGE III

This stage is similar to Stage I, with the addition of external retention with uḍḍīyāna.

Technique

1. Sit in any āsana, following the techniques of Paras 1 to 7 of ujjāyī, Stage V. Exhale whatever breath is in the lungs (Pl. 96).

2. Inhale through the right nostril, slowly, deeply and fully, following the techniques of Paras 2, 3 and 4 of Stage I (Pl. 111).

3. Completely block the right nostril, partially release the left and exhale through it slowly and deeply (Pl. 112), following the techniques given in Paras 5 and 6 of Stage I.

4. When the lungs feel completely empty, block both the nostrils and do external retention with uḍḍīyāna bandha to your capacity without strain (Pl. 146).

5. External retention takes longer to master than the internal one. Hence, gradually increase the duration of external retention by one or two seconds. When this becomes stabilised, continue increasing the length of retention without disturbing the flow and the smoothness of the in and out breaths.

6. This completes one cycle. Repeat for ten to fifteen minutes, inhale with open nostrils, then lie in śavāsana (Pl. 182).

STAGE IV

This stage combines Stages II and III. It is for highly advanced students and should be attempted only after perfecting Stages II and III.

Technique

1. Sit in any āsana, following the techniques of Paras 1 to 7 of ujjāyī, Stage V. Exhale whatever breath is in the lungs (Pl. 96).

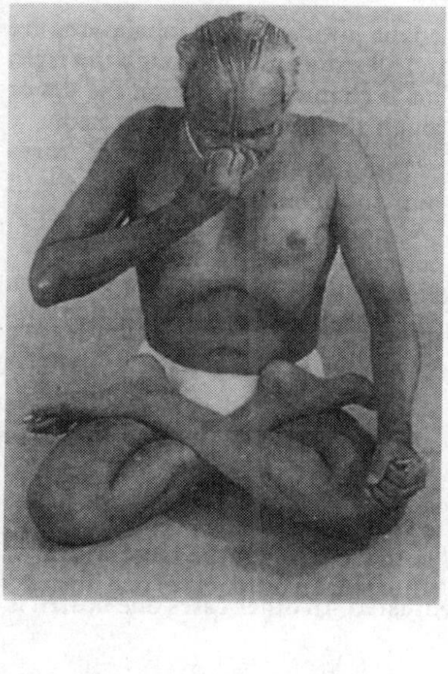

Pl. 146

2. Inhale, following the techniques given in Paras 2 and 3 of Stage II (Pl. 111), ending with mūla bandha (Pl. 145).

3. Then exhale, following the techniques given in Paras 3 and 4 of Stage III (Pl. 112) and ending with uḍḍiyāna bandha (Pl. 146).

4. Do retentions at the end of each inhalation as well as each exhalation, starting with shorter retentions and gradually increasing their length as the lung capacity develops. Do not exceed eight to ten seconds in uḍḍīyāna bandha.

5. This completes one cycle. Practise as many cycles as you comfortably can without strain, or for ten to fifteen minutes. Inhale with open nostrils, then lie in śavāsana (Pl. 182).

Effects of Sūrya Bhedana Prāṇāyāma
This increases heat in the body and digestive power. It soothes and invigorates the nerves and cleanses the sinuses. It is good for persons suffering from low blood pressure.

CHANDRA BHEDANA PRĀNĀYĀMA

This prāṇāyāma has been described in *Yoga Chūdāmaṇi Upaniṣad* (95–97) without mentioning the name chandra bhedana, but giving only the method.

Chandra is the moon. In chandra bhedana prāṇāyāma all inhalations are done through the left nostril (Pl. 112) and all exhalations through the right (Pl. 111). Prāṇic energy in all inhalations is channelled through the iḍā or chandra nāḍī. All exhalations pass through the pingalā or sūrya nāḍī.

Chandra bhedana is done in four stages, similar to those of sūrya bhedana.

Technique
Follow the same techniques as are given in all the stages of sūrya bhedana, reading the word 'right' for 'left' and vice versa. Complete the practice with śavāsana (Pl. 182).

Effects
The effects are similar to those of sūrya bhedana, except that this prāṇāyāma cools the system.

Notes for Sūrya and Chandra Bhedana Prāṇāyāma
1. Sometimes the passages of the two nostrils have not the same width. In that case the digital pressure has to be adjusted. In other cases one nostril is

all but completely blocked (for example, if there is a polyp or if the nose has been fractured), while the other is clear. If this happens, inhale through the clear side and exhale as best as you can through the blocked side. In course of time, due to digital manipulation, the blocked nostril becomes clear and inhalation through it becomes possible.

2. If the cartilage of the nasal bone is not straight, learn to manipulate the cartilage of the septum up and towards the nasal bone. Then the blocked passage opens and digital prāṇāyāma is possible (Pls 140 and 141).

3. Never perform sūrya bhedana and chandra bhedana prāṇāyāma on the same day.

4. In both prāṇāyāmas interrupted (viloma) breathing may be incorporated, bringing the number of possible stages to sixteen. The possible number of permutations and combinations is however enormous:

Stage V: Interrupted inhalation, long exhalation
VI: Long inhalation, interrupted exhalation
VII: Interrupted inhalation, interrupted exhalation
VIII: Interrupted inhalation, internal retention, long exhalation
IX: Long inhalation, internal retention, interrupted exhalation
X: Interrupted inhalation, internal retention, interrupted exhalation
XI: Interrupted inhalation, long exhalation, external retention
XII: Long inhalation, interrupted exhalation, external retention
XIII: Interrupted inhalation, interrupted exhalation, external retention
XIV: Interrupted inhalation, internal retention, long exhalation, external retention
XV: Long inhalation, internal retention, interrupted exhalation, external retention
XVI: Interrupted inhalation, internal retention, interrupted exhalation, external retention

Table of Sūrya Bhedana Prāṇāyāma

Stage	*Pūraka* *RN*	*Antara Kumbhaka* *MB*	*Rechaka* *LN*	*Bāhya Kumbhaka* *UB*
I	√		√	
II	√	15–20 sec	√	
III	√		√	ALAP
IV	√	15–20 sec	√	8–10 sec

Table of Chandra Bhedana Prāṇāyāma

Stage	*Pūraka* *LN*	*Antara Kumbhaka* *MB*	*Rechaka* *RN*	*Bāhya Kumbhaka* *UB*
I	√		√	
II	√	15–20 sec	√	
III	√		√	ALAP
IV	√	15–20 sec	√	8–10 sec

ALAP = As long as possible
LN = Left nostril
MB = Mūla bandha
RN = Right nostril
UB = Uḍḍiyāna bandha

Chapter 28

Nāḍī Śodhana Prāṇāyāma

Nāḍī is a tubular organ for the passage of prāṇa or energy carrying cosmic, vital, seminal and other energies, as well as sensation, intelligence and consciousness in the causal, subtle and physical bodies (see Ch. 5 for details). Śodhana means purifying or cleansing. The term nāḍī śodhana means the purification of the nerves. A slight obstruction in the nervous system may cause great discomfort and even paralyse a limb or organ.

The *Haṭha Yoga Pradīpikā* (II, 6–9, 19–20), *Śiva Saṁhitā* (III, 24, 25), *Gheraṇḍa Saṁhitā* (V, 49–52) and *Yoga Chūḍāmaṇi Upsaniṣad* (V. 98–100) describe a type of Prāṇāyāma which cleanses the nāḍīs. The texts mention the technique and describe its beneficial effects, specifically stating that they are 'due to cleansing of the nāḍīs' ('nāḍī śodhanāt').

Though all Yoga texts describe various types of prāṇāyāma by their titles, yet none mention the name of chandra bhedana or nāḍī śodhana prāṇāyāma.

This prāṇāyāma, described in detail below, combines the technique of exhalation (rechaka) as in anuloma, and of inhalation (pūraka) as in pratiloma prāṇāyāma. It also has another unique feature: The cycle of sūrya bhedana prāṇāyāma consists of inhalation through the right nostril and exhalation through the left, while in chandra bhedana inhalation is through the left nostril and exhalation through the right. Nāḍī śodhana prāṇāyāma combines both these into one cycle. The process has been described in the texts quoted above.

The brain is divided into two hemispheres, the left controlling the right side of the body, and the right the left. Again, it is said that the brain has two parts, the more primitive or back brain at the base of the skull, which is considered to be the contemplative brain, the seat of wisdom, while the frontal one is the active and calculating brain that deals with the external world.

The yogis realised the various disparities in the structures of the brain, lungs and other parts of the body. They adopted āsanas for even development, equal extension and attention to both sides of the body. They discovered and introduced nāḍī śodhana prāṇāyāma for the prāṇa of the in and out breaths to pass through each nostril in turn, thus revitalising both the hemispheres of the brain as well as the front and the back. By thus changing the sides for inhalation and exhalation, the energy reaches the remotest parts of the body and brain through the nāḍīs criss-crossing the chakras. The sādhaka gains the secret of even and balanced action in all the quarters of the brain, and thus experiences peace, poise and harmony.

Nāḍī śodhana prāṇāyāma requires constant meticulous attention and firm determination. Its energies have to be channelled into disciplining the breath with refinement and sensibility, so that breath, body and mind can be spiritualised.

Nāḍī śodhana prāṇāyāma is one of delicate adjustments. The brain and the fingers must learn to act together in channelling the in and out breaths while in constant communication with each other. The brain should not be dull, hard and insensitive, otherwise the fingers will be rough, broad and not sensitive enough to refine the flow of breath. The brain and the fingers must be alert to perceive any alteration in the rhythm or disturbance in the flow of breath. This study helps to adjust the fingers on the outer nostrils and make them passive, thus allowing the correct amount of breath to pass in and out. If the fingers lose their sensitivity, the brain sends a message to recall them to attention. If the brain is inattentive, the fingers lose their awareness and allow a larger volume of breath to flow through the nostrils, which alerts the brain once more.

During the processes of inhalation and exhalation the sound, resonance and flow of breath have to be constantly measured and adjusted with minute attention and delicate manipulation of the top and bottom ends of the nasal passages. This helps the sādhaka to trace the exact path of the flow of breath through the nostrils and to focus attention on balancing the finger-tips correctly on the relevant locations. If the sound is rough, then the brain is active elsewhere and the finger-tips insensitive. If the breath is smooth, the brain is quiet and watchful, and the finger-tips are sensitive. Feel the cool, moist fragrance of the inhalation and the hot exhalation, which is without fragrance. This sensitivity should be developed, as without it the practice of Prāṇāyāma is mechanical and ineffective.

Nāḍī śodhana prāṇāyāma, therefore, is the most difficult, complex and refined of all prāṇāyāmas. It is the ultimate in sensitive self-observation and control. When refined to its subtlest level it takes one to the innermost self. Hence this prāṇāyāma, by its fine concentration and minute attention leads first to dhāraṇā, and then to dhyāna.

Do not attempt nāḍī śodhana until your nasal membranes develop sensitivity and your fingers dexterity by practising the Prāṇāyāmas described earlier.

The inner corners of the tips of the fingers are used during inhalation to channel the in-breath, and the outer corners are used during exhalation to channel the out-breath. However, do not release the pressure on the outer corners during inhalation and on the inner corners during exhalation (see Paras 28 to 30 of Ch. 22 on digital prāṇāyāma (Pl. 139).

The fingers are kept on the nostrils throughout.

In the advanced stages of nāḍī śodhana prāṇāyama, kumbhakas (internal as well as external retentions) and bandhās are introduced.

As nāḍī śodhana is a highly contemplative prāṇāyāma, pay special attention to lowering the head more by gently pulling the nose downwards; do not disturb the fingers on the nostrils, nor lose contact with the nasal bone. While the head is being lowered, the chest caves in unconsciously. Do not allow this to happen. Remain alert and move the chest up as the head comes down.

This further lowering of the head will make the sādhaka realise whether or not the lungs are filled to the brim. If the tops of both feel empty, draw in more breath to fill them completely.

When the head is gently brought down and the chest is lifted up, the calculative frontal brain becomes silent and the contemplative back brain becomes active.

During internal retention, if the sādhaka feels a disturbance in the state of silence it means that his capacity for retention is over, or the chin has moved up, or some breath has escaped unnoticed through the blocked nostrils. If any of these are felt, draw the breath in again, lower the head further and then hold the breath. This makes the sādhaka's body dynamic and his mind contemplative. His pride is humbled and his intellect surrenders to his Self (Ātmā). On the other hand, external retention done with uḍḍīyāna makes the sādhaka's body as well as his mind dynamic, vibrant and alert, whereas external retention without uḍḍīyanā makes both of them quiet and contemplative.

STAGE Ia

Here both nostrils are kept partially open in inhalation and exhalation.

Technique

1. Sit in any āsana, following the techniques given in Paras 1 to 7 of ujjāyī, Stage V.

2. Bring the right hand to the nostrils as explained in Paras 12 to 22 of Ch. 22 on digital prāṇāyāma, and narrow both the nasal passages with the thumb, ring and little fingers (Pl. 110). Exhale completely through the narrowly open, but controlled nostrils.

3. Now inhale, but do not disturb the width of the passages; keep the septum and the fingers stable to prevent the head from tilting.

4. Maintain an even flow of breath in both nostrils, synchronising it with the movement of the chest. The breath should be soft, slow and smooth. Fill the lungs to the brim.

5. Then hold the breath for a second or two in order to adjust the fingers for exhalation.

6. Exhale softly, slowly and smoothly, maintaining an even rhythm. Synchronise the flow of the exhalation with release of the extension and expansion of the rib-cage. In other words, do not allow the chest to collapse suddenly.

7. As practice improves, narrow the passages more and more, so that the breath flows finer and finer. The narrower the passages the better the control of the breath.

8. One inhalation and one exhalation completes one cycle. Repeat for ten to fifteen minutes and end with an in-breath. Lower the hand, raise the head and then lie in śavāsana (Pl. 182).

Effects

This exhilarating prāṇāyāma trains the fingers and nasal membranes to become more and more sensitive for finer adjustment. The mind is engaged in concentrating on the fingers, the nasal passages and the breath, and so becomes one-pointed.

STAGE Ib

This stage is a combination of sūrya bhedana and chandra bhedana prāṇāyāma, without retentions. Here, the in and out breaths are done through alternate nostrils, which are digitally controlled.

Technique

1. Sit in any āsana, following the techniques given in Paras 1 to 7 of ujjāyi, Stage V.

2. Bring the right hand to the nostrils as explained in Paras 12 to 22 of Ch. 22 on digital prāṇāyāma.

3. Block the left nostril completely, without disturbing the septum or the passage on the right. Narrow the right nostril, bringing its outer portion closer towards the septum, without disturbing the position of the nose (Pl. 111).

4. Exhale through the right nostril.

5. Inhale through it slowly and steadily, without disturbing the width of its passage. Keep the septum and the fingers stable. Do not allow any breath to enter through the left nostril.

6. Maintain a fine flow of breath through the right nostril, synchronising it with the movements of the chest.

7. When the lungs are full, block the right nostril completely, without moving the septum or the left nostril.

8. Hold the breath for a second or two to prepare and adjust the fingers for exhalation.

9. Exhale slowly and steadily through the left nostril, synchronising the flow of out-breath with the gradual release of the extension and expansion of the rib-cage (Pl. 112).

10. When the lungs feel completely empty, hold the breath for a second to prepare and adjust the fingers for inhalation through the left nostril.

11. Block the right nasal passage without disturbing the septum or the passage on the left, and narrow the left passage (Pl. 112).

12. Now inhale through the left nostril as described in Paras 4 and 6 above, but reading the word 'right' for 'left' and vice versa.

13. When the lungs are full, block the left nostril completely, without disturbing the septum or the passage on the right.

14. Hold the breath for a second or two as in Para. 8 above.

15. Exhale through the right nostril (Pl. 111) as described in Para. 9 above. See that no breath escapes through the left nostril.

16. When the lungs feel completely empty, hold the breath for a second or two, to prepare and re-adjust the fingers for inhalation, then repeat from Para. 3 above.

17. The breath sequence is as follows: (a) exhale whatever breath is in the lungs through the right nostril; (b) breathe in through the right nostril; (c) out through the left; (d) in through the left; (e) out through the right; (f) in through the right; (g) out through the left, and so on.

18. The cycle commences at (b) and ends at (e). Repeat for ten to fifteen minutes, ending with inhalation through the right nostril. Then lie in śavāsana (Pl. 182).

Effects

Since the work of delicate fingering and narrowing of passages requires concentration, the practice of this stage prepares the sādhaka for dhāranā

STAGE IIa

This stage is similar to stage Ia, with the addition of internal retention with mūla bandha.

Technique

1. Sit in any āsana, following the techniques given in Paras 1 to 7 of ujjāyī, Stage V.

2. Inhale, following the techniques given in Paras 2 to 4 of Stage Ia (Pl. 110).

3. Block both nostrils completely to prevent escape of breath, and hold the breath for twenty seconds with mūla bandha (Pl. 145).

4. Re-adjust the fingers for exhalation following the technique given in Para. 6 of Stage Ia to empty the lungs.

5. If the flow, rhythm or timings for in and out breaths are disturbed, it means you have exceeded your capacity, or have allowed breath to escape during retention. If the former reduce the time of retention, if the latter make sure that both nostrils are properly blocked during retention.

6. One inhalation, one internal retention and one exhalation completes one cycle. Repeat for ten to fifteen minutes, ending with inhalation. Lower the hand, raise the head and lie in śavāsana (Pl. 182).

STAGE IIb

This stage is similar to Stage Ib, with the addition of internal retention and mūla bandha.

Technique

1. Sit in any āsana, following the techniques given in Paras 1 to 7 of ujjāyī, Stage V.

2. Bring the right hand to the nostrils as described in Paras 12 to 22 of Ch. 22 on digital prāṇāyāma.

3. Block the left nostril. Partially open the right, make it as narrow as you can (Pl. 111), and inhale through it, following all the instructions given in Paras 3 to 6 of Stage Ib.

4. When the lungs are full, block both nostrils and hold the breath with mūla bandha for twenty seconds (Pl. 145).

5. Adjust the fingers for exhalation through the left nostril. Block the right nostril, partially open the left and make the passage as narrow as you can (Pl. 112).

6. Exhale through the left nostril and empty the lungs as described in Para. 9 of Stage Ib. No breath should escape through the right nostril.

7. When the lungs feel completely empty, hold the breath and proceed as in Paras 10 to 11 of Stage Ib to prepare for inhalation through the left nostril.

8. Now inhale through the left nostril as described in Paras 3 to 5 above, but reading the word 'right' for 'left' and vice versa.

9. When the lungs are full, block both nostrils and hold the breath as in Para. 4 above (Pl. 145).

10. Adjust the fingers for exhalation through the right nostril, following the techniques given in Para. 5 above, but reading the word 'right' for 'left' and vice versa.

11. Exhale through the right nostril as in Para. 9 of Stage Ib. No breath should escape through the left nostril.

12. When the lungs feel completely empty, hold the breath for a few seconds, re-adjust the fingers, then repeat from Para. 3 above.

13. The breath sequence is as follows: (a) exhale whatever breath is in the lungs through the right nostril; (b) breathe in through the right nostril; (c) internal retention with mūla bandha; (d) breathe out through the left nostril; (e) in through the left; (f) internal retention with mūla bandha; (g) breathe out through the right nostril; (h) in through the right and so on.

14. The cycle commences at (b) and ends at (g). Repeat for ten to fifteen minutes, ending with an in-breath through the right. Then lie in śavāsana (Pl. 182).

Effects
This stage prepares the sādhaka for dhyāna.

STAGE IIIa

This stage is similar to Stage Ia, with the addition of external retention with uḍḍīyāna.

Technique

1. Sit in any āsana, following the techniques given in Paras 1 to 7 of ujjāyī, Stage V.

2. Bring the right hand to the nostrils and narrow both the nasal passages with the thumb, ring and little fingers and exhale through both nostrils narrowly closed (Pl. 110).

3. Inhale, following the techniques of Paras 3 and 4 of Stage Ia above.

4. Then exhale, following the techniques of Paras 5 and 6 of Stage Ia.

5. When the lungs feel empty, block both nostrils and do external retention with uḍḍīyāna for fifteen seconds, or for as long as you can (Pl. 146).

6. Release the uḍḍīyāna grip, readjust the fingers and follow the processes of inhalation and exhalation as described in Paras 3 and 4 above. Then repeat an external retention with uḍḍīyāna.

7. Here the sequence of breath is: (a) exhale deeply through both nostrils; (b) breathe in through both passages; (c) out through both; (d) external retention with uḍḍīyāna; (e) breathe in through both passages; (f) out through both; (g) external retention with uḍḍīyāna; and so on.

8. One inhalation, one exhalation and one external retention with uḍḍīyāna completes one cycle of this stage. Repeat for ten to fifteen minutes, ending with inhalation. Then lie down in śavāsana (Pl. 182).

STAGE IIIb

This stage is similar to Stage Ib, with the addition of external retention with uḍḍīyāna.

Technique

1. Sit in any āsana, following the techniques given in Paras 1 to 7 of ujjāyī, Stage V.

2. Bring the right hand to the nostrils as explained before and inhale, following the techniques given in Paras 3 to 6 of Stage Ib (Pl. 111).

3. When the lungs are full, block the right nostril and hold the breath for a second as explained in Paras 7 and 8 of Stage Ib.

4. Exhale through the left nostril as described in Para. 9 of Stage Ib (Pl. 112). No breath should escape through the right nostril.

5. When the lungs feel empty, block both nostrils and do external retention with uḍḍīyāna for fifteen seconds, or for as long as you can (Pl. 146).

6. Then release the uḍḍīyāna grip, block the right nostril, and readjust the fingers for inhalation through the left (Pl. 112).

7. Narrow the passage of the left nostril and inhale slowly, softly and smoothly.

8. When the lungs are full, readjust the fingers. Block the left nostril and exhale through the right (Pl. 111).

9. When the lungs feel empty, block both nostrils, and do external retention with uḍḍīyāna for fifteen seconds, or for the same length of time as before (Pl. 146). Then release the uḍḍīyāna grip.

10. Readjust the fingers for inhalation through the right nostril, blocking the left completely and repeat the sequence.

11. The breath sequence is as follows: (a) exhale deeply through the right nostril; (b) breathe in through the right nostril; (c) out through the left; (d) external retention with uḍḍīyāna; (e) breathe in through the left; (f) out through the right; (g) external retention with uḍḍīyāna; (h) breathe in through the right, and so on.

12. The cycle starts at (b) and ends at (g). Repeat for ten to fifteen minutes, starting with exhalation and ending with inhalation through the right nostril. Then lie down in śavāsana (Pl. 182).

Effects

Due to the uḍḍīyāna grip, the abdominal organs are revitalised, and the apāna vāyu unites with the prāṇa vāyu to improve the assimilation of food and distribution of energy throughout the body.

STAGE IVa

This is an advanced prāṇāyāma. It combines Stages IIa and IIIa.

Technique

1. Sit in any āsana following the techniques given in Paras 1 to 4 of Stage Ia above.

2. When the lungs are completely full, block both nostrils and do internal retention with mūla bandha for twenty seconds (Pl. 145).

3. Readjust the fingers for exhalation, and exhale following the technique given in Para. 6 of Stage Ia.

4. When the lungs feel empty, block both nostrils. Do external retention with uḍḍīyāna for fifteen seconds (Pl. 146).

5. Then release the uḍḍīyāna grip and inhale as in Para. 1.

6. The breath sequence is as follows: (a) exhale through both nostrils; (b) breathe in through both nostrils; (c) internal retention with mūla bandha; (d) breathe out through both nostrils; (e) external retention with uḍḍīyāna; (f) breathe in through both nostrils; and so on.

7. Here the cycle commences at (b) and ends at (e). Repeat for ten to fifteen minutes, ending with inhalation. Then lie in śavāsana (Pl. 182).

STAGE IVb

This is the most advanced prāṇāyāma in the series. It is a combination of Stages IIb and IIIb with retention after each in and out breath.

Technique

1. Sit in any āsana following the techniques given in Paras 1 to 6 of Stage Ib, keeping the left nostril blocked (Pl. 111).

2. When the lungs are completely full, block both nostrils and do internal retention with mūla bandha for twenty, twenty-five or thirty seconds (Pl. 145).

3. Readjust the fingers for exhalation, block the right nostril and keep the left narrow (Pl. 112). Exhale through the left nostril, making the passage as narrow as you can, following the technique of Para. 9 of Stage Ib.

4. When the lungs feel empty, block both nostrils and do external retention with uḍḍīyāna for fifteen seconds (Pl. 146). Then release the uḍḍīyāna grip, and readjust the fingers for inhalation.

5. Now block the right nostril and narrow the left (Pl. 112). Inhale slowly, softly and smoothly through the left.

6. When the lungs are completely full, block both nostrils and do internal retention with mūla bandha for twenty to thirty seconds (Pl. 145).

7. Prepare for exhalation and readjust the fingers. Block the left nostril. Release the grip of the thumb-tip and narrow the right nostril (Pl. 111). Exhale until the lungs are empty.

8. When the lungs feel empty, block both nostrils and do external retention and uḍḍīyāna for fifteen seconds (Pl. 146). Then release the uḍḍīyāna grip and readjust the fingers for inhalation.

9. Block the left nostril and inhale through the right as described in Para. 1 above, and continue in the same way.

10. The breath sequence is: (a) exhale through the right nostril; (b) breathe in through the right nostril; (c) internal retention with mūla bandha; (d) breathe out through the left nostril; (e) external retention with uḍḍīyāna; (f) in through the left nostril; (g) internal retention with mūla bandha; (h) out through the right nostril; (i) external retention with uḍḍīyāna; (j) in through the right nostril, and so on.

11. The cycle in this stage commences at (b) and ends with (i). Repeat for ten to fifteen minutes, ending with inhalation through the right nostril. Then lie down in śavāsana (Pl. 182).

Effects

The practice of mūla and uḍḍīyāna bandhās during retentions cleanses and strengthens the sādhaka's nerves to withstand the vicissitudes of life and prepares him for dhyāna.

In nāḍī śodhana prāṇāyāma, due to the deep penetration of prāṇa, the blood receives a larger supply of oxygen than in other types of prāṇāyāma. The nerves are calmed and purified, and the mind becomes still and lucid.

Its practice keeps the body warm, destroys diseases, gives strength and brings serenity.

The vital energy drawn in from the cosmic energy through inhalation passes close to vital chakras and feeds the glands. The respiratory control centre of the brain is stimulated and becomes fresh, clear and tranquil. The light of intelligence is lit simultaneously in the brain as well as in the mind. This leads to right living, right thinking, quick action and sound judgement.

Table of Nāḍī Śodhana Prāṇāyāma

Stage		Pūraka BNPC	Antara Kumbhaka MB	Rechaka BNPC	Bāhya Kumbhaka UB
I	A	√		√	
II	A	√	20 sec	√	
III	A	√		√	15 sec
IV	A	√	20 sec	√	15 sec

Stage		Pūraka RN	AK	Rechaka LN	BK	Pūraka LN	AK	Rechaka RN	BK
I	B	√		√		√		√	
II	B	√	20 sec	√		√	20 sec	√	
III	B	√		√	15 sec	√		√	15 sec
IV	B	√	20 sec	√	15 sec	√	20 sec	√	15 sec

AK = Antara kumbhaka
BK = Bāhya kumbhaka
BNPC = Both nostrils partially closed
LN = Left nostril
MB = Mūla bandha
RN = Right nostril
UB = Uḍḍīyāna bandha

Part Two

Freedom and Beatitude

Chapter 29

Dhyāna (Meditation)

1. Dhyāna means absorption. It is the art of self-study, reflection, keen observation, or the search for the Infinite within. It is the observation of the physical processes of the body, study of mental states and profound contemplation. It means looking inwards to one's innermost being. Dhyāna is the discovery of the Self.

2. When the powers of the intellect and the heart are harmoniously blended, this is dhyāna. All creativity proceeds from it, and its good and beautiful results benefit mankind.

3. Dhyāna is like deep sleep, but with a difference. The serenity of deep sleep comes as a result of unconsciously forgetting one's identity and individuality, whereas meditation brings serenity which is alert and conscious throughout. The sādhaka remains a witness (sākṣī) to all activities. Chronological and psychological time have no existence in deep sleep or in total absorption. In sleep the body and mind recover from wear and tear and feel fresh upon waking. In meditation the sādhaka experiences illumination.

4. Dhyāna is the full integration of the contemplator, the act of contemplation and the object contemplated upon becoming one. The distinction between the knower, the instrument of knowledge and the object known vanishes. The sādhaka becomes vibrant, alert and poised. He becomes free from hunger, thirst, sleep and sex as well as from desire, anger, greed, infatuation, pride and envy. He is unassailable by the dualities of body and mind, or mind and self. His vision reflects his true self like a well-polished mirror. This is Ātma-Darśana, the reflection of the Soul.

5. Jesus said that man does not live by bread alone, but by every word that proceeds out of the mouth of God. Pondering upon the meaning of life, man is convinced that there dwells within his soul a force or light far greater than himself. Yet in his walk of life he is beset by many cares and doubts. Being caught in the environment of artificial civilisation he develops a false sense of values. His words and actions run counter to his thoughts. He is bewildered by these contradictions. He realises that life is full of opposites – pain and pleasure, sorrow and joy, conflict and peace. Seeing these

polarities, he strives to attain a balance between them and to find a state of stability so that he can experience freedom from pain, sorrow and conflict. In his search he discovers the three noble ways of word (jñāna), work (karma) and worship (bhakti), which teach him that his inner light is the only guide leading to mastery over his own life. To reach this inner light he turns to meditation or dyhāna.

6. To have a clear notion of the true natures of man, of the world and of God, the sādhaka should study the sacred books (Śāstras). Then he can distinguish the real from the unreal. Knowledge of these three truths (tattva traya) – the soul (chit), the world (achit) and God (Īśvara) – is essential for him who seeks liberation. Such knowledge gives him insight into life's problems and their solution, and strengthens his spiritual sādhana. Yet knowledge acquired by reading alone will not lead to liberation. It is by having courage and unshakable faith in the teachings contained in the sacred books and by putting them into practice till they become a part of his daily life that the sādhaka gains freedom from the domination of his senses. Knowledge of the sacred books and sādhana are the two wings by which the sādhaka flies towards liberation.

7. Man is drawn between two paths: one drags him downwards towards fulfilment of voluptuous desires and sense gratifications, leading to bondage and destruction; the other guides him upwards towards purity and realisation of his inner Self. Desires fog his mind and veil his true Self. It is the mind alone which leads to bondage or to liberation. It is his reason or intelligence which either controls his mind or allows itself to be dominated.

8. An untrained mind flies aimlessly in all directions. The practice of meditation brings it to a state of stability and then directs it to proceed from imperfect knowledge to perfection. The sādhaka's mind and intelligence work as an integrated team led by his will-power. He finds harmony between his thoughts, speech and actions. His stilled mind and intelligence burn like a lamp in a windless place with simplicity, innocence and illumination.

9. Man has great potentialities that lie dormant within him. His body and mind are like fallow land lying untilled and unsown. A wise farmer ploughs his land (kśetra), provides it with water and fertiliser, plants the best seeds, carefully tends the crops and ultimately reaps a good harvest. To the sādhaka, his own body, mind and intellect are the field which he ploughs with energy and right action. He sows with the finest seeds of knowledge, waters it with devotion and tends them with unrelenting spiritual discipline to reap the harvest of harmony and peace. He then becomes the wise owner (kśetrajna) of his field, and his body becomes a sacred place. The

germination of the seeds of good thoughts (savichāra), planted by sound logic (savitarka), brings clarity to his mind and wisdom to his intellect (sāsmita). He becomes an abode of joy (ānanda) as his whole being is filled with the Lord.

10. The journey to the moon and outer space demanded years of rigorous training and discipline, deep study, research and preparation. The inward journey of man to reach his inner Self demands the same type of relentless effort. Years of discipline and long uninterrupted practice of the moral and ethical principles of yama and niyama, training of the body by āsanas and prāṇāyāma, restraint of the senses by pratyāhāra and dhāraṇā, ensure the growth of the mind and of inner awareness – dhyāna and samādhi.

11. Dhāraṇā (derived from the root dhṛ, meaning to hold, or concentration) is like a lamp which is covered and does not light up the area outside. When the cover is removed, the lamp lights up the whole area. This is dhyāna, which is the expansion of consciousness. Then the sādhaka acquires a unified mind and maintains a dynamic unfading awareness in its pristine purity. Like oil in seeds and fragrance in flowers, the soul of man permeates his whole body.

12. The lotus is symbolic of meditation. It symbolises purity. Its quiet beauty has given it a prime place in Indian religious thought. It is connected with most of the Hindu deities and their seats in the chakras. The stage of meditation is like that of a lotus bud hiding its inner beauty while awaiting transformation into a full blown lotus. As the bud opens to reveal its resplendent beauty, so also the sādhaka's inner light is transformed and transfigured by meditation. He becomes an enlightened soul (siddha) and an inspired sage. He lives in the eternal now – the present, without yesterdays and tomorrows.

13. This state of the sādhaka is one of passivity known as manolaya (manas meaning mind, and laya, meaning absorption or merging). He has fully marshalled his intelligence (prajñā) and energy (prāṇa) to prevent the intrusion of external thoughts. His state is full of dynamic alertness. When both the internal and external thoughts are stilled and silenced, there is no waste of physical, mental or intellectual energy.

14. Dhyāna is a subjective experience of an objective state. It is difficult to describe the experience in words, for words are inadequate to do so. The delight experienced at the first bite of a delicious mango is indescribable. So it is with meditation. In meditation there is no seeking or searching, as the soul and goal have become one. The nectar of infinity must be tasted, the abundant grace of the Lord within must be experienced. Then the

individual soul (jīvātmā) becomes one with the Universal Soul (Paramātmā). The sādhaka experiences the fullness sung by the *Upanisads:* That is full; this is full. Fullness comes out of fullness. Even after fullness is taken from the full, fullness yet remains.

SABĪJA OR SAGARBHA DHYĀNA

15. In meditation chanting of mantras is sometimes given to the beginner to steady his wandering mind and to keep him away from worldly desires. At first the mantra has to be recited aloud, then it is said mentally; lastly comes silence. This is known as sabīja or sagarbha dhyāna (bīja meaning seed, garbha meaning embryo). Sitting in meditation without reciting mantras is known as nirbīja or agarbha dhyāna. (The prefixes 'nir' and 'a' denote the absence of something, and mean without, see Ch. 17.)

16. Before proceeding to the techniques of dhyāna, one should be careful to differentiate between the emptiness and tranquillity of the senses on the one hand, and the illumination and serenity of the spirit on the other. Meditation (dhyāna) has three categories: sāttvic, rājasic and tāmasic. In the Uttara Kāṇḍa of the epic *Rāmāyāna* it is told that King Rāvaṇa and his two brothers Kumbhakarṇa and Vibhīṣaṇa spent many years in acquiring sacred knowledge. Kumbhakarṇa's effort made him fall into a death-like torpor, for his meditation had been tāmasic. Rāvaṇa became engulfed in amorous pursuits and ambitions, for his had been rājasic. Only Vibhīṣaṇa remained truthful and righteous and abstained from sin, for his meditation had been sāttvic.

Technique

1. Meditation is the technique of inter-penetrating the five sheaths (kośas) of the Sādhaka to blend them into one harmonious whole.

2. The body is known as the city of Brahmā (Brahmapuri) with nine gates. These gates are the eyes, ears, nostrils, mouth, anus and the reproductive organ. Some add the navel and the crown of the head and say that the body has eleven gates. All these have to be closed in meditation. The city is controlled by the ten winds (vāyus), five organs of perception (jñānendriyas), five organs of action (karmendriyas) and seven chakras or inner chambers. As pearls are strung together on a thread to make a necklace, so have the chakras to be connected to the self to make an integrated person.

3. In meditation, the brain has to be well balanced in relation to the spine. Any unevenness in its position disturbs the quietness of meditation. The energies of the left and the right hemispheres of the brain have to be brought to the centre. The thinking activity of the brain ceases. Just as one

withdraws energy from a particular limb or part of the body to make it passive, so also the flow of energy to the brain must be reduced and directed towards the heart – the seat of the soul. The key to the technique of meditation lies in keeping the brain as a passive observer.

4. The various preparatory techniques of yama, niyama, āsana and prāṇāyāma mould the body and mind, pacify and balance them. In a steady and stable posture, free from physical and mental disturbances, an even circulation of arterial and venous blood, lymphatic and cerebro-spinal fluid is maintained through the head and spinal column. Stimulation is kept minimal and as symmetrical as possible. This evenness of circulation and stimulation allows the brain and mind to attain a unification of knowledge and experience.

5. The brain is divided into three main portions: the cerebral cortex, the hypothalamus and the cerebellum. The cerebral cortex functions in the process of thinking, speech, memory and imagination. The hypothalamus regulates the activities of the internal organs and imprints emotional reactions of pleasure and pain, joy and sorrow, contentment and disappointment. The cerebellum is the centre of muscular co-ordination. The back brain is regarded as that which functions in meditation; it is the seat of wisdom and clarity.

6. The art of sitting correctly and silently is essential to achieve physical and mental harmony while practising meditation.

7. Any comfortable position may be assumed for sitting, though padmāsana (Pl. 13) is ideal.

Alignment of the Body

8. Without performing the jālandhara bandha, follow correctly the instructions given in Ch. 11 on the Art of Sitting.

9. Raise the front and back portions of the body evenly, attentively and rhythmically, without jerking.

10. Keep the spine erect and the chest lifted up. This slows down the flow of breath, lessens the activity of the brain and leads to the cessation of all thoughts.

11. Keep the body alert, with razor-sharp awareness. Keep the brain passive, sensitive and silent, like the thin end of a leaf, which shakes even in a gentle breeze.

Pl. 147

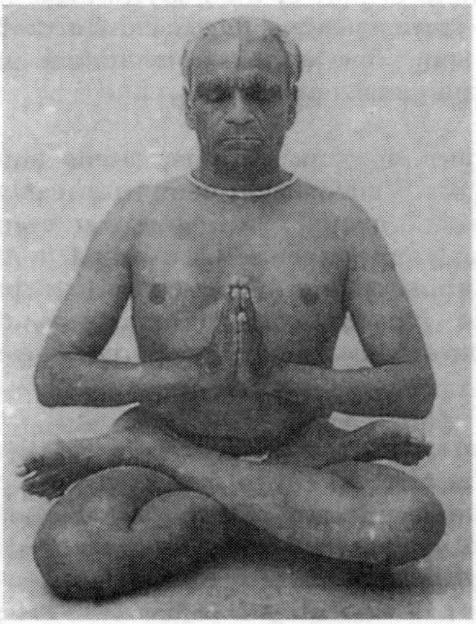

Pl. 148

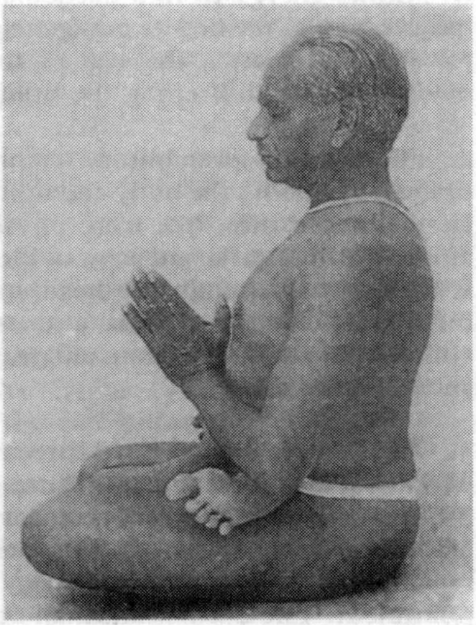

12. Collapse of the body brings intellectual dullness and a distracted mind disturbs the steadiness of the body. Avoid both.

The Head

13. Keep the crown of the head parallel to the ceiling without tilting the head to the right or the left, forwards or backwards, up or down.

14. If the head is down, the sādhaka is brooding on the past, the mind is dull and tāmasic. If it moves up, he is wandering in the future, which is rājasic. When the head is held level, he is in the present, and this is a pure (sāttvic) state of mind.

Eyes and Ears

15. Close the eyes and look within. Shut your ears to outward sounds. Listen to the inner vibrations and follow them until they merge in their source. Any absent-mindedness or lack of awareness in the eyes and ears creates fluctuations in the mind. The closure of the eyes and ears directs the sādhaka to meditate upon Him who is verily the eye of the eye, the ear of the ear, the speech of speech, the mind of the mind and the life of life.

16. Flex the arms at the elbows, raise the hands and fold the palms in front of the chest with the thumbs pointing towards the sternum. This is called ātmāñjali or hṛdayāñjali mudrā (Pls: front view 147, and side view 148).

17. Intelligence oscillating between the head and the heart creates multiple thoughts. When the mind oscillates, press the palms to bring back the attention of the mind on the Self. If the pressure of the palms becomes loose, it is a sign that the mind is wandering. Again join them firmly to recollect the Self.

18. Dhyāna is the integration of the body, mind, intelligence, will, consciousness, ego and the self. The body is the external layer of the mind, mind of the intelligence, intelligence of the will, will of consciousness, consciousness of the 'I' or ego and the 'I' of the pure Self (Ātmā). Dhyāna is the process of inter-penetration of all these sheaths, a merging of all that is known into unknown, or of the finite into the Infinite.

19. The mind acts as the subject and the Self object; yet in reality the Self is the subject. The end of meditation is to make the mind submerge in the Self so that all seeking and searching comes to an end. Then the sādhaka experiences his own universality, timelessness and fullness.

20. Stay in meditation for as long as you can, without allowing the body to collapse. Then do śavāsana (Pl. 182).

Notes

1. Do not sit for meditation immediately after doing āsanas and prāṇāyāma. Only those who can sit steadily for a long period can do prāṇāyāma and dhyāna together. Otherwise the limbs will ache and disturb mental equilibrium.

2. The best time to meditate is when one is fresh in body and mind, or at the time of going to bed when one feels peaceful.

3. Do not allow the eyes to look upwards, for this leads to retention of breath and creates tension in the nerves, muscles, blood vessels, head and brain.

4. Only people who are easily dejected or distressed and who have dull or weak minds are advised to direct the gaze at the centre between the eyebrows (Pls 149 and 150) with closed eyes for short periods of time. This should be done four or five times during meditation, with an interval between each attempt. This practice brings about mental stability and intellectual sharpness. However, people with hyper-tension should not follow this procedure.

5. Stop meditation the moment the body starts swaying forwards, backwards or sideways or if faintness is felt. Do not persist when this happens, as

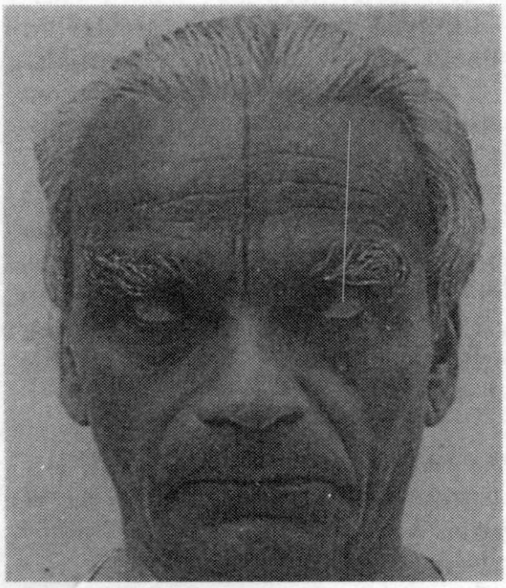
Pl. 149

Pl. 150
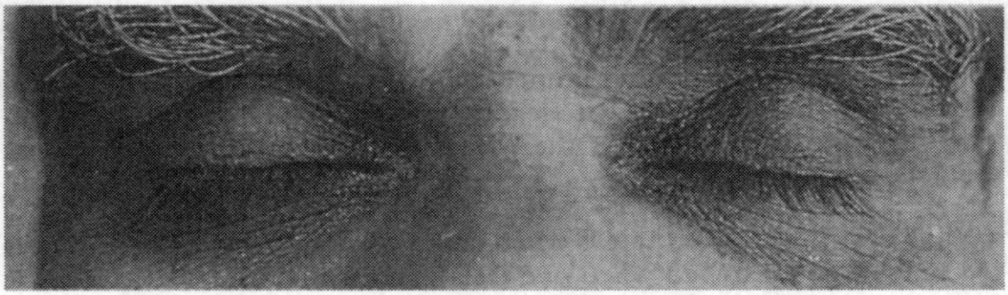

it means that the time for meditation is over for the day. If you persist, it may lead to mental imbalance.

Effects of Meditation

1. In meditation the mind traces its origin and comes to rest there as a child rests on the lap of the mother. The yogi, having found his own resting place and spiritual haven, sees the underlying reality around and within him.

2. Meditation abolishes the polarity between the analytical dominant consciousness of the front brain and the receding sub-consciousness or unconsciousness of the back brain. It controls and slows down certain automatic physical functions which normally stimulate the brain, such as intestinal contractions, breathing, and the heart beat. All external stimuli

which normally disturb human consciousness through the various sense organs are cut off as the nine gates of the body are closed in dhyāna.

3. In meditation mind and matter are fused. This fusion burns out all distracting thoughts. The sādhaka becomes dynamic, creative and supremely attentive. He has inexhaustible reserves of energy and engages himself in bettering humanity.

4. He experiences a new dimension wherein his senses and his chitta become crystal clear. He sees things as they are and is free from prejudices and delusions. This is the Jāgṛtāvasthā, a state of watchful awareness. His soul is awake, but his senses are under control. He is full of knowledge (prajñā), understanding, precision, freedom and truth. Illumined by the divine fire within, he radiates joy, unity and peace.

5. The sādhaka progressively attains the seven states of higher consciousness. These are right desire (śubhechhā), right reflection (vichāraṇā), disappearance of the mind (tanumānasā), self-realisation (sattavāpatti), non-attachment (asaṁsakta), non-perception of objects (padārthābhāva), and the experience of a state which is beyond words. It is the sum total of all knowledge: knowledge (jñāna) of the body (śarīra), breath (prāṇa), mind (manas) and intelligence (vijñāna); knowledge gained by experience (ānubhavika), by digesting the various sentiments and flavours that life offers (rasātmaka), and knowledge of the Self (Ātmā-jñāna).

6. His senses are drawn in. His thoughts are pure. Free from attachment and delusions, he has become stable and a jīvana-mukta (free from the bondages of life).

The state of a jīvana-mukta is described thus in the *Bhagavad Gītā* (Chapter XVIII, 53–56): 'He has left behind him vanity, violence and arrogance. He has gone beyond lust, anger and greed. He has become selfless and tranquil – he is fit to be one with the Eternal. He who dwells with the Eternal and is tranquil in spirit, neither grieves nor desires. His love is the same for all creation; he has supreme love for the Lord.'

7. Thus, the Sādhaka begins his journey from bondage to freedom of the spirit. From conquest of the body, he proceeds to master the breath (bio-energy). After the mastery of the breath, he controls the movements of the mind. From stability of mind, he develops sound judgement. By sound judgement, he does right actions and gains total awareness and becomes illumined. This illumination (prajñā) leads to Supreme knowledge (para-jñāna). With this knowledge, he surrenders his very soul (ātmā) to the Lord (Paramātmā). This is Śaraṇāgati yoga – the Yoga of Surrender.

Chapter 30

Śavāsana (Relaxation)

1. Śava in Sanskrit means a corpse, and āsana a posture. Thus śavāsana is a posture that simulates a dead body, and evokes the experience of remaining in a state as in death and of ending the heart-aches and the shocks that the flesh is heir to. It means relaxation, and therefore recuperation. It is not simply lying on one's back with a vacant mind and gazing, nor does it end in snoring. It is the most difficult of yogic āsanas to perfect, but it is also the most refreshing and rewarding.

2. A perfect śavāsana needs perfect discipline. It is easy to relax for a few minutes, but to do so without physical movement or without wavering of the intellect requires long training. At the start, a prolonged stay in śavāsana is not only very uncomfortable to the brain, but makes the body feel like a piece of dry, dead wood. Pricking sensations are felt on the skin along the limbs and they grow more acute if the pose is continued.

Rhythm

3. When śavāsana is well performed the breath moves like a string holding the pearls of a necklace together. The pearls are the ribs which move slowly, very steadily and reverently, reverent because when one is in that precise state, the body, the breath, the mind and the brain move towards the real self (Ātmā), like a spider returning to the centre of its web. At this juncture a state of samāhita chitta (equanimity of the mind, the intellect and the self) is felt.

4. In the beginning, the ribs do not relax, the breath is rough and uneven, while the mind and intellect waver. The body, the breath, the mind and the intellect are not united with the Ātmā or the Self. For correct śavāsana there must be unity of the body, the breath, the mind and the intellect where the Self holds the reins. All four bow down respectfully to the Ātmā. Then the chitta (that is, manas, buddhi and ahaṁkāra or ego, which is the state that ascertains that 'I know') becomes samāhita chitta, in which the mind, the intellect and the ego are balanced. This is a state of stillness.

5. This state is achieved by controlled discipline of the body, the senses and the mind. It should not, however, be mistaken for silence. In stillness there is rigidity due to force of will. Here the attention is focused to keep

the consciousness (chitta) still (dhāraṇā), whereas in silence that attention is expanded and released (dhyāna) and the will is submerged in the Atmā. This subtle distinction between stillness and silence can be known only by experience. In śavāsana the attempt is to achieve silence in all the five sheaths or kośas: the annamaya (anatomical), the Prāṇamaya (physiological), the manomaya (mental or emotional), the vijñānamaya (intellectual) and the ānandamaya (the body of bliss), which envelop the person from the skin to the self.

6. A star pulsates with energy and the energy is translated into light rays, which may take many light-years to reach human eyes on earth. The Ātman is like such a star and it transmits and imprints its likes and desires on the mind. These latent desires, like stellar energy translated into light, may resurface to the mind level, breaching the silence.

7. First, learn to achieve the silence of the body. Then control the subtle movements of the breath. Next learn about the silence of the mind and the emotions and then of the intellect. From there proceed to learn and study about the silence of the Self. It is not until then that the ego or small self (ahaṃkāra) of the practitioner can merge with his Self (Ātman). The fluctuations of the mind and the intellect cease, the 'I' or ego disappears and Śavāsana provides an experience of unalloyed bliss.

Stages of Consciousness

8. Yoga teaches four main states of consciousness. The three normal ones are the state of deep sleep or spiritual ignorance (suśupti), the dreamy or indolent state (svapna) and lastly the state of watchfulness or awareness (jāgṛta). There are varying stages between them. The fourth (turīya) has a different dimension in which the sādhaka is spiritually illumined. Some call it the Eternal Now, beyond space and time. Others call it the soul becoming one with the Creator. This can be experienced in perfect śavāsana when the body is at rest as in deep sleep, the senses as in a dream but the intellect alert and aware. Such perfection, however, is rarely achieved. The sādhaka is then born anew or emancipated (siddha). His soul sings the words of Śankarāchārya:

> I was, I am, I shall be, so why fear birth and death?
> Whence pangs of thirst and hunger? I have no life no breath.
> I am neither mind nor ego, can delusion or sorrow grind me?
> I am but the instrument, can actions free or bind me?

Techniques

1. It is necessary to describe in great detail the technique for practising śavāsana. However, a beginner need not be discouraged about mastering the details. When first learning to drive a car, he gets confused. Yet with

help from an instructor he gradually learns to master the intricacies until they all become instinctive. It is the same with śavāsana, except that the working of the human body is more intricate than that of any car.

2. Śavāsana is difficult to learn as it involves stilling the body, the senses and the mind while keeping the intellect alert. The seeker approaches it by studying the various aspects of his being – the body, the senses, the mind, the intellect and the Self. Scholastic knowledge is not enough. Correct practice is essential to master śavāsana.

3. Before starting the practice remove constricting garments, belts, glasses, contact lenses, hearing aids and so on.

Time and Place

4. Although śavāsana can be done at any time, it is advisable to do it during the quiet hours. In large cities and industrial areas it is difficult to find an atmosphere free from smoke, smog or chemical pollution. Choose a clean level place, free from insects, noise and unpleasant smells. Do not practice on a hard floor, or on an unyielding surface or on a soft mattress, as the body sinks into it unevenly.

Pl.151

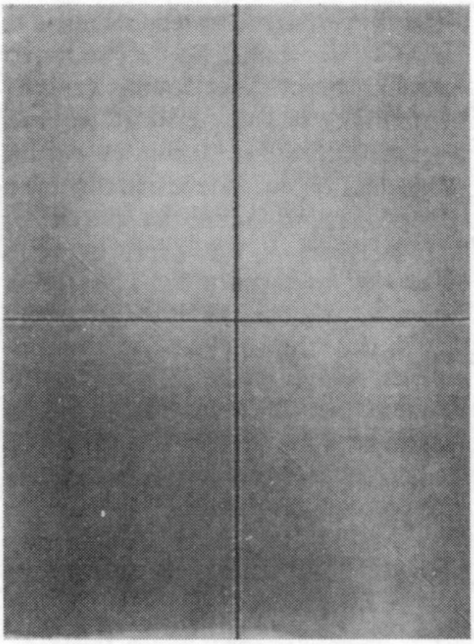

Pl.152

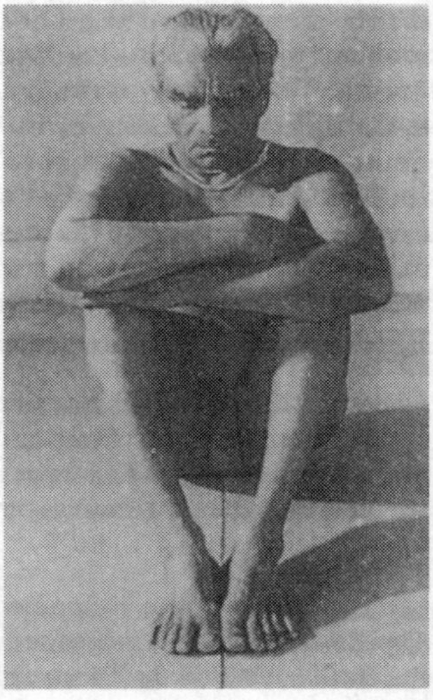

Alignment

5. Śavāsana is performed lying down full length on the back on a blanket spread on the floor. Draw a straight line there to position the body correctly (Pl. 151). Sit on the drawn line with the knees drawn up and the feet together. (Pl. 152). Gradually lower the back vertebra by vertebra along

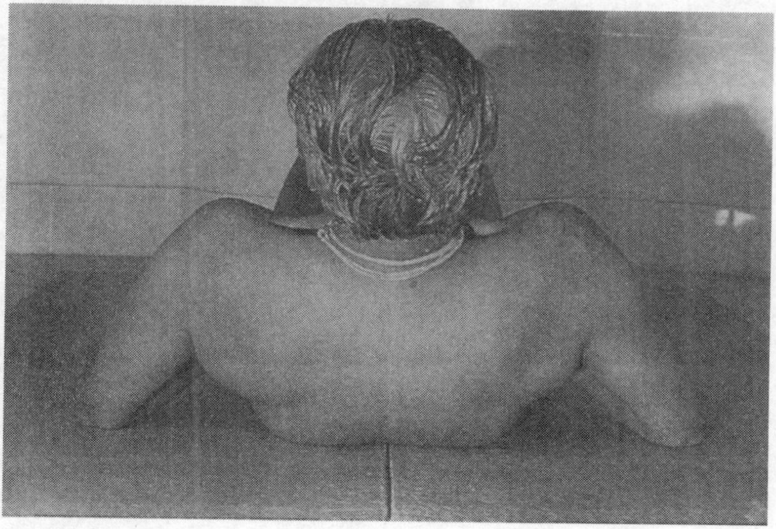

Pl. 153

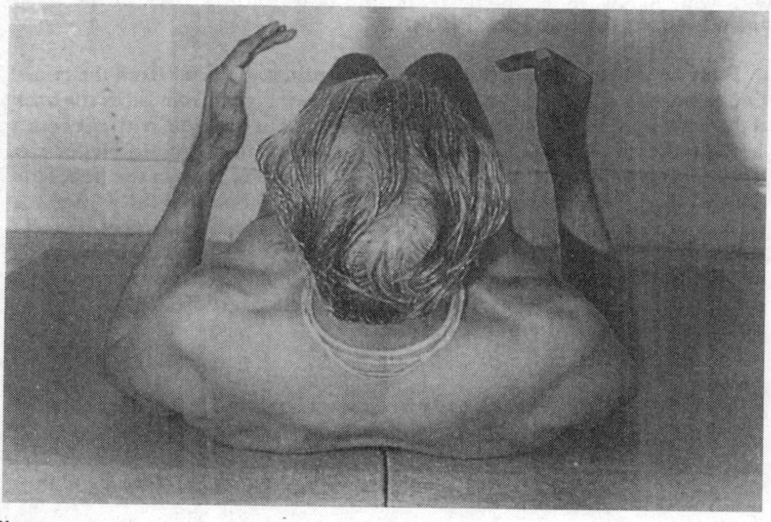

Pl. 154

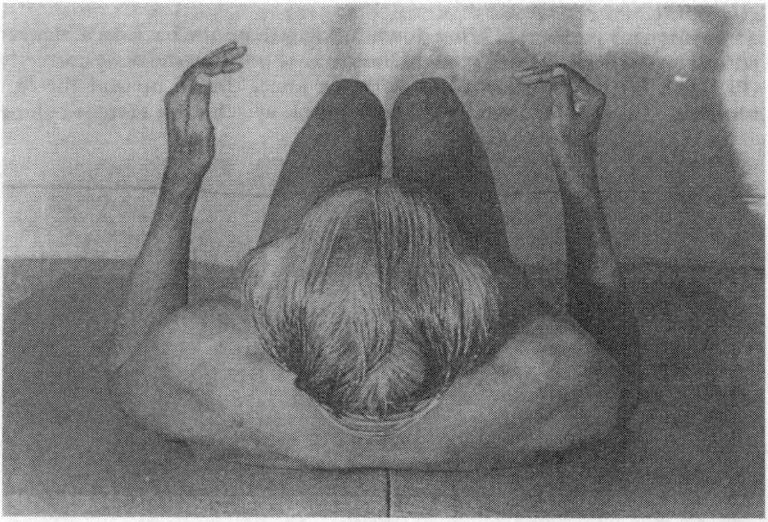

Pl.155

the drawn line on the floor or on the blanket. Place the body accurately so that the middle of the spine lies exactly on the straight line drawn on the floor or blanket (Pls 153 to 155).

6. Press the feet on the floor, lift the hips as well as the sacroiliac region, and with your hands, move the flesh and the skin from the back of the waist down towards the buttocks (Pl. 156).

7. First adjust the back of the body. Then adjust the head from the front. The reason for adjusting the head from the front is that from birth the back of the head becomes uneven, because babies lean to one side, with the result that one side of the head gets more compressed than the other. Hence it is important to adjust the head from the front and feel it from the back (Pls 157 and 158). Then extend first one leg and then the other fully. (See Pls 47–49). Join both the heels and knees. The joined heels, knees, crotch, centre of the coccyx, the spinal column and base of the skull should rest exactly on the straight line (Pl. 159). Then adjust the front of the body, keeping the centre of the eye-brows, the bridge of the nose, chin, sternum, navel and centre of the pubis in line.

Balance

8. To prevent any tilt of the body keep it straight and level. To check the

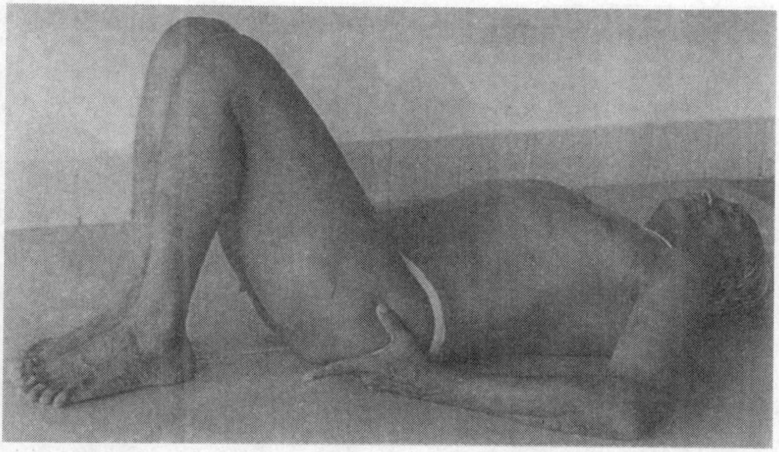

Pl. 156

Pl. 157

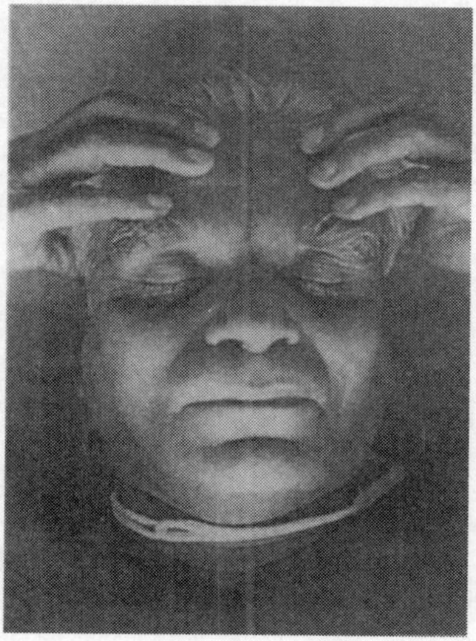

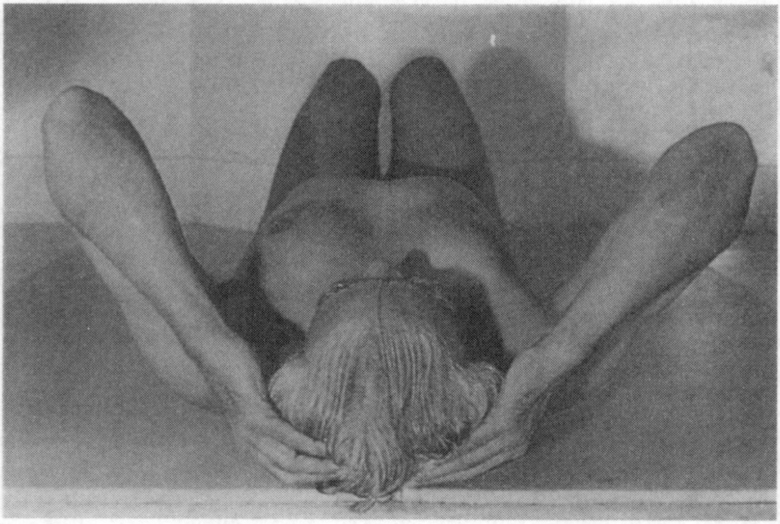

Pl.158

Pl.159

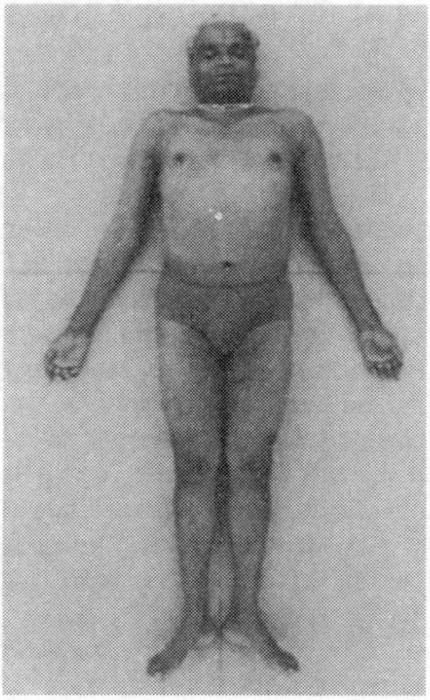

former draw an imaginary line straight along the centre of the forehead, eye-brows, root of the nose, middle of the lips, chin, throat and sternum, centre of the diaphragm, navel and pubis, and then through the space between the inner sides of the thighs, knees, calves, ankles and heels. Then check that the body is level, starting with the head, keeping the two ears, outer corners of the eyes, the lips and the base of the jaw-bone parallel to the floor (Pls 160 and 161). Finally stretch and adjust the back of the neck, so that it is centrally placed on the floor (Pl. 162).

Torso

9. Pin the apex (inner point) of each shoulder blade to the floor (Pls 163 and 164). Roll the skin of the top chest from the collar-bones towards the shoulder blades and adjust the back to rest perfectly on the blanket (Pl. 165). See that the dorsal and lumbar areas of the spine rest evenly on either

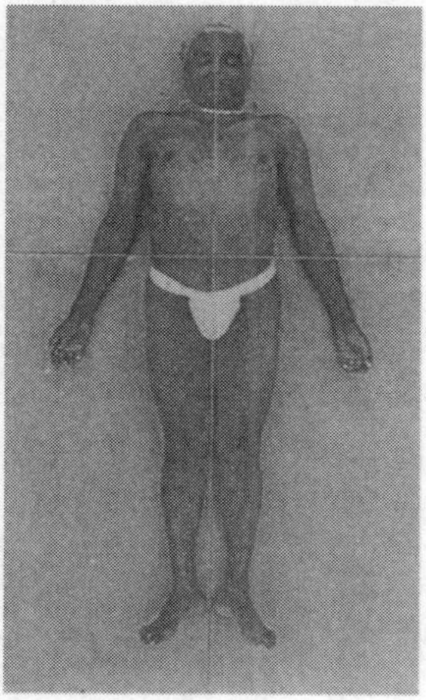

Pl. 160

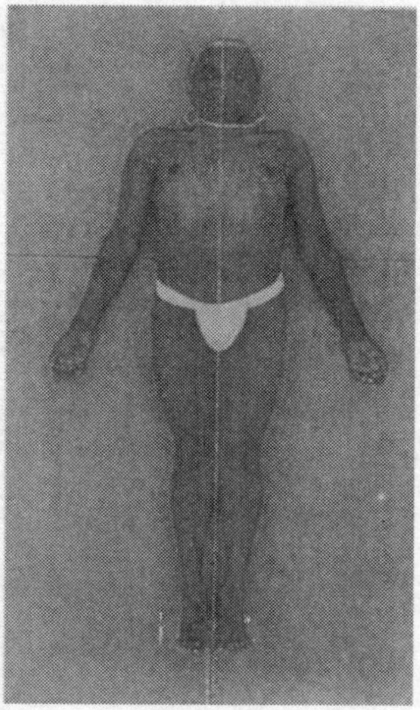

Pl. 161

side and that the ribs spread out uniformly. About ninety-nine per cent of people do not rest evenly on both buttocks, but rest on one of them. Rest the centre of the sacrum on the floor so that the buttocks relax evenly. Draw a line between the nipples, floating ribs (Pls 160 and 161) and pelvic bones to keep them parallel to the floor.

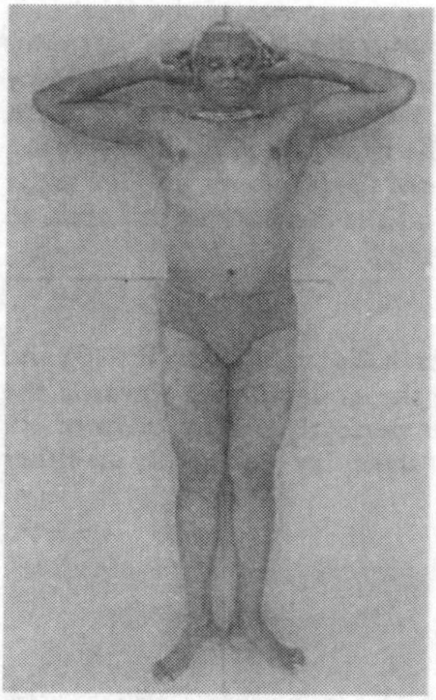

Pl. 162

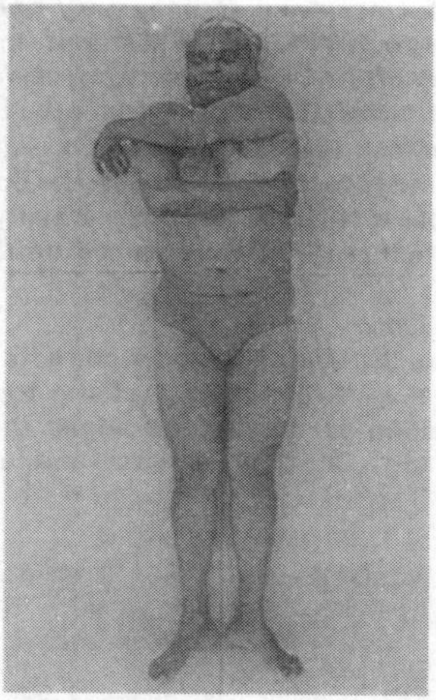

Pl. 163

Pl. 164

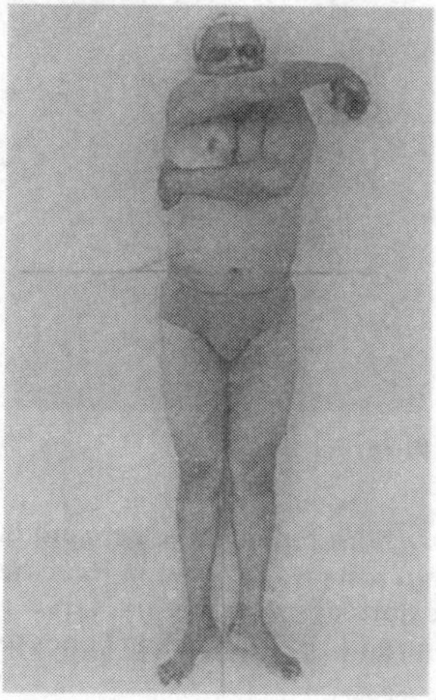

Pl. 165

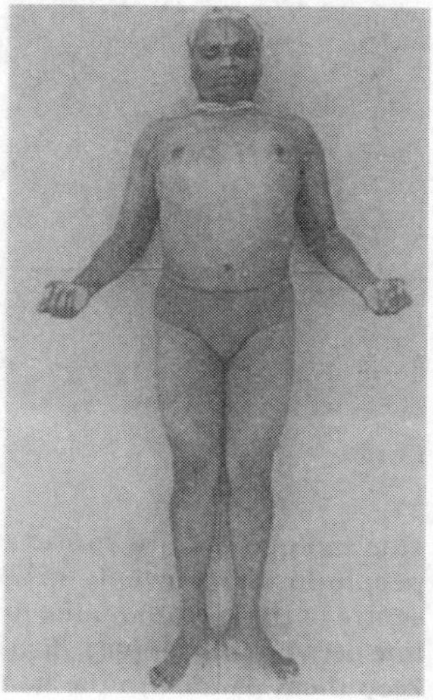

Pl. 166

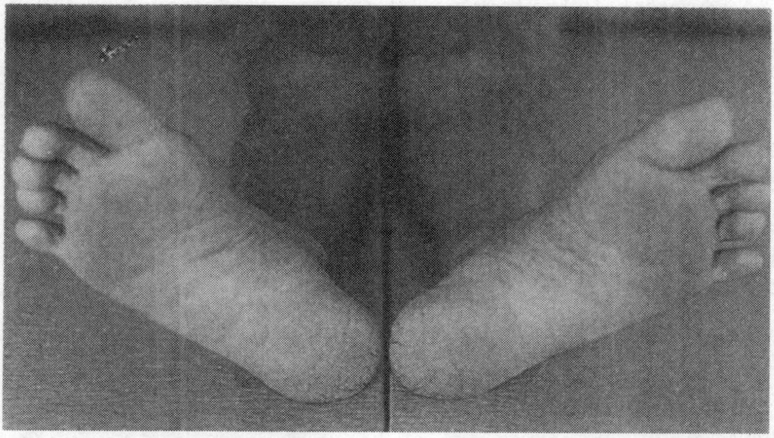

Feet

10. Keep the feet together and stretch the outer edges of the heels (Pl. 160); then let the feet fall outwards evenly (Pl. 166). The big toes should feel weightless and non-resistant (Pl. 167). It is wrong to force the little toes to touch the floor. Persons with stiff legs may keep their feet about a yard apart, as this will enable them to keep the back rested on the floor (Pl. 168). Keep the back outer corner of the knees touching the floor. If they cannot rest use a folded blanket or pillow behind them (Pl. 85). If the legs do not feel relaxed, place weights on the upper thighs (25 to 50 lbs) (Pl. 169). This removes tension or hardness in the muscles and keeps the legs quiet.

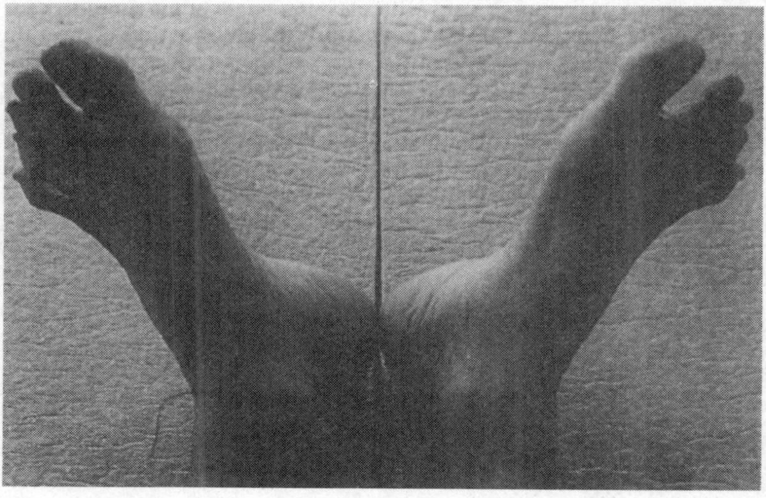

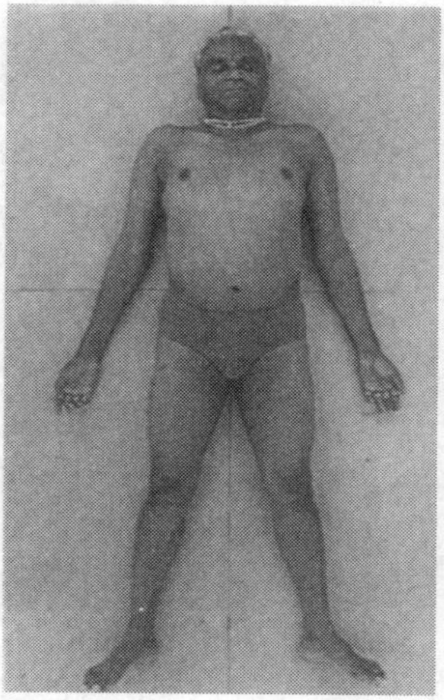

Pl. 168

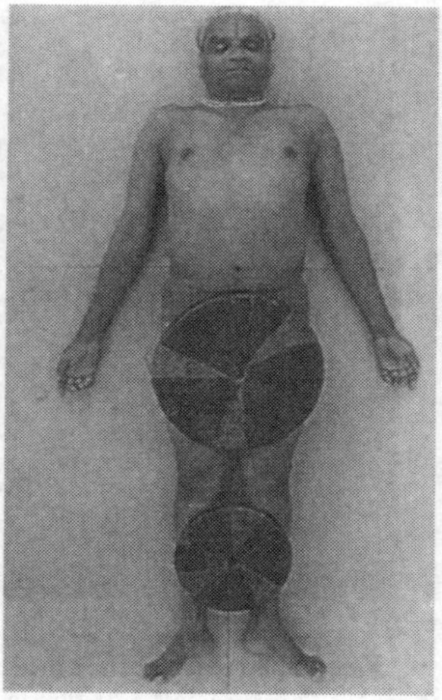

Pl. 169

Hands

11. Keep the hands away from the body, forming an angle of fifteen to twenty degrees at the armpits. Bend the arms at the elbows, touching the shoulder tops with the fingers (Pl. 170). Extend the triceps at the back portion of the upper arms and take the elbows as far as you can towards the feet. Keep the whole upper arms with the outer edges of the shoulders and elbows on the floor (Pl. 171). Do not disturb the elbow points. Lower the forearms. Extend the hands from the wrists to the knuckles, palms facing upwards (Pls 172 and 173). Keep the fingers passive and relaxed, with the backs of the middle fingers touching the floor up to the first knuckles (Pl. 174). See that the median plane of the arms, elbows, wrists and palms are in contact with the floor. If the arms are kept close to the body and the body does not rest properly, and hardness is felt in the arms or in the muscles of the trunk at the back, spread the arms to the level of the shoulders (Pl. 175). The feeling of lying on the floor should be as though the body is sinking into Mother Earth.

Unconscious Tensions

12. One may be unaware of tension in the palms, the fingers, the soles of the feet or the toes (Pls 176 and 177). Watch for and release this tension when and where it occurs and drop these parts back to their correct positions.

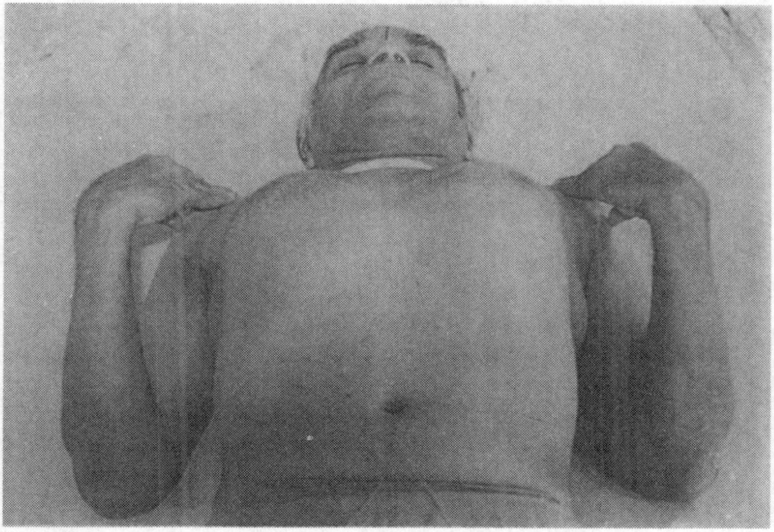

Pl. 170

Pl. 171

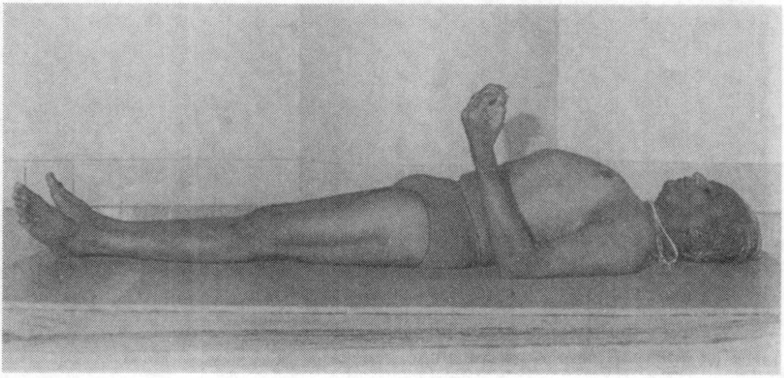

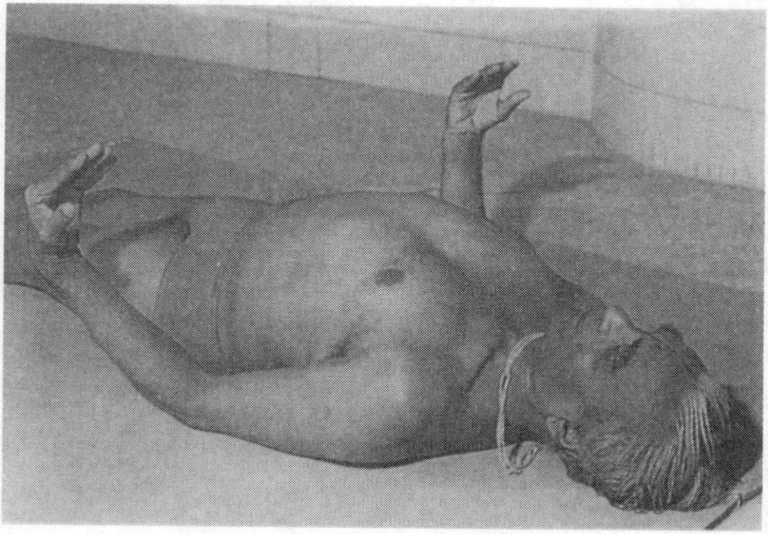

Pl. 172

Pl. 173

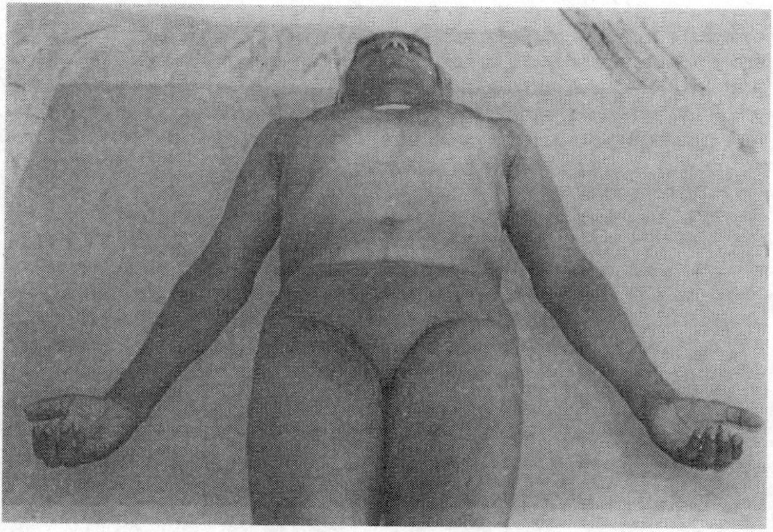

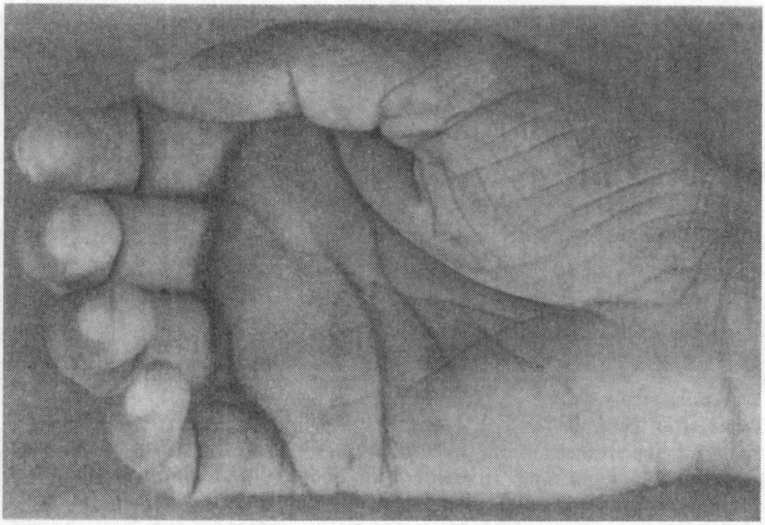

Pl. 174

Pl. 175

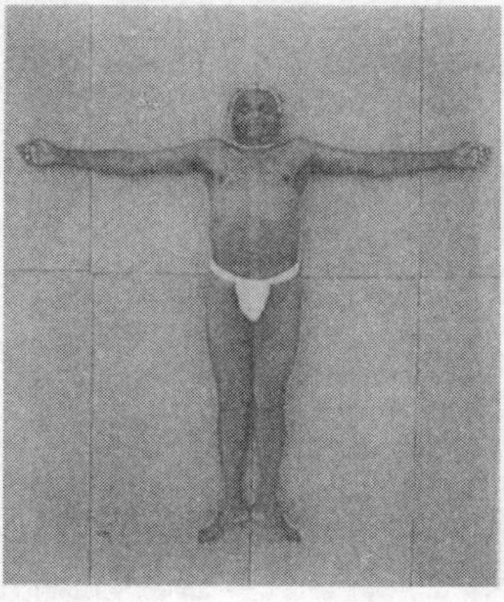

Pl. 176

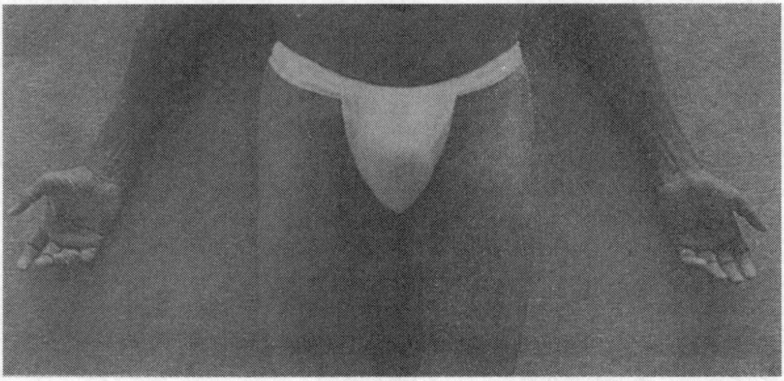

Removal of Tension

13. First, learn to relax the back of the body from the trunk to the neck, arms and legs. Next relax the front of the body from the pubis to the throat, where emotional upheavals take place, and then from the neck to the crown of the head. In this way learn to relax the entire body.

Pl. 177

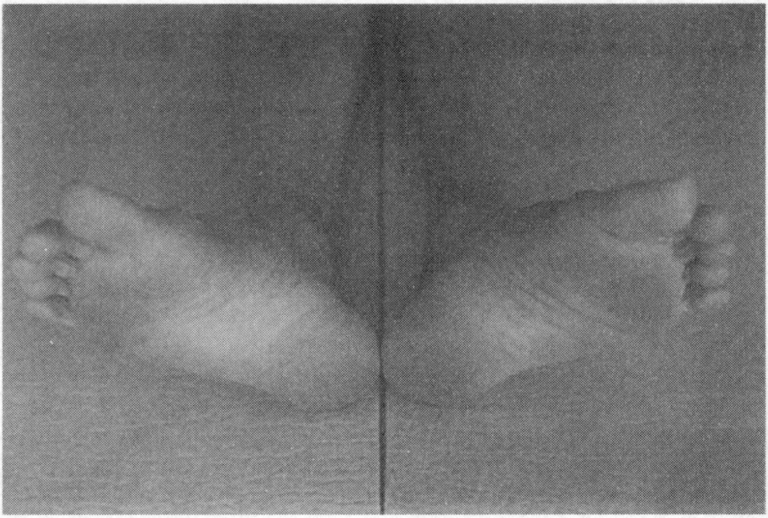

14. Experience the feeling of non-existence or emptiness in the pits of the arms, the inner pits of the groin, diaphragm, lungs, spinal muscles and the abdomen. The body then feels like a discarded stick. In correct śavāsana the head feels as if it has shrunk.

15. Learn to silence the tissues of the physical body before dealing with the mind. The gross physical body (annamaya kośa) should be brought under control before one proceeds to quieten the subtler mental (manomaya) and intellectual bodies (vijñānamaya kośas).

16. Complete serenity of the body is the first requisite, and it is the first sign of attaining spiritual tranquillity. There is no emancipation of the mind unless there is a feeling of serenity in all parts of the body. Silence in the body will bring about silence in the mind.

The Senses

17. *Eyes.* In śavāsana the sādhaka turns his gaze inwards and looks within himself. This introspection prepares him for pratyāhāra, the fifth of the eight steps of Yoga, where the senses are withdrawn inwards, and he begins the journey to the source of his being, his Ātmā.

18. The eyes are the windows of the brain. Each has lids, which act as shutters. The iris surrounding the pupil serves as an automatic regulator of the amount of light reaching the retina. The iris reacts automatically to the intellectual and emotional states of the person. By closing the lids he can shut out all that is outside and become aware of what is within. If he closes them too tightly the eyes are squeezed causing colours, lights and shadows to appear and distract him. Gently move the upper lids towards the inner corners of the eyes. This relaxes the skin just above them and creates space

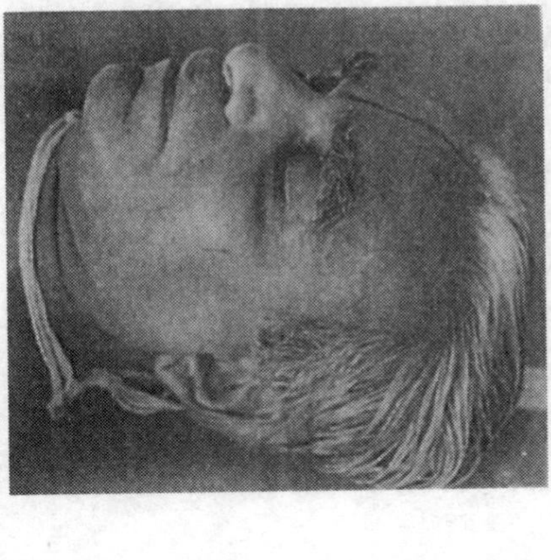

Pl. 178

between the eye-brows. Treat the eyes gently like petals of a flower. Raise the eyebrows just enough to release any tightness of the skin in the forehead (Pl. 178).

19. *Ears.* These play an important part both in śavāsana and in Prāṇāyāma. While the eyes are kept passive, the ears should be quiet and receptive. Tension or relaxation in either affects the mind in the same way and vice versa. The seat of the intellect is in the head, while the mind is rooted in the heart. When there are thought waves, the inner ears lose their receptivity. By careful training, the process can be reversed and the ears can send messages back to stop the fluctuations so that the mind will quieten. If the eyes are kept tense the ears become blocked, and if they are relaxed so are the ears.

20. *Tongue.* Keep the root of the tongue passive as in sleep and resting on the lower palate. Any movement or pressure of the tongue on the teeth or upper palate indicates a fluctuating mind. If it moves to one side, the head does the same, making total relaxation difficult. Keep the corners of the lips relaxed by stretching them sideways.

21. *Skin.* The skin which covers the body provides the structure for what is perhaps the most important of the senses. The five organs of knowledge are the eyes, ears, nose, tongue and skin. The subtle primary elements of light, colour, sound, smell, taste and touch (the tanmātras) leave their impressions on the organs of sense. These in turn send messages to the brain and receive them back for response and challenge. The nerves controlling the senses are relaxed by releasing the tension from the facial muscles, while the brain is freed from contact with the organs of knowledge. Pay special attention to the areas of the temples, the cheekbones and the lower jaw. This will enable you to sense a feeling of quietness between the upper palate and the root of the tongue. In śavāsana the muscles relax and the pores of the skin shrink and the relevant nerves are at rest.

Breathing

22. See that the breath flows evenly on either side of the nostrils. Start by inhaling normally, but exhale softly, deeply and longer. For some, deep inhalation creates disturbance in the head and trunk, with tautness in the legs and arms. For them normal inhalations with deep and soft exhalations are recommended. This quietens the nerves and the mind. For those who become restless the moment śavāsana is attempted, they should perform deep, slow and prolonged in and out breaths until quietness is attained. The moment quietness is felt, they should stop deep breathing and let the breath flow by itself. When the art of exhalation is perfected, one feels as if the breath is oozing from the pores of the skin on the chest, which is a sign of

perfect relaxation. Each out-breath takes the sādhaka's mind towards his own self and purges his brain of all its tensions and activities. Exhalation is the best form of surrender by the sādhaka of his all – his breath, life and soul – to his Creator.

Head

23. Make sure that the head is straight and parallel to the ceiling. If it tilts up (Pl. 179) the mind dwells in the future. If down (Pl. 180), it broods in the past. If it leans to one side (Pl. 181), the innner ear (the vestibular apparatus, utricle saccule and semi-circular canals) follows. This affects the mid-brain and one tends to fall asleep and lose awareness. Learn to keep the head level with the floor so that the mind remains always in the present (Pl. 182). Correction of any tilt will help to bring that balance '(samatva) between the two hemispheres of the brain and the body which is one of the gateways to divinity.

24. At the beginning the chin moves up and down unconsciously in respiration. Check this by consciously keeping the back of the head parallel to the floor by stretching it from the neck towards the back of the crown (Pl. 182).

Brain

25. If the brain or mind is tense, so is the skin and vice versa. Learn to discipline yourself from the pores of the skin to the Self as well as the other

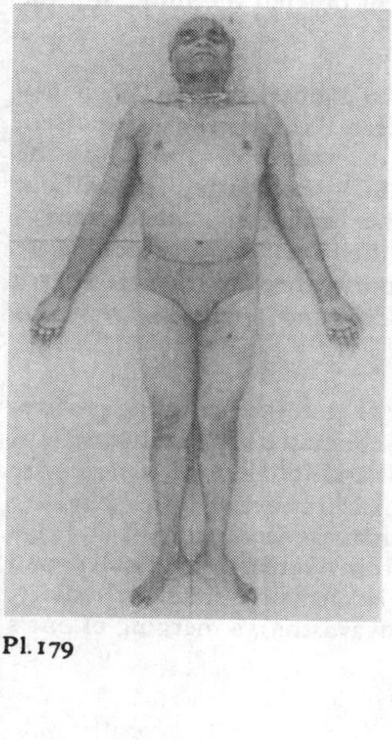

Pl. 179

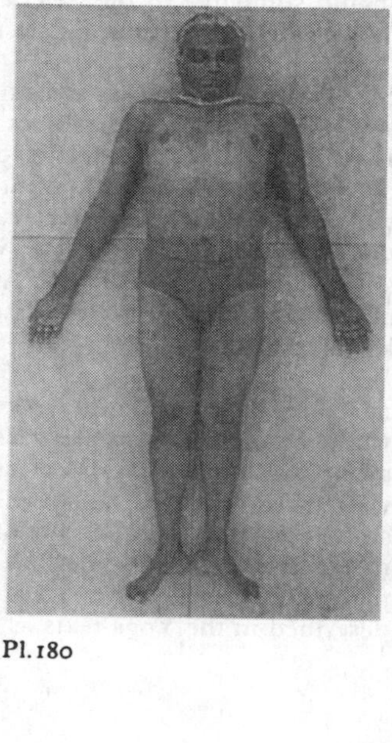

Pl. 180

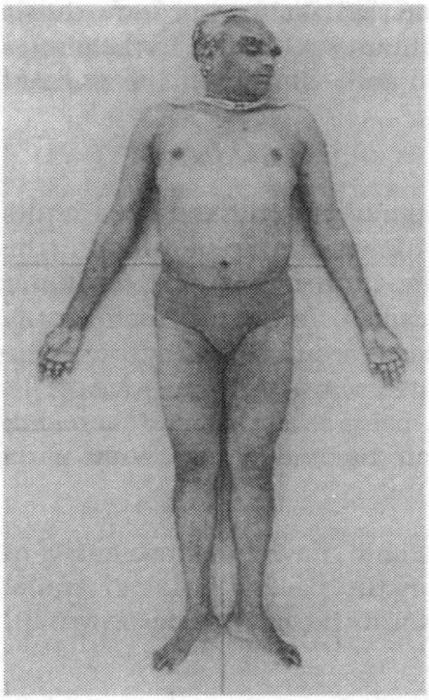

Pl. 181

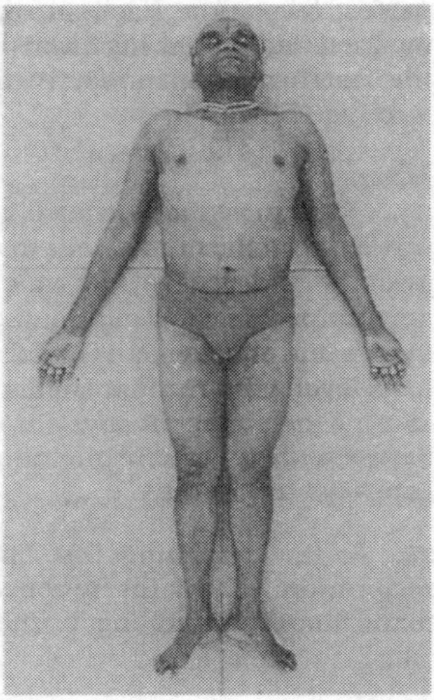

Pl. 182

way round. The total energy of the body, the mind and the intelligence should submerge in the Self. Use the will to quieten the mind and the intellect. Ultimately sublimate the will.

26. As long as the senses are active, the Ātmā remains dormant. When they are stilled and silenced, it shines forth as the clouds of desires are dispersed. Like the darting movements of a fish in the water of a pond are the movements of the mind and intellect (buddhi) – both within and without the body. When the water is unruffled, the image reflected therein is unbroken and still. When the waverings of the mind and the intellect are stilled, the image of the Self (Ātmā) rises undisturbed to the surface, free of desires. This desireless state of simplicity and purity is known as kaivalyāvasthā.

27. The aim in śavāsana is to keep the body at rest, the breathing passive, while the mind and intellect are gradually sublimated. When fluctuations take place internally and externally, mental and intellectual energies are wasted. In śavāsana the internal or emotional upheavals in the mind are stilled, bringing about a state of manolaya (manas meaning mind and laya meaning immersion). Then the mind, free from fluctuations, dissolves and merges in the self, like a river in the sea. It is a negative state of passivity, described in the Yoga texts as 'empty' (śūnyāvasthā), a merging of one's

identity at the emotional level. Then the sādhaka prevents the incoming thoughts which distract and dissipate his intellectual energy. At this level he experiences a state of clarity where the intellect is in full command and does not allow invading thoughts to disturb it. This state is known as an aśūnyāvasthā (A meaning not, śūnya meaning empty). When he gets mastery over mind and brain, he reaches a new positive state beyond both manolaya and amanaskatva, which is pure being.

28. Manolaya or śūnyāvasthā may be compared to the new moon, where the moon, though rotating round the earth, is not visible. The states of amanaskatva or aśūnyāvasthā may be compared to the full moon, reflecting the light of the sun, the Ātmā. In both śūnyāvasthā or aśūnyāvasthā, the sādhaka's body, mind and intellect are well balanced and radiate energy. He attains equipoise between the two tides of emptiness of emotion and fullness of intellect.

29. To achieve this state, the sādhaka must develop discrimination. This in turn will lead to clarity and enable him to relax better. When clarity is gained, doubts vanish, bringing illumination. His being then gets merged in the Infinite (Paramātmā). This is the experience of the sādhaka, the nectar of śavāsana.

30. Practise śavāsana for some ten to fifteen minutes to experience a sense of timelessness. The slightest thought or movement will break the spell and you are once more in the world of time, with a beginning and an end.

31. Getting back to normal from a successful śavāsana requires time. Between two breaths and two thoughts there is a varying gap of time, as there is between an active and a passive state. Śavāsana being a passive

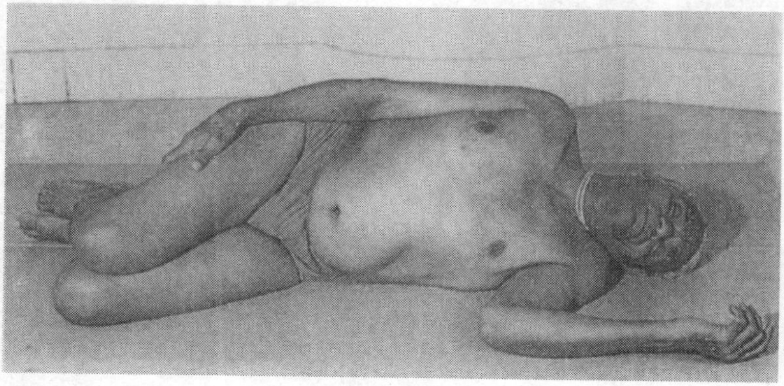

Pl. 183

state, the sādhaka should remain a silent observer until normal activity creeps into the brain and body. After successful śavāsana the nerves feel shrunken on returning to normal, while the back of the brain seems dry and heavy and the front empty. Therefore do not raise your head quickly, as you may black out or feel heavy. Gradually and gently open your eyes, which are at first unfocused. Remain in that state for a while. Then bend the knees, turn the head and body to one side (Pl. 183) and stay for a minute or two in that position. Repeat this on the other side. As a result you will feel no strain when getting up.

Special Precautions

Those suffering from hyper-tension, high blood pressure, heart disease, emphysema or restlessness should lie on wooden planks and place pillows under the head (Pls 80–82).

Tense and restless people should place weights (of about 50 lbs) on their upper thighs and 5 lbs on the palms. (Pl. 184). They should do ṣaṇmukhī mudrā (Pl. 185) or wrap a long soft and thin piece of folded cloth about three inches wide around the head and over the eyes and temples. Start from the eye-brows, without blocking the nose; tuck in the ends, either at the temple above or at the sides of the nose below. The cloth should be neither too tight nor too loose (Pl. 186). When the brain is active, movements of the temples and tension in the eye-balls will push the cloth

Pl. 184

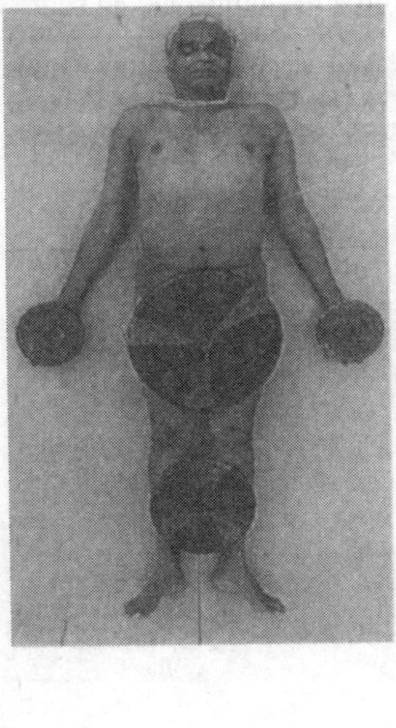

Pl. 185

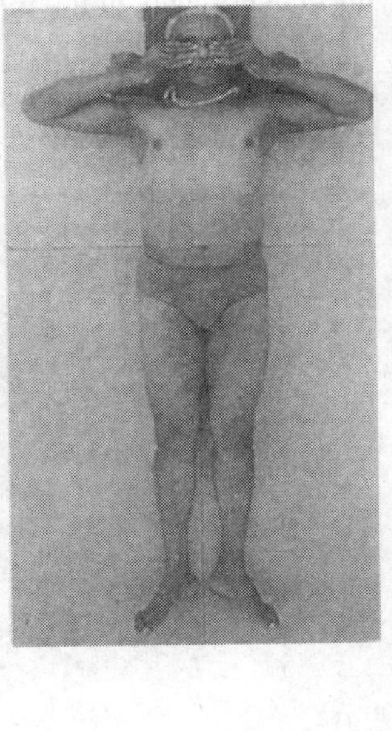

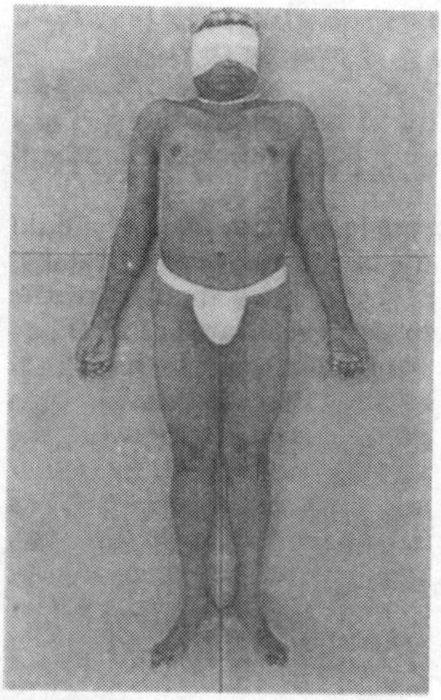

Pl. 186

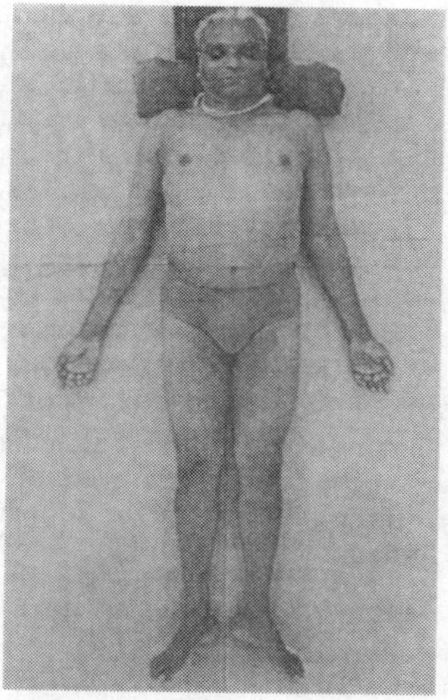

Pl. 187

Pl. 188

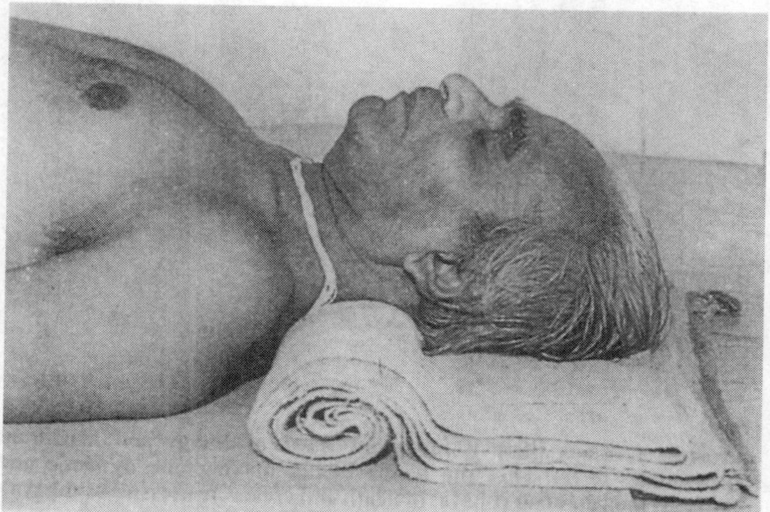

outwards. When the skin there relaxes, you no longer feel to be in contact with the cloth. This is a sign that the brain is beginning to relax.

Those with painful necks, due to cervical spondylitis or sprain, will find it difficult to stretch the back of the neck and to rest comfortably. They should insert a towel or a folded cloth between the base of the neck and skull as illustrated (Pls 187 and 188).

Highly nervous people, or those suffering from loss of confidence, should lie in śavāsana, directing the gaze at the middle of the eye-brows (trāṭaka) (Pl. 149), close the eyes and gaze inwardly (Pl. 150). They should breathe deeply, holding the breath for a second or two after each inhalation. They should practise śavāsana only after doing sarvāngāsana, which is described in *Light on Yoga*. The deep inhalation and exhalation enable such persons to relax, after which they need no longer focus the gaze between the eye-brows nor concentrate on deep breathing.

If the gap between the floor and the waist is too great, use a soft pillow or a folded blanket to fill it. This support rests the lumbar back (Pl 189). Persons with backache should keep a weight (25–50 lbs) on the abdomen. This eases the pain (Pl. 190).

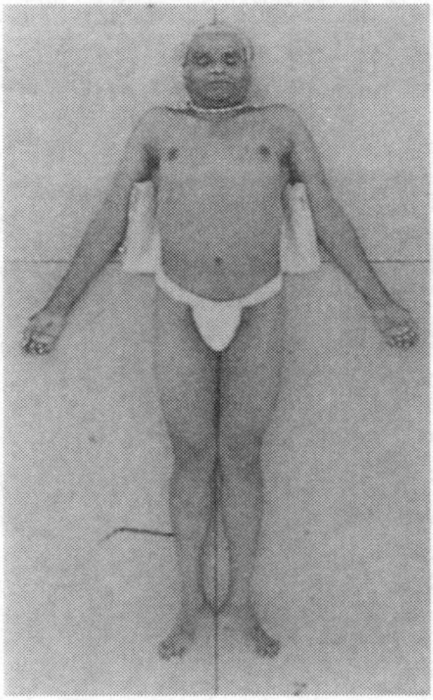

Pl. 189

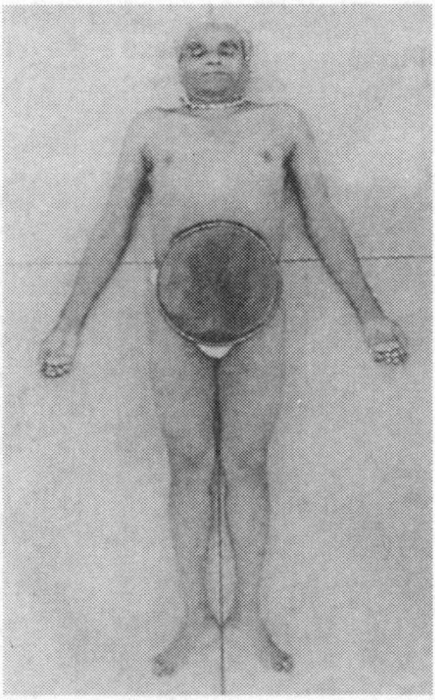

Pl. 190

Effect

In correct śavāsana there is minimum waste of energy and maximum recuperation. It refreshes the whole being, making one dynamic and creative. It banishes fear (bhaya) of death and creates fearlessness (abhaya). The sādhaka experiences a state of serenity and inner oneness.

Appendix

Prāṇāyāma Courses

Prāṇāyāma is here divided into five groups: preparatory, primary, intermediate, advanced and highly intense courses. This series of prāṇāyāmas is given for daily practice, with indication of the time it may take to gain some control in all courses. The mastering of each stage depends upon the sādhaka's dedication to the art and devotion to the practice.

First the courses are divided for easy reference before dealing with week-to-week practices.

1. PREPARATORY COURSE	STAGES
(a) Ujjāyī prāṇāyāma	I to VII
(b) Viloma prāṇāyāma	I and II

2. PRIMARY COURSE	
(a) Ujjāyī prāṇāyāma	VIII to X
(b) Viloma prāṇāyāma	III to V
(c) Anuloma prāṇāyāma	Ia and Ib Va and Vb
(d) Pratiloma prāṇāyāma	Ia and Ib
(e) Sūrya bhedana prāṇāyāma	I
(f) Chandra bhedana prāṇāyāma	I

3. INTERMEDIATE COURSE	
(a) Ujjāyī prāṇāyāma	XI
(b) Viloma prāṇāyāma	III, VI and VII
(c) Anuloma prāṇāyāma	IIa and IIb VIa and VIb
(d) Pratiloma prāṇāyāma	IIa and IIb
(e) Sūrya bhedana prāṇāyāma	II
(f) Chandra bhedana prāṇāyāma	II
(g) Nāḍī sodhana prāṇāyāma	Ia and Ib

4. ADVANCED COURSE

(a)	Ujjāyī prāṇāyāma	XII
(b)	Viloma prāṇāyāma	VIII
(c)	Anuloma prāṇāyāma	IIIa, IIIb VIIa, VIIb
(d)	Pratiloma prāṇāyāma	IIIa, IIIb
(e)	Sūrya bhedana prāṇāyāma	III
(f)	Chandra bhedana prāṇāyāma	III
(g)	Nāḍī śodhana prāṇāyāma	IIa, IIb

5. HIGHLY INTENSE COURSE

(a)	Ujjāyī prāṇāyāma	XIII
(b)	Viloma prāṇāyāma	IX
(c)	Anuloma prāṇāyāma	VIII
(d)	Pratiloma prāṇāyāma	IV
(e)	Sūrya bhedana prāṇāyāma	IV
(f)	Chandra bhedana prāṇāyāma	IV
(g)	Nāḍī śodhana prāṇāyāma	IIIa, IIIb IVa, IVb

Śītalī and śītakārī may be done with or without digital control, as well as with or without internal and external retention, for a few minutes once in a while. It is advisable during hot weather to do them before sunrise or after sunset, and when one feels over-heated.

Bhrāmarī and mūrchha may be done merely to learn the method, since their effects are covered by the other major prāṇāyāmas given in table form.

Kapālabhāti and bhastrikā are dealt with in the text. Any one of them may be added to the daily practices for a few minutes just to cleanse the nostrils and to refresh the brain, adjusting the stages in a way congenial to the body and to the nostrils.

Limited time has been given to retentions (kumbhakas) but none for in- and out-breaths; this is because on one day the sādhaka can concentrate on increasing the length of time for the in and out breaths, on other days for internal and on some for external retentions.

When sufficient control has been acquired, vṛtti prāṇāyāma ratios may be attempted, but only at the sādhaka's own risk.

COURSE ONE (PREPARATORY)

Weeks	*Prāṇāyāma*	*Stages*	*Time in Minutes*
1 and 2	Ujjāyī	I and II	7–8 each
3 and 4	Ujjāyī	II and III	8 ,,
5 and 6	Ujjāyī	II and III	5 ,,

Weeks	*Prāṇāyāma*	*Stages*	*Time in Minutes*
	Viloma	I and II	5 each
7 and 8	Ujjāyī	I, II, III	5 ,,
	Viloma	I and II	5 ,,
9 and 10	Ujjāyī	IV and V	5 ,,
	Viloma	IV	5 ,,
	Viloma	I	5 ,,
11 and 12	Ujjāyī	V and VI	5 ,,
	Viloma	IV	10 ,,
13 to 15	Ujjāyī	V, VI, VII	5 ,,
	Viloma	II	10 ,,
16 to 18	Ujjāyī	VI and VII	5 ,,
	Viloma	I and II	5 ,,
19 to 22	Repeat and consolidate, and get accustomed to the series.		
23 to 25	Ujjāyī	VI and VII	8 ,,
	Viloma	IV and V	8 ,,

Important stages in Course One:

Ujjāyī II, III, IV, VI and VII.
Viloma I and II.

COURSE TWO (PRIMARY)

26 to 28	Ujjāyī	VIII	10
	Viloma	III	10
29 to 31	Ujjāyī	IX	10
	Anuloma	Ia	10
	Viloma	II	5
32 to 34	Viloma	III	5–8
	Anuloma	Ib	5–8
	Ujjāyī	IX	5
35 to 38	Anuloma	Ia	10
	Pratiloma	Ia	10
	Ujjāyī	IV	as long as you can
39 to 42	Ujjāyī	X	8–10
	Anuloma	Ib	6–8
	Pratiloma	Ib	6–8
	Viloma	III	as long as you can
43 to 46	Repeat and consolidate the above stages.		
47 to 50	Repeat important stages from Course One and practise whatever you can from Course Two according to the time at your disposal.		

Weeks	*Prāṇāyāma*	*Stages*	*Time in Minutes*
51 to 54	Anuloma	Va	5
	Pratiloma	Ia	5
	Sūrya bhedana	I	10
55 to 58	Anuloma	Vb	5
	Pratiloma	Ib	10
	Chandra bhedana	I	5
59 to 62	Repeat Course Two and consolidate, adjusting the practice according to the time at your disposal.		

Important stages in Course Two:

Ujjāyī X, viloma III, anuloma Ib, pratiloma Ib, sūrya bhedana I and chandra bhedana I.

COURSE THREE (INTERMEDIATE)

63 to 67	Viloma	III	5
	Ujjāyī	XI	5–8
	Viloma	VI	5
	Anuloma	IIa	5
	Pratiloma	IIa	5
	Anuloma	VIa	5
	Sūrya bhedana	II	5
	Chandra bhedana	II	5

Here the sādhaka may do ujjāyī XI, anuloma IIa, pratiloma IIa, and sūrya bhedana II on one day, and the others on alternate days.

68 to 72	Viloma	VII	5
	Anuloma	IIb	6–8
	Pratiloma	IIb	6–8
	Nāḍī śodhana	Ia	10
73 to 75	Ujjāyī	VIII	5
	Anuloma	VIb	6
	Pratiloma	II	6
	Nāḍī śodhana	Ib	10

If Anuloma is done one day, Pratiloma may be done on the next day.

76 to 80	Anuloma	IIb	10
	Pratiloma	IIb	10
	Sūrya bhedana	II	10
	Chandra bhedana	II	10
	Nāḍī śodhana	II	10

If anuloma, sūrya bhedana and nāḍī śodhana are done on the first day, do the rest on the second, and so on.

81 to 85	Consolidate the practice.

Weeks	*Prāṇāyāma*	*Stages*	*Time in Minutes*
Important stages in Course Three:			
	Ujjāyī XI, viloma VII, anuloma IIb, pratiloma IIb, sūrya bhedana II, chandra bhedana II and nāḍī śodhana II.		
86 to 90	Do important prāṇāyāmas from Courses One, Two and Three.		

Now begin practising one stage at a stretch every day, so that each division in Courses One, Two and Three are learnt well before proceeding to the Advanced Course. For example:

91 to 120

First Week

Monday	Ujjāyī	VIII	20–25
Tuesday	Sūrya bhedana	I	20–25
Wednesday	Anuloma	Ib	20–25
Thursday	Viloma	I and II	20–25
Friday	Pratiloma	Ib	20–25
Saturday	Nāḍī śodhana	Ib	20–25
Sunday	Viloma	II	20–25

Second Week

Monday	Chandra bhedana	I	20–25
Tuesday	Anuloma	IIa	20–25
Wednesday	Pratiloma	IIb	20–25
Thursday	Ujjāyī	X	20–25
Friday	Nāḍī śodhana	Ib	20–25
Saturday	Viloma	Vb	20–25
Sunday	Viloma	III	20–25

Third Week

Monday	Sūrya bhedana	II	20–25
Tuesday	Chandra bhedana	II	20–25
Wednesday	Viloma	VII	20–25
Thursday	Anuloma	Vb	20–25
Friday	Pratiloma	Ia	20–25
Saturday	Nāḍī śodhana	Ia	20–25
Sunday	Ujjāyī	X	20–25

Now each sādhaka may prepare his or her own schedule for the succeeding days, until all the Prāṇāyāmas given in the three courses have been covered, then start again with the first week given above. Make sure each principal prāṇāyāma is represented every week, and do not repeat any stages in any three consecutive weeks. Rest on Sundays or do a simple and restful prāṇāyāma.

If you find that a scheduled prāṇāyāma does not seem right on a particular day, choose another from the same week.

If for physical reasons you are unable to do any prāṇāyāmas in the three courses, prepare your own schedule out of those which you can do.

With regard to the few minor prāṇāyāmas where it has been said that they should only be done for a few minutes, do not attempt to do these for twenty to twenty-five minutes stated here. They may however, be done, by way of experiment, on the last Saturday of every month for not more than five minutes.

COURSE FOUR: ADVANCED

Weeks	*Prāṇāyāma*	*Stages*	*Time in Minutes*
121 to 125	Sūrya bhedana	I	5
	Ujjāyī	XII	10
	Viloma	VIII	10
126 to 130	Chandra bhedana	I	5
	Anuloma	IIIa	10
	Pratiloma	IIIa	10
	Viloma	VIII	5
131 to 136	Anuloma	VIIa	10
	Nāḍī śodhana	IIa	10
	Viloma	VIII	5
137 to 142	Sūrya bhedana	II	10
	Nāḍī śodhana	IIb	15
143 to 148	Chandra bhedana	II	10
	Nāḍī śodhana	Ib	15
149 to 155	Sūrya bhedana	III	10
	Anuloma	IIIb	8
	Pratiloma	IIIb	8
156 to 160	Chandra bhedana	III	10
	Anuloma	VIIb	8
	Pratiloma	IIIa	8
	Nāḍī śodhana	IIb	8–10

Important stages in Course Four:

Anuloma IIIb, pratiloma IIIb, sūrya bhedana III, chandra bhedana III and nāḍī śodhana IIb.

161 to 170 Repeat all the important prāṇāyāmas of the above courses.

COURSE FIVE: HIGHLY INTENSE

171 to 175	Nāḍī śodhana	Ib	8–10
	Ujjāyī	XIII	10
	Anuloma	VIIIa	10

Weeks	*Prāṇāyāma*	*Stages*	*Time in Minutes*
176 to 180	Viloma	IX	10
	Pratiloma	IVa	10
181 to 185	Nāḍī śodhana	IIIa	10
	Anuloma	VIIIb	10
	Ujjāyī	XII (lying)	8
186 to 190	Sūrya bhedana	IV	10
	Nāḍī śodhana	IIIb	15
	Ujjāyī	II (lying)	10
191 to 195	Chandra bhedana	IV	10
	Pratiloma	IVb	10
	Viloma	II (lying)	8–10
196 to 200	Nāḍī śodhana	IVa	10
	Nāḍī śodhana	IVb	10
	Ujjāyī	II (lying)	10

Important stages in Course Five:

Sūrya bhedana IV, chandra bhedana IV, and nāḍī śodhana IVb.

WEEKLY PRACTICE

The cycles or sequences may be altered as desired.

Monday	Nāḍī śodhana	Ib	15–20
	Ujjāyī	XI	15–20
	Śavāsana		10
Tuesday	Viloma	V and VI	15–20
	Sūrya bhedana	II and III	15–20
	Śavāsana		10
Wednesday	Nāḍī śodhana	IIb	15–20
	Anuloma	VIIb	15–20
	Śavāsana		10
Thursday	Chandra bhedana	II and III	15–20
	Pratiloma	IIIb	15–20
	Śavāsana		10
Friday	Ujjāyī	VIII	20
	Nāḍī śodhana	IVb	20
	Śavāsana		10
Saturday	Viloma	VII	10
	Nāḍī śodhana	Ib	20
	Śavāsana		10

After finishing the main prāṇāyāma, bhastrikā may be done before śavāsana for two or three minutes, with or without blocking the nasal passages.

Glossary

A	Negative particle meaning 'non', as in non-violence.
Abhaya	Freedom from fear.
Abhiniveśa	Instinctive clinging to life and the fear that one may be cut off from all by death.
Abhyāsa	Constant study and disciplined practice.
Achala	Immovable.
Achalatā	Immovability.
Achit	That which is not 'chit' (chit = the animating principle of life).
Adhama	The lowest, the meanest.
Adhamādhama	The lowest of the low.
Adhamamadhyama	The lowest of the middling.
Adhamottama	The best among the low.
Ādhāra	A support.
Ādi Śeṣa	The primeval serpent, said to have a thousand heads, and represented as forming the couch of Viṣṇu or as supporting the entire world on his head.
Agarbha dhyāna	Garbha means a foetus, an embryo. Dhyāna means meditation. Dhyāna is the seventh stage of Yoga mentioned by Patanjali. In meditation a beginner is given a mantra (sacred thought or prayer) to bring his wandering mind to a state of steadiness and to keep him from worldly desires. This is known as sabīja or sagarbha (sa = with; bīja = seed; garbha = embryo) dhyāna. Sitting in meditation without recitation of mantras is known as nirbīja or agarbha dhyāna. The prefixes 'nir' and 'a' denote absence of something, and 'a' means without.
Agni	Fire or digestive faculty.
Ahaṁkāra	Ego or egoism; literally 'the I-maker', the state that ascertains 'I know'.
Ahiṁsā	Non-violence. The word has not merely the negative and restrictive meaning of 'non-killing' or 'non-violence', but the positive and comprehensive meaning of 'love embracing all creation'.
Āhuti	Offering an oblation to a deity, any solemn rite accompanied with oblations.

Ājñā chakra	The nervous plexus situated between the eyebrows, the seat of command (ājñā = command).
Ākāśa	The sky, ether (considered as the fifth element), free space.
Alabdha Bhūmikatva	Failure to attain firm ground or continuity in practice, feeling that it is not possible to see reality.
Ālambusā nāḍī	Name of one of the nādīs, which are tubular organs of the subtle body through which energy flows. Ālambusā is said to connect the mouth and the anus.
Ālasya	Idleness, sloth, apathy.
Amanaskatva	The aim of Yoga is to sublimate the mind and the intellect gradually. When fluctuations take place internally and externally, mental and intellectual energies get wasted. When the internal or emotional upheavals of the mind are stilled, the state experienced is that of manolaya (manas = mind; laya = immersion), where the mind is free from fluctuations, dissolves and merges in the Self, like a river in the sea, a merging of one's identity at the emotional level. Where the intellect is in full command and does not allow invading thoughts to disturb it, the state experienced is that of amanaskatva, of being without the organ of desires or thoughts. It is a state of intellectual clarity. (Amanaskatva = A state (tva) of being without the organ of desires or thoughts (amanaska).
Anāhata chakra	The nervous plexus situated in the cardiac region.
Ānanda	Happiness, joy, bliss.
Ānandamaya kośa	The sheath (kośa) of joy (ānanda) enveloping the soul.
Anavasthitattva	Inability to continue the practices, feeling that it is no longer necessary, since the aspirant believes he has reached the highest state of samādhi.
Anna	Food (in general). Also, food as representing the lowest form in which the Supreme Soul is manifested.
Annamaya kośa	The gross material body, the sthūla (gross) śarīra (frame), which is sustained by food, and which is the outer vesture or wrapper or sheath of the soul. It is also the material world, the coarsest or lowest form in which Brahma is considered as manifesting itself in worldly existence.
Antaḥkaraṇa	The heart, soul, the seat of thought and feeling, the thinking faculty, mind, conscience. (anta = last or extreme point, final limit; karaṇa = an organ of sense, an instrument or means of action.)

Antara — The interior, inside, internal.

Antara kumbhaka — Suspension of breath after full inhalation.

Antarātmā — The inmost spirit or soul; the inherent supreme spirit or soul residing in the interior of man.

Ānubhavika jñāna — Knowledge (= jñāna) gained by experience (= anubhava).

Anuloma — Anu means with, along with or connected. Anuloma means 'with the hair' (loma), with the grain, along with the current, regular. In a natural order.

Anuloma prāṇāyāma — In anuloma prāṇāyāma, inhalation is done through both nostrils and exhalation is done alternately through either nostril.

Anusandhāna — Close scrutiny, examination; also suitable connection.

Anuṣṭhana — Regular spiritual practices.

Ap — Water, one of the five elements of creation.

Apāna vāyu — One of the vital airs (vāyu) which move in the sphere of the lower abdomen and control the function of elimination of urine and faeces.

Aparigraha — Freedom from hoarding or collecting.

Ārambhāvasthā — The state (= avasthā) of commencement (= ārambha). This is the first state of prāṇāyāma mentioned in the *Śiva Saṁhitā*.

Arjuna — A Pāndava prince, the mighty bowman and hero of the epic *Mahābhārata*.

Āroha — Ascent, rising, elevation.

Artha — Meaning, sense, signification, import. Also, wealth as one of the objects of human pursuit.

Artha bhāvanam — A feeling of devotion or faith (bhāvanā) arising as a result of contemplation upon the meaning (artha) of a mantra or name of the Lord.

Asaṁsaktā — Indifferent (= asakta) to praise or revilement (= śaṁs).

Āsana — Posture, the third stage of Yoga.

Asat — Non-existent, unreal.

Asmitā — Egoism.

Aśokavana — The grove of Aśoka trees in Laṅkā, where the demon king Rāvana had kept captive Sītā, who remained loyal to her husband Rāma.

Asteya — Non-stealing.

Asthi — A bone.

Aśūnya — Not (A) empty (śunya). Fulfilled.

Aśūnyāvasthā — A state (= ąvasthā) of clarity where the intellect is in full command and does not allow invading thoughts to disturb it.

Aśva — Horse.

Aśvini Mudrā	Contraction of the anal sphincter muscles.
Ātmā	The Supreme Soul or Brahman.
Ātma darśana	Seeing (darśana) oneself (Ātmā) as being a part of the Supreme Soul. A vision (darśana) of the Self (= Atmā).
Ātmānusandhāna	The quest of the self.
Ātma-sādhana	Self-culture.
Ātmāhuti	An oblation of oneself. Self-sacrifice.
Ātma jaya	The conquest of oneself.
Ātma jñāna	Self-knowledge, spiritual knowledge, knowledge of the soul or the Supreme Spirit. True wisdom.
Ātmānjali mudrā	Folding the palms in front of the chest in salutation to the soul within.
Āuṁ	Like the Latin word *Omne*, the Sanskrit word Āuṁ means 'all' and conveys the concepts of omniscience, omnipresence and omnipotence.
Āuṁ namo Nārāyaṇāya / *Āuṁ namaḥ Śivāya*	Since the word Āuṁ is one of great power, it is recommended that its power be diluted, by adding to it the names of deities like Nārāyana or Śiva, to enable the seeker to repeat it and grasp its true significance.
Avasthā	State or condition of the mind.
Avidyā	Ignorance, especially in the spiritual sense.
Avirati	Sensuality.
Āyāma	Length, expansion, extension. It also conveys the idea of restraint, control and stopping.
Āyurveda	The science of health or medicine.
Baddha Koṇāsana	One of the postures recommended for the practice of prāṇāyāma or dhyāna.
Bāhya kumbhaka	Suspension of breath after full exhalation, where the lungs are completely empty.
Bandha	Bondage or fetter. It means a posture where certain organs or parts of the body are contracted and controlled.
Bhadrāsana	One of the postures recommended for the practice of Prāṇāyāma or dhyāna.
Bhagavad-Gītā	The Song Divine, the sacred dialogues between Kṛṣna and Arjuna. It is one of the source books of Hindu philosophy, containing the essence of the *Upaniṣads*.
Bhakti	Worship, adoration.
Bhakti mārga	The way or path to salvation through adoration of a personal God.
Bhastrikā	A bellows used in a furnace. Bhastrikā is a type of prāṇāyāma where air is forcibly drawn in and out or blasted as in a furnace.
Bhava vairāgya	Absence of worldly desires.

Bhāvanā	A feeling of devotion or faith.
Bhāvanam	Perception, faith, understanding.
Bhaya	Fear.
Bhedana	Piercing, breaking through, passing through.
Bhoga	Enjoyment of worldly pleasures.
Bhramara	A large black bee.
Bhrāmarī	A type of prāṇāyāma where during exhalation a soft humming sound like the murmuring of a bee is made.
Bhrānti-darśana	Erroneous (bhrānti) vision or knowledge (darśana), delusion.
Bhuh	The earth, the first of the three worlds, the other two being ether and the sky or heaven. It is also a mystic word, one of the first giving rise to speech.
Bhuvaḥ	The atmosphere or ether, the second of the three worlds, the one immediately above the earth. It is also a mystic word, one of the first in the creation of speech.
Bīja	A seed or germ.
Bīja mantra	In meditation the chanting of mantras is sometimes given to the beginner to bring his wandering mind to a state of steadiness and keep him away from worldly desires. A bīja mantra is a mystic syllable with a sacred prayer repeated mentally during prāṇāyāma or dhyāna, and the seed thus planted in the mind germinates into one-pointedness.
Bindu	A drop, small particle, a dot, a point.
Brahmā	The Supreme Being: the Creator.
Brahmacharya	A life of celibacy, religious study and self-restraint.
Brahman	The Supreme Being, the cause of the universe, the all-pervading spirit of the universe.
Brahma nāḍī	Another name for suṣumṇa-nāḍī, the main channel of energy running through the centre of the spinal column. When prāṇa (energy) enters it, it takes the seeker to Brahman, the final beatitude. Hence the name.
Brahmapurī	The city (purī) of Brahman, the human body.
Brahmarandhra	The aperture (randhra) in the crown of the head through which the soul is said to leave the body on death.
Brahma vidyā	The knowledge of the Supreme Spirit.
Buddha	Founder of Buddhism.
Buddhi	Intellect, reason, discrimination, judgement.
Chakra	Literally, a wheel or circle. Energy (prāṇa) is said to flow in the human body through three main channels (nāḍīs), namely, suṣumṇā, pingalā and iḍā. Suṣumṇā is situated inside the spinal column. Pingalā and iḍā start

respectively from the right and left nostrils, move up to the crown of the head and course downwards to the base of the spine. These two nāḍīs intersect with each other and also with the suṣumṇā. These junctions of the nāḍīs are known as chakras or the fly-wheels which regulate the body mechanism. The important chakras are: (a) mūlādhāra (mūla = root, source; ādhāra = support, vital part) situated in the pelvis above the anus; (b) svādhiṣṭhāna (sva = vital force, soul; adhiṣṭhāna = seat or abode) situated above the organs of generation; (c) maṇipūraka (maṇipūra = navel) situated in the navel; (d) manas (= mind) and (e) sūrya (= the sun), situated in the region between the navel and the heart; (f) anāhata (= unbeaten), situated in the cardiac area; (g) viśuddhi (= purity), situated in the pharyngeal region; (h) ājñā (= command) situated between the eyebrows; (i) soma (= the moon), situated in the centre of the brain; (j) lalāṭa (= forehead), which is at the top of the forehead; and (k) sahasrāra (sahasra = thousand) which is called the thousand-petalled lotus in the cerebral cavity.

Chakṣu — The eye.

Chāndogyopaniṣad — One of the principal *Upaniṣads*.

Chandra — The moon.

Chandra bhedana prāṇāyāma — Chandra is the moon. Bhedana, derived from the root 'bhid', means to pierce, to break or pass through. In chandra bhedana prāṇāyāma the breath is inhaled through the left nostril, and prāṇa passes through the iḍā or chandra nāḍī and is then exhaled through the right nostril, which is the path of the piṅgalā or sūrya nāḍī.

Chandra nāḍī — The nāḍī of the moon; another name of Iḍā nāḍī.

Charaka Saṁhitā — A treatise on the Indian system of medicine.

Chidātmā — The thinking principle or faculty, pure intelligence, the Supreme Spirit.

Chit — Thought, perception, intellect, mind. The soul, spirit, the animating principle of life. Universal consciousness.

Chitrā nāḍī — One of the nāḍīs emanating from the heart, through which the creative energy (śakti) of Kuṇḍalinī passes to reach the sahasrāra.

Chitta — The mind in its total or collective sense, being composed of three categories: (a) mind (manas) having the faculty of attention, selection and rejection; (b) reason

	(buddhi), the decisive state which determines the distinction between things, and (c) ego (ahaṁkāra), the I-maker.
Dairghya	Horizontal expansion.
Dala	A large number.
Darśana	A vision, discernment. Also, a system of philosophy.
Daurmanasya	Despair.
Deśa	Place or state.
Devadatta vāyu	One of the vital airs which provides for the intake of extra oxygen in a tired body by causing a yawn.
Dhamana	Blowing as with a bellows.
Dhamanī	A tubular organ or duct within the physical or subtle body conveying energy in different forms.
Dhanañjaya vāyu	One of the vital airs which remains in the body even after death and sometimes bloats a corpse.
Dhāraṇā	Concentration or complete attention. The sixth stage of Yoga mentioned by Patanjali.
Dharma	Derived from the root 'dhṛ', meaning to uphold, maintain, support, sustain; dharma means religion, law, moral merit, righteousness, good works. It is the code of conduct that sustains the soul and produces virtue, morality or religious merit, leading towards the development of man. It is regarded as one of the four ends of human existence.
Dharma Kṣetra	Name of a plain, the scene of the great battle between the Kauravas and the Pāṇḍavas in the Mahābhārata War. It is the battlefield where Kṛṣṇa expounded the *Bhagavad Gītā* to the Pāndava prince Arjuna and urged him to do his duty as a warrior.
Dhātu	An element. A humour or affection of the body like vāta (= wind), pitta (= bile) and kapha (phlegm).
Dhṛ	To hold or concentrate.
Dhyāna	Meditation. The seventh stage of Yoga mentioned by Patanjali.
Doṣa	A fault or defect, a noxious quality, disorder of the three humours of the body.
Duḥkha	Sorrow and pain.
Dvāra-pāla	Guardian or keeper (pāla) of the gate (dvāra).
Dveṣa	Hatred, enmity.
Ekāgra	(Eka = one; agra = foremost). Fixed on one object or point only; closely attentive, where the mental faculties are all focused on a single point.
Gandha	Smell.
Gāndhārī nāḍī	Name of one of the nāḍīs said to be located behind the

	idā nāḍī, terminating near the left eye, regulating the function of sight.
Garbha	A foetus or an embryo.
Gautama	Name of the propounder of the Nyāya system of philosophy.
Gāyatri mantra	A vedic hymn composed on the wife of Brahmā – the mother of the vedas.
Ghaṭa	A large earthen water pot, an intense effort.
Ghaṭāvasthā	The second stage (avasthā) of prāṇāyāma discussed in the *Śiva Saṁhitā*, where the body like an earthen pot (ghaṭa) has to be baked hard in the fire of prāṇāyāma to gain stability.
Gheraṇḍa Saṁhitā	A classical work on haṭha yoga.
Gu	First syllable in the word 'guru', meaning darkness.
Guṇa	A quality, an ingredient or constituent of nature. One of the three constituents of cosmic substance (prakṛti), illuminating (sattva), activating (rajas) and restraining (tamas).
Guṇātīta	One who is freed from and gone beyond or has crossed the three guṇas of sattva, rajas and tamas.
Guru	Spiritual preceptor, one who illumines the darkness of spiritual doubt.
Hanumān	A powerful monkey chief of extraordinary strength and prowess, whose exploits are celebrated in the epic *Rāmāyaṇa*. He was the son of Añjanā and Vāyu, the god of wind. He is regarded as one of the immortals in the Hindu pantheon and a master of prāṇāyāma and a champion of athletes.
Hastijihvā nāḍī	Name of one of the nāḍīs, located in front of the iḍā nāḍī, terminating near the right eye, regulating the function of sight.
Haṭha yoga	The way towards realisation through rigorous discipline.
Haṭha-yoga-pradīpikā	A celebrated text book on Haṭha Yoga written by Svātmārāma.
Hiraṇyagarbha	Name of Brahman, as born from a golden egg (hiraṇya = gold; garbha = embryo, egg). It also means the soul invested by the subtle body (sūkṣma = subtle; śarīra = body).
Hṛdayam	The heart, soul, mind. The interior or essence of anything.
Hṛdayāñjali mudrā	Folding of hands in front of the heart in respectful salutation to the dweller within.
Ichhā	Wish, desire, will.

Iḍā nāḍī — A nāḍi or channel of energy starting from the left nostril, then moving to the crown of the head and thence descending to the base of the spine. In its course it conveys lunar energy and is therefore called chandra nāḍī (channel of lunar energy).

Indriyas — Senses of perception and action.

Iṣṭadevatā — Chosen deity.

Īśvara — The Supreme Being. God.

Īśvara praṇidhāna — Dedication to the Lord of one's actions and one's will.

Jābāli — Name of a sage, son of Jābālā, a serving woman. As a boy he had confessed that he was not aware of his parentage and was accepted by the sage Gautama, who was impressed by his innocence and truthfulness. Gautama named him Satyakāma-Jābāli (satyakāma = lover of truth; Jābāli = son of Jābālā).

Jāgṛta — Awake, watchful.

Jāgṛtāvasthā — The state (avasthā) of watchfulness, awareness.

Jāgṛti — Watchfulness, awareness.

Jāla — A net, lattice. Also a collection, number, mass.

Jālandhara bandha — Jālandhara is a posture where the neck and throat are extended and the chin is rested in the notch between the collar-bones at the top of the breastbone, stimulating the pharyngeal plexus.

Japa — Prayer.

Jāṭarāgni — Digestive fire.

Jaya — Conquest, success.

Jitēndriya — One who has conquered his passions or subdued his senses.

Jīva — A living being, a creature. An individual soul, as distinguished from the universal soul.

Jīvana mukta — A person who is emancipated during his lifetime by true knowledge of the Supreme Spirit.

Jīvātmā — The individual or personal soul.

Jñāna — Sacred knowledge derived from meditation on the higher truths of religion and philosophy, which teaches a man how to understand his own nature.

Jñāna chakṣu — The eye (chakṣu) of intelligence, the mind's eye, the intellectual vision (as opposed to the eye of the flesh).

Jñāna mārga — The path of knowledge by which man finds realisation.

Jñāna mudrā — The gesture of the hand where the index finger and the thumb tip are brought in contact, while the remaining three fingers are kept extended. The gesture is the symbol of knowledge (jñāna). The index finger is the

	symbol of the individual soul, the thumb signifies the Supreme Universal, and the union of these two symbolises true knowledge.
Jñānendriya	The senses of knowledge, hearing, touch, sight, taste and smell.
Jvalanti	Blazing or shining.
Kaivalyāvasthā	Kaivalya is perfect isolation, exclusiveness or detachment of the soul from matter, identification with the Supreme Spirit. Kaivalyāvasthā is the state (= avasthā) of final emancipation or beatitude.
Kāla	Time.
Kāla chakra	The wheel of time.
Kāma	Desire, lust.
Kanda	A bulbous root, a knot. The kanda is of a round shape of about four inches, situated about twelve inches above the anus and near the navel, where the three main nāḍīs – suṣumṇā, iḍā and pingalā – unite and separate. It is covered as if with a soft white piece of cloth.
Kandasthāna	The place or position of the kanda.
Kapāla	Skull.
Kapāla-bhāti	Kapāla = skull; bhāti = light. Kapāla-bhāti is a process of clearing the sinuses. It is a milder form of bhastrikā prāṇāyāma.
Kapha	Phlegm.
Kāraṇa śarīra	The inner rudiment of the body (śarīra), the causal (= kāraṇa) frame. It is the spiritual sheath of joy (ānandamaya kośa). The experience of being aware of it is felt when one is totally absorbed in the object of one's meditation or awakes from refreshing sleep.
Karma	Action.
Karma mārga	The way of an active man towards realisation through action.
Karma mukta	One who is liberated from the results or fruits of action.
Karma phalatyāgi	One who has abandoned or renounced (tyāgi) the fruits or rewards (phala) of action (karma) done in life.
Karmendriya	Organs (indriya) of action, of excretion, generation, hands, feet and speech.
Kaṭhopaniṣad	One of the principal *Upaniṣads* in verse and in the form of a dialogue between the seeker Nachiketā and Yama, the god of Death.
Kauśiki nāḍī	One of the nāḍīs, terminating at the big toes.
Kauṣītaki Upaniṣad	One of the *Upaniṣads*.
Kevala kumbhaka	When the practices of kumbhaka (respiratory pro-

cesses) become so perfect that they are instinctive, they are known as kevala (pure or simple) kumbhaka.

Kośa — A sheath, a case. According to Vedantic philosophy, there are three types of body (śarīra) enveloping the soul. These three types or frames of the body consist of five inter-penetrating and inter-dependent sheaths or cases (kośas). The five kośas are: (a) annamaya or anatomical sheath of nourishment; (b) prāṇamaya or physiological sheath, including the respiratory and other systems of the body; (c) manomaya or psychological sheath, affecting awareness, feeling and motivation not derived from subjective experience; (d) vijñānamaya or intellectual sheath, affecting the process of reasoning and judgement derived from subjective experience; and (e) ānandamaya, or the spiritual sheath of joy. Annamaya kośa forms the sthūla śarīra, the gross body. The prāṇamaya, manomaya and vijñānamaya kośas form the sūkṣma śarīra, the subtle body. The ānandamaya kośa forms the kārana śarīra, the causal body.

Kriyā — An expiatory rite, a cleansing process.

Kṛkara vāyu — One of the five subsidiary vāyus, which, by making one sneeze or cough, prevent substances passing up the nasal passages and down the throat

Krodha — Anger.

Kṛṣṇa — The Lord of all Yogas (Yogeśvara). The most celebrated hero in Hindu mythology. The eighth incarnation of Viṣṇu.

Kṣetra — The body regarded as the field of activity.

Kṣetrajña — The husbandman. The knower of the body, the soul.

Kṣipta — Distracted, neglected.

Kuhū — Name of one of the nāḍīs, said to be located in front of the suṣumṇā, and its function is to evacuate faeces.

Kulāla chakra — The wheel (chakra) of a potter (kulāla).

Kumbha — A water pot, a pitcher, a chalice.

Kumbhaka — Kumbhaka is the interval of time or retention of breath after full inhalation or after full exhalation. The imagery of the lungs being completely full or completely empty like a full or empty water pot.

Kumbhakarṇa — Pitcher-eared. The name of a gigantic demon, brother of Rāvaṇa, ultimately slain by Rāma. He practised most rigid austerities to humiliate the gods. Brahmā was about to grant him a boon, when the gods requested Saraswatī, goddess of speech to sit on his

	tongue and deflect it. When Kumbhakarna went to Brahmā, instead of asking Indrapada (the status of *Indra*, the king of gods) he asked Nidrapada (the status of sleep = nidra), which was readily granted. His effort made him fall into death-like torpor, for his meditation and austerities had been tāmasic.
Kuṇḍalinī	The kuṇḍalinī (kuṇḍala = the coil of a rope; kuṇḍalinī = a coiled female serpent) is divine cosmic energy. The force or energy is symbolised by a coiled and sleeping serpent lying dormant in the lowest nerve centre at the base of the spinal column, the mūlādhāra chakra. This latent energy has to be aroused and made to ascend the main spinal channel, the suṣumnā piercing the chakras right up to the sahasrāra, the thousand-petalled lotus in the head. Then the yogi is in union with the Supreme Universal Soul.
Kūrma nāḍī	Name of one of the subsidiary nāḍīs, whose function is to stabilise the body and the mind.
Kūrma vāyu	It is the name of one of the subsidiary vital airs whose function is to control the movements of the eyelids to prevent foreign matter or too bright a light entering the eyes.
Kuru Kṣetra	Name of an extensive plain near Delhi, the scene of the Mahābhārata War between the Kauravas and the Pāṇḍavas. The human body is compared to this field of conflict between the powers of evil and of good, or between self-interest and duty.
Kuśa	Sacred grass used at the time of religious ceremonies.
Lalāṭa chakra	Lalāṭa means the forehead. The lalāṭa chakra is located at the top of the forehead.
Lanka	Ceylon, Republic of Śri Lanka.
Laya	Dissolution; absorption of the mind or devotion.
Lobha	Greed.
Loma	Hair
Mada	Pride, lust.
Madhyama	Middling, average, mediocre.
Mahānārāyaṇopaniṣad	Name of one of the *Upaniṣads*.
Mahā tapas	Great (mahā) austerities (tapas).
Mahā vidyā	Great knowledge, exalted knowledge.
Mahā vṛta	A great vow or fundamental duty.
Mahat	The unevolved primary germ of the productive principle whence all phenomena of the material world are developed. In Sāṁkhya philosophy, it is the great

	principle, the intellect (distinguished from manas), the second of the twenty-five elements or tattvas recognised by the Sāṁkhyas.
Majjā	Marrow.
Māṁsa	Flesh.
Manana	Reflection, meditation.
Manas	The individual mind, having the power and faculty of attention, selection and rejection. The ruler of the senses.
Manas chakra	Nervous plexus situated between the navel and the heart.
Maṇipūraka chakra	The nervous plexus situated in the region of the navel.
Manojñāna	Knowledge of the working of the mind and emotions.
Manomaya kośa	One of the sheaths (kośa) enveloping the soul. The manomaya kośa affects the functions of awareness, feeling and motivation not derived from subjective experience.
Manolaya	Manolaya (manas = mind; laya = immersion) is the state where the internal or emotional upheavals of the mind are stilled. Then the mind, free from fluctuations, dissolves and merges in the self, like a river in the sea, losing its individual identity.
Mantra	Vedic hymn.
Mātsarya	Envy.
Medas	Fat.
Merudaṇḍa	Spinal column.
Mīmāṁsā	Examination. Also systems of Indian philosophy. Pūrva mīmāṁsā deals with the general conception of the Deity, but stresses the importance of action (karma) and rituals. Uttara mīmāṁsā accepts God on the basis of the Vēdas, but lays special stress on spiritual knowledge (jñāna).
Moha	Infatuation.
Mokṣa	Liberation; final emancipation of the soul from recurring births.
Muḍha	Dull.
Mudrā	A seal; a sealing posture.
Mukta	Liberated.
Mukti	Release, liberation, final absolution of the soul from the chain of birth and death.
Mūla	The root, base.
Mūla bandha	A posture where the body from the anus to the navel is contracted and lifted towards the spine.
Mūlādhāra chakra	Nervous plexus situated in the pelvis above the anus at

	the base or root of the spine; the main support of the body.
Mūrchhā prāṇāyāma	A type of prāṇāyāma where breath is held almost to the point of swooning (mūrchhā).
Nachiketa	Name of the seeker and one of the principal characters in the Kaṭhopaniṣad. His father Vājaśravas wanted to give away all his possessions so as to acquire religious merit. Nachiketa felt puzzled when his father started giving away old and barren cattle and asked him again and again: 'To whom will you give me?'. His father said: 'I give you to Yama (the God of Death)'. Nachiketa went to the realm of Death and obtained three boons, the last of which was the knowledge of the secret of life after death. Yama tried to divert Nachiketa from obtaining his wish by offering the greatest earthly pleasures, but Nachiketa was not swayed from his purpose and ultimately Yama gave him the knowledge desired.
Nāda	Inner mystical sound.
Nādānusandhāna	Anusandhāna is examination, planning, arrangement or suitable connection. Nādānusandhāna is close scrutiny of the sound of rhythmic patterns of breath during the practice of prāṇāyāma and total absorption in the sound, like a master musician in his music.
Nādarūpiṇi	Sound incarnate.
Nāḍī	A tubular organ of the subtle body through which energy flows. Nāḍīs are ducts or channels which carry air, water, blood, nutrients and other substances throughout the body. They channel cosmic, vital, seminal and other energies as well as sensations, consciousness and spiritual aura.
Nāḍī chakra	Ganglia or plexuses in the gross, subtle and causal bodies.
Nāḍikā	Small nāḍī.
Nāḍī śodhana prāṇāyāma	Prāṇāyāma done for the purification or cleansing of the nāḍīs. It is the highest and most difficult type of prāṇāyāma.
Nāga vāyu	One of the five subsidiary vāyus which relieves abdominal pressure by belching.
Nārada	Name of a divine sage. He is represented as a messenger between the gods and men. He is said to be the inventor of the lute (vīṇā). He was a great devotee of Viṣṇu and author of the *Bhakti Sūtras* (Aphorisms on

	Divine Love) and also a code of laws which goes by his name.
Narāyaṇa	Another name for Lord Viṣṇu.
Nididhyāsana	Profound and repeated meditation, constant musing.
Nidrā	Sleep.
Nirbīja	Bīja is a seed or germ. A bīja mantra is a mystical syllable or sacred prayer repeated mentally during prāṇāyāma or dhyāna to bring the wandering mind to a state of steadiness. With practice the seed planted in the mind germinates into one-pointedness. Gradually the practice becomes nirbīja (nir = without; bīja = seed) where the practitioner does not have to resort to the bīja mantra.
Nirbīja dhyāna	Dhyāna, where the practitioner does not have to resort to the bīja mantra.
Nirbīja prāṇāyāma	Prāṇāyāma, where the practitioner does not have to resort to the bīja mantra.
Niruddha	Restrained, checked, controlled.
Nirvāṇa	Eternal bliss; liberated from existence.
Nirviṣaya	Without sensuality.
Niṣpatti	Perfection, ripeness.
Niṣpatti avasthā	The state of perfection or ripeness. Consummation.
Nivṛtti mārga	The path of realisation by abstaining from worldly acts, and being uninfluenced by worldly desires.
Niyama	Self-purification by discipline. The second stage of Yoga mentioned by Patanjali.
Nyāya	A system of Indian philosophy stressing logic and primarily concerned with the laws of thought relying on reason and analogy.
Ojas	Vitality, lustre, splendour.
Padārthābhāva	Non-existence or absence (abhāva) of things or objects (padārtha). The absence of the phenomenal creation. The final emancipation of the purusa or soul (the twenty-fifth tattva) from the bonds of worldly existence – the fetters of phenomenal creation – by conveying the correct knowledge of the twenty-four other tattvas and by properly discriminating the soul from them.
Padmāsana	The lotus pose, sitting cross-legged on the floor with the spine erect. The pose is ideal for practice of prāṇāyāma and dhyāna.
Panchamahābhūtas	Five gross elements, namely earth, water, fire, air and aether.
Parā	Supreme.

Parabrahman	The highest or supreme (para) spirit (Brahman).
Para-jñāna	The supreme knowledge, absolute knowledge.
Paramātmā	The supreme (parama) spirit (Atmā).
Parā nāḍī	Supreme nāḍī or nerve.
Paratattva	Beyond (para) the elements or primary substances (tattva); the Supreme Universal Spirit, which is beyond the material world, pervading the universe.
Parichaya	Acquaintance, intimacy, frequent repetition. Intimate knowledge.
Parichayāvasthā	The stage of intimate knowledge (parichaya). This is the third stage of Prāṇāyāma mentioned in the *Śiva Saṁhitā*.
Paśchimottānāsana	Intense posterior stretch from the heels to the head.
Patanjali	Name of a philosopher, the propounder of Yoga philosophy, the author of the *Yoga Sūtras*. He created serenity of mind by his work on Yoga, clarity of speech by his work on grammar, and purity of body by his work on medicine. He is the reputed author of the *Mahābhāśya*, the great commentary on Pāṇini's Sūtras on grammar.
Payaswini nāḍī	Name of one of the nāḍīs, terminating at the right big toe. It is said to be located between the pūṣā (which is behind the pingalā nāḍī) and the saraswati nāḍī (which is behind the suṣumnā nāḍī).
Pingalā nāḍī	A nāḍī or channel of energy, starting from the right nostril, then moving to the crown of the head and thence downwards to the base of the spine. As the solar energy flows through it, it is also called the sūrya nāḍī. Pingalā means tawny or reddish.
Pitta	Bile, one of the humours of the body, the other two being vāta (wind) and kapha (phlegm).
Plāvinī prāṇāyāma	Plāvana means swimming, overflowing, flooding. Plāvinī Prāṇāyāma is said to help one to float or swim. Except for the name there is hardly any mention of this type of prāṇāyāma in the Yoga texts.
Prajāpati	The Lord of created beings.
Prajñā	Intelligence, wisdom.
Prakṛti	Nature, the original source of the material world, consisting of the three qualities, sattva, rajas and tamas.
Pramāda	Indifference, insensibility.
Prāṇa	Breath, respiration, life, vitality, wind, energy, strength. It also connotes the soul.
Prāṇa jñāna	The knowledge of breath and life.
Prāṇa vāyu	The vital air which pervades the entire human body. It moves in the region of the chest.

Prāṇamaya kośa — The physiological (prāṇamaya) sheath (kosá), which along with the psychological (manomaya) and the intellectual (vijñānamaya) sheaths make up the subtle body (sūksma śarīra) enveloping the soul. The prāṇamaya kośa includes the respiratory, circulatory, digestive, endocrine, excretory and genital systems.

Praṇava — Another word for the sacred syllable AUM.

Prāṇāyāma — Rhythmic control (āyama) of breath. The fourth stage of Yoga. It is the hub around which the wheel of Yoga revolves.

Prāṇāyāma vidyā — Knowledge, learning, lore or science (vidyā) of Prāṇāyāma.

Praśṇopaniṣad — Name of one of the major *Upaniṣads*.

Pratiloma prāṇāyāma — Pratiloma means against the hair, against the grain, against the current. In this type of prāṇāyāma inhalation is controlled digitally through either nostril alternately, followed by exhalation through open nostrils.

Pratyāhāra — Withdrawal and emancipation of the mind from the domination of the senses and sensual objects. The fifth stage of Yoga.

Pravṛtti marqa — Path of action.

Pṛtvi — Earth.

Pṛtvi tattva — Element of earth.

Pūraka — Inhalation or the filling of the lungs.

Puruṣa — Universal psychic principle.

Puruṣārthās — Four aims of life in man. They are dharma (duty), artha (acquisition), kāma (pleasures) and mokṣa (liberation).

Pūrva Mīmāṁsā — One of the systems of Indian philosophy which deals with the concept of Deity but lays special stress on actions and rituals.

Rāga — Attachment.

Rajas — Action, passion, emotion.

Rakta — Blood.

Rāma — The seventh incarnation of Lord Viṣṇu.

Rāmāyaṇa — The celebrated epic story of Rāma.

Randra — Aperture.

Rasa — Taste.

Rasātmaka — Experiences of various sentiments and flavours that life offers.

Ratna — Jewel.

Ratnākara — The ocean, producer of jewels. Also the name of a robber who later became the sage Vālmīki, celebrated author of the epic *Rāmāyaṇa*. One day the robber held up the sage Nārada, whom he asked on pain of death to deliver up his possessions. Nārada told the robber to go home and ask his wife and children if they were ready to become his partners in the innumerable iniquities which he had committed. The robber went home and returned chastened at hearing their unwillingness to become his partners in sin. Nārada told the robber to repeat the name of Rāma, but when the robber declined, requested him to repeat 'marā' (which is Rāma inverted) continuously and then disappeared. Ratnākara kept on repeatedly saying 'marā' and became so absorbed in it and in thinking of Rāma that his body was covered up with ant-hills (vālmīka). Nārada returned and got the robber-turned-saint out, and as he came out of the shell of ant-hills, he was called Vālmīki. When Sītā was pregnant and abandoned he gave her shelter in his hermitage and brought up her twin sons, later restoring them all to Rāma.

Ratnapūrita dhatu — Elements filled with essential ingredients (jewels).

Rāvaṇa — Name of the demon king of Laṅkā, who abducted Sītā, wife of Rāma, and was consequently slain by Rāma. Rāvaṇa was highly intellectual and had prodigious strength. He was an ardent devotee of Śiva and well versed in the Vedas, and is reputed to have given the accents to the Vedic texts so that they have remained unchanged.

Rechaka — Exhalation; emptying of the lungs.

Retas — Semen.

Ṛg Veda — Name of the first of the four *Vedas*, the sacred books of the Hindus.

Ru — The second syllable in the word 'guru', meaning light.

Rudra — Formidable, terrible. Also, name of Śiva.

Rūpa — Form.

Sa — A prefix. Compounded with nouns, it forms adjectives and adverbs in the sense of (a) with, together with, along with, accompanied by, having; (b) similar, like; (c) same.

Śabda — Sound, word.

Sabīja — Bīja is a seed or germ. Sabīja means accompanied by a seed. In prāṇāyāma and dhyāna the chanting or mental repetition of a bīja mantra, a sacred prayer, is given to the beginner to bring his wandering mind to a steady condition.

Sabīja dhyāna	Dhyāna performed with the mental repetition of a sacred prayer.
Sabīja prāṇāyāma	Prāṇāyāma performed with the mental repetition of a sacred prayer.
Sad-asad-viveka	Discrimination (viveka) between the true (sad) and the untrue (asad).
Sādhaka	A seeker, an aspirant.
Sādhana	Practice, quest.
Sagarbha dhyāna	Garbha is a foetus or embryo. Sagarbha dhyāna is meditation practised together with a sacred prayer, which like an embryo germinates in the mind and brings it to a state of steadiness.
Sahasrāra chakra	The thousand petalled lotus in the cerebral cavity.
Sahasrāra dala	'Dala' means a heap, a large number, a detachment or a body of troops. Sahasrāra dala is another name for sahasrāra chakra.
Sahasrāra nāḍī	This nāḍī is the seat of the Supreme Spirit, and the gateway to it.
Sahita kumbhaka	'Sahita' means 'accompanied by' or 'attended by' or 'together with'. An intentional suspension of breath.
Sākṣi	A witness or seer. The Supreme Being which sees but does not act.
Śakti	Power, energy, capacity, strength, representing the power of consciousness to act. Śakti is portrayed as the female aspect of the Ultimate Principle and deified as the wife of Śiva.
Śakti chālana	Ascendance of divine energy or kuṇḍalinī.
Sāma Veda	Name of one of the four Vedas, containing priestly chants.
Samādhi	A state in which the aspirant is one with the object of his meditation, the Supreme Spirit pervading the universe, where there is a feeling of unutterable joy and peace. The eighth and highest stage of Yoga.
Samāhita chitta	The state wherein the mind, intellect and ego are evenly balanced and well disposed. A well-balanced personality.
Samāna vāyu	One of the vital airs which aids digestion for a harmonious functioning of the abdominal organs.
Samavṛtti prāṇāyāma	Of equal movement or duration in inhalation, exhalation and suspension of breath in Prāṇāyāma.
Saṁkalpa	Intention, mental resolve, determination.
Śaṁkhiṇī nāḍī	Name of a nāḍī, located between the iḍā and the suṣumṇā, terminating at the genital organs. Its function is to carry the essence of food.

Saṃkhyā Number, enumeration, calculation.

Sāṃkhya One of the schools of Hindu philosophy, founded by Kapila, giving a systematic account of cosmic evolution. It is so called because it enumerates twenty-five tattvas (categories). These are: Puruṣa (cosmic spirit), Prakṛti (cosmic substance), mahat (cosmic intelligence), ahaṁkāra (individuating principle), manas (cosmic mind), indriyas (ten abstract sense-powers of cognition and of action), tanmātras (five subtle elements – sound, touch, form, flavour and odour, which are the subtle objects of the sense powers) and mahābhūtas (five sense particulars – the great elements of ether (space), air, fire, water and earth).

Saṁśaya Doubt.

Samskāra Mental impression of the past.

Saṁyama Restraint, check, control.

Śankarāchārya A celebrated teacher of the doctrine of Advaita (non-dualism). Within a short life span of about thirty-two years he wrote authoritative commentaries, numerous philosophical poems, and founded four monasteries (maṭhas), at Śṛṅgeri in the south, Badrināth in the north, Pūri in the east, and Dwārkā in the west.

Ṣaṇmukhī mudrā A sealing posture where the apertures in the head are closed and the mind is directed inwards to train it for meditation.

Sanskṛt A refined language.

Santoṣa Contentment.

Śaraṇāgati Surrender, to take refuge.

Saraswatī Goddess of learning and speech. Also, name of a nāḍī located behind the suṣumṇā, terminating at the tongue, controlling speech and keeping the abdominal organs free from disease.

Śarīra The body enveloping the soul. According to Vedantic philosophy there are three frames or types of the body (śarīra), consisting of five inter-penetrating and inter-dependent sheaths (kośas). The three śarīraṣ are: (a) sthūla, the gross frame, consisting of the anatomical sheath of nourishment (annamaya kośa); (b) sūkṣma, the subtle frame, consisting of the physiological sheath (prāṇamaya kośa including the respiratory, circulatory, digestive, nervous, endocrine, excretory and genital systems), the psychological sheath (manomaya kośa, affecting the functions of awareness, feeling, and motivation not derived from subjective experience), and the intellectual sheath (vijñānamaya kośa, affect-

	ing the intellectual processes of reasoning and judgement derived through subjective experience); and (c) the kāraṇa, the causal frame, consisting of the spiritual sheath of joy (ānandamaya kośa).
Śarīra jñāna	Knowledge of the body. One of the benefits of meditation is a thorough grasp of the three frames or types of the body (śarīra) and the five sheaths (kośas).
Sarvāngāsana	Sarvānga (sarva = all, whole, entire, complete; anga = limb or body) means the entire body or all the limbs. In this posture (āsana) the whole body benefits from its performance, hence the name.
Sāsmita	With (sa) egoism (asmitā). Sāsmita samādhi is one of the types of profound meditation where the ego of the aspirant is not completely forgotten.
Śāstra	Any manual or compedium of rules, any book or treatise, especially religious or scientific treatise, any sacred book or composition of divine authority. The word śāstra is normally found after the word denoting the subject of the book or is applied collectively to departments of knowledge, for example, Yoga śāstra, a work on Yoga philosophy or the body of teaching on the subject of Yoga.
Sat	Being, real, truth, Brahman, or the Supreme Spirit.
Ṣaṭ-Chakra-Nirūpaṇa	Name of a Yoga text dealing with kuṇḍalinī śakti and its arousal from the mūlādhāra to reach the sahasrāra, piercing the six (ṣaṭ) chakras on its way up.
Sattva	The illuminating, pure and good quality of everything in nature.
Sattvāpatti	Self-realisation.
Sāttvic prajñā	Illuminated wisdom
Satya	Truth.
Satyakāma Jābāla	Name of a sage. See Jābāli.
Śaucha	Cleanliness, purity.
Śava	A dead body, a corpse.
Śavāsana	The pose of the dead. In this āsana the object is to simulate the dead. Once life has departed, the body remains still and no movements are possible. By remaining motionless for some time, and by keeping the mind still while one is fully conscious, one learns to relax. This conscious relaxation invigorates and refreshes both body and mind. It is harder to keep the mind still than the body. Hence this apparently easy posture is one of the most difficult to master.
Savichāraṇā	Right (sa) reflection (vichāraṇā)

Savitarka	Sound or right (sa) reasoning, logic or deliberation (vitarka).
Setu-Bandha-sarvāngāsana	Setu means a bridge. Setu bandha means construction of a bridge. In this position, the body is arched and supported on the shoulders at one end and heels at the other. The arch is supported by the hands at the waist.
Siddha	A sage, seer or prophet; also a semi-divine being of great purity and holiness.
Siddhāsana	In this sitting posture the legs are crossed at the ankles, the body is at rest and the erect back keeps the mind attentive and alert. This āsana is recommended for the practice of Prāṇāyāma and for medititation.
Siddhi	Accomplishment, success. It also means superhuman powers.
Sirā	A tubular organ in the body distributing vital seminal energy throughout the subtle body.
Śīrsāsana	Head balance.
Śiṣya	A pupil, a disciple.
Sītā	Name of the wife of Rāma, the heroine of the epic *Rāmāyāṇa*.
Śītakārī and Śītalī	Types of prāṇāyāma which cool the system.
Śiva saṁhitā	A classical text book on Hatha yoga.
Śiva Svarodaya	A Haṭha yoga text.
Śleṣma	Phlegm.
Smṛti	Memory, a code of law.
Soham	'He am I', the unconscious repititive prayer that goes on with every respiration within every living creature throughout life.
Soma	The moon.
Soma chakra	A nervous plexus located in the centre of the brain.
Soma nāḍī	Another name for idā nāḍī, which in its course conveys lunar energy and is therefore called chandra or soma nāḍī (channel of lunar energy).
Sparśa	The subtle element (tanmātra) of touch.
Srota	A rapid stream. Also a canal of nutriment in the body.
Śravaṇa	Hearing, the first stage of self-culture.
Śrī	Auspicious, beautiful.
Sthiratā	Firmness, steadiness, stability, fortitude, constancy, fixity.
Sthita prajñā	Firm in judgement or wisdom, free from any hallucination.
Sthūla śarīra	The gross (sthūla) body (śarīra), the material or perishable body which is destroyed at death.
Styāna	Langour, sloth.

Śubha — Good, virtuous, auspicious; also name of a nāḍī.

Śubhechhā — Good desire or intention (ichhā).

Śukra — Semen, virile.

Sūkṣma — Subtle.

Sūkṣma śarīra — Subtle body heaving and sighing; inhalation and exhalation.

Śūnya — Empty, void, lonely, desolate, non-existent, blank, zero.

Śūnya deśa — A desolate or lonely place. The state of aloneness.

Śūnyāvasthā — The state (avasthā) when the internal and emotional upheavals are stilled. It is a negative state of passivity, when the mind is empty (śūnya) and, free from fluctuations, dissolves and merges in the self, losing its identity like a river in the sea.

Śūrā nāḍī — Name of a nāḍī located between the eye-brows.

Sūrya — The sun.

Sūrya bhedana prāṇāyāma — Piercing or passing through (bhedana) the sun. Here the inhalation is done through the right nostril, from where the pingalā nāḍī or Sūrya nāḍī starts. Exhalation is done through the left nostril, from where the iḍā nāḍī or chandra nāḍī starts.

Sūrya chakra — Nervous plexus situated between the navel and the heart.

Sūrya nāḍī — The nāḍī of the sun. Another name for pingalā nāḍī.

Suṣumṇā nāḍī — The main channel of energy situated inside the spinal column.

Suṣupti-avasthā — The state of the mind in dreamless sleep.

Svādhiṣṭhāna chakra — The nervous plexus situated above the organs of generation.

Svādhyāya — Education of the self by study of divine literature.

Svaḥ — The sky.

Svapnāvasthā — The state of the mind in a dream.

Svātmārāma — Author of *Haṭha Yoga Pradīpikā*, a classical text book on Hatha Yoga.

Śvāsa-praśvāsa — Heaving and sighing; inhalation and exhalation.

Śvetaketu — Son of the sage Uddālaka, who gave him instruction concerning the key to all knowledge. Their dialogue forms part of *Chāndogya Upaniṣad*.

Śvetāśvetaropaniṣad — Name of one of the principal Upanisads.

Swastikāsana — Sitting cross-legged, with back erect. One of the postures for the practice of Prāṇāyāma or dhyāna.

Tāḍāsana — A standing pose where one stands firm and erect as a mountain (tāḍa).

Taittirīyopaniṣad	Name of one of the principal Upaniṣads.
Tamas	Darkness or ignorance, one of the three qualities or constituents of everything in nature.
Tāmasic	Having the quality of darkness or ignorance (tamas).
Tanmātra	The subtle elements, namely, the essence of sound (śabda), touch (sparśa), form (rūpa), flavour (rasa) and odour (gandha). They are subtle objects of the sense powers (indriyas), namely, the powers of hearing (śrota), feeling (tvak), seeing (chakṣu), tasting (rasanā) and smelling (ghrāna).
Tantra	A class of works teaching magical and mystical formulas.
Tanumānasā	Disappearance of the mind.
Tapas	A burning effort which involves purification, self-discipline and austerity.
Tattva	'Thatness'. The true or first principle, an element or primary substance. The real nature of the human soul or the material world and the Supreme Universal Spirit pervading the universe.
Tattvamasi	That thou art.
Tattva-traya	The three essential elements, namely, (a) being (sat), (b) non-being (asat) and (c) the supreme being, the Creator of all (Iśvara).
Tejas	Lustre, brilliance, majesty.
Trāṭaka	Gazing fixedly at an object.
Turīyāvasthā	The fourth state of the soul, combining yet transcending the other three states of waking, dreaming and sleeping – the state of samādhi.
Tyāgi	One who renounces.
Uḍ	Upwards, expansion.
Uddālaka	Name of a sage who instructed his son Śvetaketu concerning the key to all knowledge. The instruction forms part of the *Chāndogyopaniṣad*.
Udāna vāyu	One of the vital airs which pervades the human body, filling it with vital energy. It dwells in the thoracic cavity and controls the intake of air and food.
Uḍḍīyāna	One of the bandhās (locks or seals). Here the diaphragm is lifted high up the thorax and the abdominal organs are pulled back towards the spine. Through the uḍḍīyāna the great bird prāṇa (life) is forced up to fly through the suṣumṇā nāḍī.
Ujjāyī	A type of prāṇāyāma in which the lungs are fully expanded and the chest is puffed out like that of a proud conqueror.
Upa-prāṇa vāyu	These are five subsidiary (upa) vital airs (prāna

vāyu). They are: nāga, which relieves abdominal pressure by belching; kūrma, which controls the movements of the eyelids to prevent foreign matter or too bright a light entering the eyes; kṛkara, which prevents substances passing up the nasal passages and down the throat forcing one to sneeze or cough; devadatta, which provides intake of extra oxygen in a tired body by causing a yawn; and dhanañjaya, which remains in the body even after death and sometimes bloats up a corpse.

Upaniṣads The word is derived from the prefixes 'upa' (near) and 'ni' (down), added to the root 'sad' (to sit). It means sitting down or near a guru to receive spiritual instruction. The Upaniṣads are the philosophical portion of the Vedas, the most ancient sacred literature of the Hindus, dealing with the nature of man and the universe and the union of the individual soul or self with the Universal Soul.

Ūrdhva Raised, elevated, tending upwards.

Ūrdhvadhanurāsana Elevated backarch like a bow.

Ūrdhva-retas (Ūrdhva = upwards; retas = semen). One who lives in perpetual celebacy and abstains from sexual intercourse. One who has sublimated sexual desire.

Ūṣṭrāsana Camel pose.

Uttama Best, excellent, first, highest.

Uttamōttama Most excellent, first amongst the best, highest of the high.

Uttara-kāṇḍa of Rāmāyaṇa The sequel to *Rāmāyaṇa*, the celebrated epic story of Rāma.

Uttara mīmāṁsa One of the systems of Indian philosophy, which accepts God on the basis of the Vedas, but lays special stress on spiritual knowledge (jñāna).

Vāc Speech.

Vairāgya Absence of worldly desires.

Vaiśeṣika One of the six systems of Indian philosophy founded by Kanāda. It is so called because it teaches that knowledge of the nature of reality is obtained by knowing the special properties (viśeṣa) or essential differences which distinguish nine eternal realities or substances (dravyas). These are: earth (pṛthvī), water (ap), fire (tejas), air (vāyu), ether (ākāṣa), time (kāla), space (dik), self (ātman) and mind (manas).

Vālmīki Name of the author of the celebrated epic *Rāmāyaṇa*. See Ratnākara.

Varāhopaniṣad	Name of one of the Upaniṣads dealing with nāḍīs.
Vāruṇī nāḍī	Name of one of the nāḍis which flows throughout the body. Its function is the evacuation of urine.
Vāsanā	Desire, inclination, longing.
Vāsudeva	Name of Lord Viṣṇu.
Vāta	Wind.
Vāyu	The wind, the vital airs.
Vāyu sādhanā	Practice or quest (sādhanā) of vital airs (vāyu). Another name for prāṇāyāma.
Veda	The sacred scriptures of the Hindus, classified as revealed literature (śruti), consisting of four collections called Ṛgveda – hymns to gods, sāmaveda – priests' chants, yajurveda – sacrificial formulae in prose, and Atharvaveda – magical chants. They contain the first philosophical insights and are regarded as the final authority. Each Veda has broadly two divisions, namely, mantras (hymns) and brāhmaṇa (precepts). The latter include āraṇyaka (theology) and upaniṣads (philosophy).
Vedanta	Literally, the end (anta) of the Vedas, popular name for the system of Indian philosophy called Uttara Mīmāṁsa, meaning the last investigation of the Vēdas, because its central theme is the philosophical teachings of the Upaniṣads. These teachings concern the nature and relationship of three principles, namely, the Ultimate Principle (Brahman), the world (jagat) and the individual soul (jīvātmā) and also includes the relationship between the Universal Soul (Paramātmā) and the individual soul.
Vibhīśaṇa	Name of the brother of Rāvaṇa, who told the latter that his conduct in abducting Rama's wife Sītā was unrighteous, and that she should be restored to her husband. Failing to persuade Rāvaṇa, Vibhīśaṇa left and joined Rāma in his battle against Rāvaṇa. After Rāvaṇa was slain, Vibhīsaṇa was crowned as the King of Laṅka. He is regarded as a model of upright conduct and one whose meditation practices were sāttvic.
Vichāraṇā	Examination, investigation, discussion, consideration.
Vidyā	Knowledge, learning lore, science.
Vijñāna	Knowledge, wisdom, intelligence, understanding, discrimination. It also means worldly knowledge derived from worldly experience as opposed to knowledge of Brahma or Supreme Spirit.
Vijñāna nāḍī	Vessels of consciousness.

Vijñānamaya kośa	The sheath of intelligence enveloping the soul, affecting the process of reasoning and judgement derived from subjective experience.
Vikṣipta	Agitated state of mind brought about by distraction, confusion or perplexity.
Viloma prāṇāyāma	Viloma means against the hair (loma), against the current, against the order of things. The particle 'vi' denotes negation or privation. In viloma prāṇāyāma the inhalation or exhalation is not one continuous process, but is done gradually with several pauses.
Viṇā	Indian lute.
Viṇādaṇḍa	Spinal column.
Vīrāsana	Vīra means a hero, warrior or champion. This sitting posture is done by keeping together the knees, spreading the feet and resting them by the side of the hips. The pose is good for meditation and prāṇāyāma.
Viśālatā	Extension, space, breadth, width.
Viṣama vṛtti prāṇāyāma	Viṣama means irregular and difficult. Viṣama vṛtti prāṇāyāma is so called because the same length of time for inhalation, retention and exhalation is not maintained. This leads to interruption of rhythm and the difference in ratio creates difficulty and danger for the pupil.
Viṣṇu	The second deity of the Hindu trinity.
Viśuddhi chakra	The nervous plexus in the pharyngeal region.
Viśvadhāriṇī	Supporter of the Universe.
Viśvodharī nāḍī	Name of one of the nāḍīs, having the function of absorption of food.
Viveka	Judgement, discrimination.
Viveka khyāti	The knowledge or faculty (khyāti) of discrimination.
Vṛtti	A course of action, behaviour, mode of being, condition or mental state.
Vṛtti prāṇāyāma	Vṛtti Prāṇāyāma are of two types – sama vṛtti prāṇāyāma and viṣama vṛtti prāṇāyāma. In the former an attempt is made to achieve uniformity in the duration of all three processes of respiration, namely, inhalation, retention and exhalation in any type of prāṇāyāma. In viṣama vṛtti prāṇāyāma there is a difference in ratio of inhalation, retention and exhalation, leading to interrupted rhythm.
Vyādhi	Sickness, disease, illness.
Vyāna vāyu	One of the vital airs, which pervades the entire body and circulates the energy derived from food and breathing all over the body.

Vyavasāyātmika-Buddhi — Industrious and persevering intellect.

Yagñā — Ritual or sacrifice.

Yājñavalkya — Name of a sage and author of a code of laws. He was spiritual preceptor to King Janaka. The dialogue between Yājñavalkya and his wife Gārgī forms a part of the *Bṛhadāraṇyaka Upaniṣad*.

Yajur Veda — Name of one of the four Vedas, which form the sacred scriptures of the Hindus.

Yama — The god of death, whose dialogue with the seeker Nachiketā forms the basis of the Kaṭhopaniṣad. Yama is also the first of the eight limbs of Yoga. Yamas are universal moral commandments or ethical principles transcending creeds, countries, age and time. These are non-violence (ahimsā), truth (satya), non-stealing (asteya), continence (brahmacharya), and non-coveting (aparigraha).

Yaśasvinī nāḍī — Name of one of the nādīs.

Yoga — Union, communion. The word 'Yoga' is derived from the root 'Yuj' meaning to join, to yoke, to concentrate one's attention on. It is one of the six systems of Indian philosophy collated by the sage Patanjali. Yoga is the union of our will to the will of God, a poise of the soul, which enables one to look evenly at life in all its aspects. The chief aim of Yoga is to teach the means by which the human soul may be completely united with the Supreme Spirit pervading the universe and thus secure absolution.

Yoga Chuḍāmaṇi Upaniṣad — Name of one of the Yoga Upaniṣads.

Yoga Sūtra — The classical work on Yoga by Patanjali. It consists of terse aphorisms on Yoga and it is divided into four parts dealing respectively with deep meditation (samādhi), the means (sādhana) by which Yoga is attained, the powers (vibhūti) the seeker comes across in his quest, and the state of absolution (kaivalya).

Yuj — To join, to yoke, to concentrate.

Index